1979

CONTEMPORARY
SOCIAL
GERONTOLOGY

CONTEMPORARY SOCIAL GERONTOLOGY

SIGNIFICANT DEVELOPMENTS IN THE FIELD OF AGING

Edited by

BILL D. BELL, Ph.D.
Gerontology Center
University of Nebraska at Omaha
Omaha, Nebraska

With a Foreword by

Erdman Palmore, Ph.D.
Center for the Study of Aging
and Human Development
Duke University
Durham, North Carolina

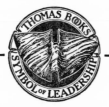

CHARLES C THOMAS · PUBLISHER
Springfield · Illinois · U.S.A.

Published and Distributed Throughout the World by

CHARLES C THOMAS • PUBLISHER

BANNERSTONE HOUSE

301-327 East Lawrence Avenue, Springfield, Illinois, U.S.A.

© *1976, by* CHARLES C THOMAS • PUBLISHER

ISBN 0-398-03464-8

Library of Congress Catalog Card Number: 75-19129

With THOMAS BOOKS *careful attention is given to all details of
manufacturing and design. It is the Publisher's desire to present
books that are satisfactory as to their physical qualities and artistic
possibilities and appropriate for their particular use.* THOMAS
BOOKS *will be true to those laws of quality that assure a good
name and good will.*

Printed in the United States of America

N-1

Library of Congress Cataloging in Publication Data

Main entry under title:

Contemporary social gerontology.

   Bibliography: p
   Includes indexes
   1. Aging—Addresses, essays, lectures. 2. Aged—United States—Ad-
dresses, essays, lectures. 3. Gerontology—Addresses, essays, lectures. I. Bell,
Bill D.
HQ1061.C65 1976   301.43'5   75-19129
ISBN 0-398-03464-8

CONTRIBUTORS

Inge M. Ahammer, Ph.D.
School of Behavioral Sciences
North Ryde, Australia

Jon P. Alston, Ph.D.
Department of Sociology and
Anthropology
University of Georgia
Athens, Georgia

Robert C. Atchley, Ph.D.
Scripps Foundation for Research in
Population Problems
Miami University
Oxford, Ohio

Paul B. Baltes, Ph.D.
Department of Psychology
West Virginia University
Morgantown, West Virginia

Bill D. Bell, Ph.D.
Gerontology Center
University of Nebraska at Omaha
Omaha, Nebraska

Vern L. Bengston, Ph.D.
Andrus Gerontology Center
University of Southern California
University Park
Los Angeles, California

James E. Birren, Ph.D.
Andrus Gerontology Center
University of Southern California
University Park
Los Angeles, California

Margaret Blenkner, D.S.W.
Regional Institute of Social Welfare
Research
School of Social Work
University of Georgia
Athens, Georgia

Martin Bloom, Ph.D.
Center for Social Work/Social Science
Interchange
Indiana University-Purdue University
at Indiana
Indianapolis, Indiana

Stanley J. Brody, M.S.W.
Departments of Community Medicine
and Psychiatry
University of Pennsylvania
Medical Center
Philadelphia, Pennsylvania

Gordon L. Bultena, Ph.D.
Department of Sociology
Iowa State University
Ames, Iowa

Frances M. Carp, Ph.D.
The Wright Institute
Berkeley, California

Albert Chevan, Ph.D.
Department of Sociology
University of Massachusetts
Amherst, Massachusetts

Margaret Clark, Ph.D.
Adult Development Research and
Training Program
Langley Porter Neuropsychiatric
Institute
University of California
School of Medicine
San Francisco, California

Jacob Cohen, Ph.D.
Department of Sociology
New York University
New York, New York

Ben M. Crouch, Ph.D.
Department of Sociology and
Anthropology
Texas A and M University
College Station, Texas

Arthur G. Cryns, Ph.D.
School of Social Policy and
Community Services
State University of New York at Buffalo
Buffalo, New York

Timothy J. Curry, Ph.D.
Department of Sociology
Ohio State University
Columbus, Ohio

Stephen J. Cutler, Ph.D.
Department of Sociology and
Anthropology
Oberlin College
Oberlin, Ohio

Elizabeth B. Douglass, M.A.
Center for the Study of Aging and
Human Development
Duke University Medical Center
Durham, North Carolina

Thomas Downs, Ph.D.
School of Public Health
University of Texas at Houston
Houston, Texas

John Edwards, Ph.D.
Department of Sociology
Virginia Polytechnic Institute and
State University
Blacksburg, Virginia

Gerda G. Fillenbaum, Ph.D.
Center for the Study of Aging and
Human Development
Duke University Medical Center
Durham, North Carolina

Norval D. Glenn, Ph.D.
Department of Sociology
The University of Texas
Austin, Texas

Jaber F. Gubrium, Ph.D.
Department of Sociology and
Anthropology
Marquette University
Milwaukee, Wisconsin

Jacquelyne J. Jackson, Ph.D.
Center for the Study of Aging and
Human Development
Duke University Medical Center
Durham, North Carolina

David L. Klemmack, Ph.D.
Department of Sociology
Virginia Polytechnic Institute and
State University
Blacksburg, Virginia

Bernard Kutner, Ph.D.
Albert Einstein College of Medicine
Bronx, New York

J. A. Kuypers, Ph.D.
Institute of Human Development
University of California
Berkeley, California

M. Powell Lawton, Ph.D.
Philadelphia Geriatric Center
Philadelphia, Pennsylvania

Bruce W. Lemon, M.A.
Department of Sociology
Los Angeles Harbor College
Los Angeles, California

Morton A. Lieberman, Ph.D.
Committee on Human Development
University of Chicago
Chicago, Illinois

Helena Z. Lopata, Ph.D.
Department of Sociology
Loyola University
Chicago, Illinois

George L. Maddox, Ph.D.
Center for the Study of Aging and
Human Development
Duke University Medical Center
Durham, North Carolina

Elliot Markus, D.S.W.
Israel Institute for Applied Social
Research
Jerusalem, Israel

Abraham Monk, Ph.D.
School of Social Policy and
Community Services
State University of New York at Buffalo
Buffalo, New York

Joan Moore, Ph.D.
Andrus Gerontology Center
University of Southern California
University Park
Los Angeles, California

John F. O'Rourke, Ph.D.
Department of Sociology
University of Massachusetts
Amherst, Massachusetts

Erdman Palmore, Ph.D.
Center for the Study of Aging and
Human Development
Duke University Medical Center
Durham, North Carolina

David A. Peterson, Ph.D.
Gerontology Center
College of Public Affairs and
Community Service
University of Nebraska at Omaha
Omaha, Nebraska

James A. Peterson, Ph.D.
Department of Sociology
University of Southern California
University Park
Los Angeles, California

Eric Pfeiffer, M.D.
Center for the Study of Aging and
Human Development
Duke University Medical Center
Durham, North Carolina

A. William Pollman, Ph.D.
Department of Economics and
Business Administration
Wisconsin State University
Main Hall
La Crosse, Wisconsin

Hans G. Proppe
Department of Sociology
University of Southern California
University Park
Los Angeles, California

Bascom W. Ratliff, M.S.W.
School of Social Work
Ohio State University
Columbus, Ohio

George G. Reader, M.D.
Cornell University Medical Center
New York, New York

Arnold M. Rose, Ph.D. (deceased)
Department of Sociology
University of Minnesota
Minneapolis, Minnesota

George S. Rosenberg, Ph.D.
Department of Sociology
Case Western Reserve University
Cleveland, Ohio

James H. Schulz, Ph.D.
Department of Welfare Economics
Brandeis University
Waltham, Massachusetts

Arthur N. Schwartz, Ph.D.
Andrus Gerontology Center
University of Southern California
Los Angeles, California

Mildred M. Seltzer, Ph.D.
Department of Sociology and
Anthropology
Miami University
Oxford, Ohio

Susan R. Sherman, Ph.D.
Mental Health Research Unit
New York State Department of
Mental Hygiene
Albany, New York

Donald L. Spence, Ph.D.
University of Rhode Island
Kingston, Rhode Island

Gary G. Stanfield, M.A.
Department of Sociology
University of Missouri
Columbia, Missouri

Margot Tallmer, Ph.D.
Post Graduate Center for
Mental Health
New York, New York

Gayle B. Thompson, Ph.D.
Division of Retirement and
Survivor Studies
Office of Research and Statistics
Social Security Administration
Washington, D.C.

Sheldon S. Tobin, Ph.D.
School of Social Service Administration
Committee on Human Development
University of Chicago
Chicago, Illinois

Barbara F. Turner, Ph.D.
Departments of Human Development
and Psychology
University of Massachusetts
Amherst, Massachusetts

C. Ray Wingrove, Ph.D.
Department of Sociology and
Anthropology
University of Richmond
Richmond, Virginia

Vivian Wood, Ph.D.
School of Social Work
University of Wisconsin
Madison, Wisconsin

Richard E. Zody, Ph.D.
Department of Political Science
Wichita State University
Wichita, Kansas

To those students of aging who see as their principal
task the expansion of human knowledge

FOREWORD

$\mathbf{I}$T FREQUENTLY HAPPENS WHEN I MEET PEOPLE. They find out I am a gerontologist and ask, "What's that?" When I reply that gerontology is the study of
aging, the next question often is, "Why do you want to study *that?*" One can
almost hear the unspoken assumptions: Aging is unpleasant, hopeless, depressing,
and the aged are boring, ugly, decrepit, senile, etc. Who would want to study
that?

Without commenting on the prejudices revealed by these assumptions, one
could simply answer that more and more people want to study aging for a wide
variety of reasons. The broadest category includes everybody of all ages who
realize that they themselves are aging and that, barring premature death, they
too will someday join the ranks of "the aged." They realize that they have a
very personal stake in understanding what this process is and how it is likely to
affect them. A second category are the more than twenty million older people
who are presently faced with the many problems and opportunities of old age
and want to know how to age "successfully." Many middle-aged and younger
people want to understand the problems and opportunities of their aged parents
and grandparents. Reformers interested in solving social problems and correcting
social inequities want to study the prejudices and discriminations against the
aged which exclude most of them from the mainstream of our society. People in
various business and service agencies want to study aging because of the unprecedented demands for services by the unprecedented numbers of aged persons.
And finally, scholars and scientists may be attracted for any of the above reasons
plus a belief that gerontology is a new and relatively uncharted field.

The statistics on the growth of gerontology are dramatic. A generation ago
there were hardly any gerontologists identified as such. Now there are about
4,000 professional members of the Gerontological Society. A generation ago there
were almost no courses offered in gerontology. Now, there are literally hundreds
of such courses in a majority of the universities and many of the colleges across
the United States. A generation ago there were no centers for the study of aging.
Now there are about two dozen centers or institutes primarily devoted to research
and training in gerontology. Even the federal government has finally established
a National Institute on Aging for gerontological research.

Considering this growth, it is surprising that there has been only one general
text and no general readers in social gerontology published in the last six years.
Clearly, there is a need for an up-to-date reader that surveys recent developments
in social gerontology. A general text by one author must necessarily be somewhat
superficial in its treatment of most topics. A reader has the advantages of utilizing

xi

the best in-depth reports of the leading authorities in each of the subspecialties.

This reader fulfills this need in an admirable way. It balances comprehensiveness with in-depth treatments by focusing on ten main areas. It emphasizes theoretical and methodological developments rather than applied problem solving. Yet it does deal with many of the basic problems of adequate housing and health care, threats of social isolation and institutionalization, and the maintenance of life satisfaction. It also focuses on *normal aging* in the sense of processes and problems common to the majority of aged persons, rather than on unusual or deviant problems confined to a few. In this sense, it complements our normal aging reports from the Duke Longitudinal Studies (Palmore, *Normal Aging I* and *II,* Durham, North Carolina: Duke University Press, 1970; 1974). Most of the articles also manage to combine rigorous scholarship and research with lucid reporting in standard English. There is a minimum of technical jargon, and where technical terms are necessary they are fully explained. Nevertheless, the reader should be warned that this book is intended for the intelligent and serious student in gerontology rather than the casual diletante.

As aids to the reader, the book contains the references of the original articles, a complete name and subject index, and introductions to each of the ten parts. These introductions survey past developments in the field during three time periods: the pre-1950s, mid-1950 to 1968, and the contemporary or post-1968 period. They highlight the significance of the selections in the volume, which are all from the contemporary time frame.

These selections explode old myths and challenge many current assumptions. They show that the aged are not a homogeneous category, rather that heterogeneity tends to increase with aging. They show that disengagement is not an inevitable and general result of aging, but it is a complex, variable phenomenon, usually resulting from stress or social breakdown, and that some dimensions of it are related to loss of life satisfaction. They show that relocation is not necessarily a negative or dangerous event for the aged and may have beneficial effects under many circumstances. Sexual interest and activity is shown to be far more widespread and to occur at later ages than generally thought. There are many problems with the idea of the aged forming a subcultural group and one is that age peer contacts do not appear to increase with advancing years. There are many arguments for and against compulsory retirement, but the facts remain that it is by definition discrimination against an age category and that it prevents millions of able older persons from continuing their contribution to our economy and from supporting themselves. Poor health appears to be declining in importance as the main reason for retirement, with compulsory retirement for older workers and attractive pension plans for early retirement increasing in importance. There may be less prejudice against the aged than currently supposed. An aggressive personality appears to aid survival in institutions. The effects of institutionalization are not necessarily good or bad, but depend on a complex of factors.

These are but a few of the highlights of this text. Other gerontologists will find this to be a useful compendium of many recent developments in these and other basic areas. Newcomers to the field will find it provides a basic orientation to the nature and directions of current advance in this new and growing science of later life.

ERDMAN PALMORE
Center for the Study of Aging
  and Human Development
Duke University

PREFACE

G ERONTOLOGY IS ONE OF THE FASTEST growing disciplines in the social sciences. As the number of older persons in the United States edges toward the 10 percent mark, the problems as well as potentialities of elderly people have become apparent. At present, it is estimated that over one-half of American universities offer at least one course in gerontology. Usually included in the curriculum is an overview of the field with special emphasis given to such questions as income, health, housing, social relations, and the like. Ironically, however, the resources in this area are relatively limited. By and large, texts in social gerontology are few in number. Those which are available tend to present the broad outlines of the dispicline with little attempt at systematic presentation. In addition, most popular works are products of the late 1950s and 1960s. The *Handbook of Aging and the Individual,* Birren, and the *Handbook of Social Gerontology,* Tibbitts, for example, were published in 1959 and 1960, respectively. *Gerontology,* Vedder, and the *Processes of Aging,* Williams *et al.,* were published in 1963. Similarly, *Middle Age and Aging,* Neugarten, and *Aging and Society,* Riley and Foner, appeared in 1968.

The year 1968 constitutes a wartermark in social gerontology. Following this date, only Atchley has addressed the discipline in totality (*The Social Forces in Later Life,* 1972). His work, however, tends to summarize rather than illustrate specific instances of theoretical and methodological development. Similarly, Riley and Foner's work is both voluminous and difficult to place in perspective. Like the writing of Neugarten, their book is also of a pre-1968 character.

The present volume, while limited in part, presents the reader with a contemporary view of social gerontology. In general, the focus is on those theoretical and methodological developments characteristic of the post-1968 era. Efforts to limit consideration to the latter time frame are rare in gerontology. In most recent publications, authors have confined their attention to specific issues within the discipline (e.g. income, retirement, and health) rather than attempting an overview of the field. This book offers a comprehensive approach to developments in several critical areas.

For the most part, the material in this text is analytical in nature. Although policy implications can and frequently are drawn from many of the writings, the primary focus is the realm of disciplinary advance. Such a view gives precedence to those empirical efforts designed to test and supplement the theories of aging. In the final analysis, emphasis is placed upon the so-called *normal aged* and their perceptions and reactions to the aging process.

In selecting the readings for this text, consideration has been given to many orientations. As a consequence, contributors have not been limited to "greats" in the field. Instead, considerable care has been exercised to select the most representative and complete works within a particular area of investigation as opposed to giving primary consideration to the reputation of specific authors. As a result, many of the names often associated with gerontology in the past may not appear in this work.

The areas selected for consideration include the demography and ecology of age; theories of aging; economics, housing, and health; work, retirement, and leisure; attitudes toward age and aging; family roles and social relations; morale, adjustment, and life satisfaction; the minority elderly; the institutionalized aged; and contemporary research strategies. These areas are deemed typical of the field and represent those facets of the aging picture which have witnessed the most dramatic development subsequent to 1968. The focal point of each section is the *process of aging* as this experience or set of experiences affects both the individual and the social structure.

In general, this book is directed toward both an undergraduate and graduate audience. As such, it is meant to partially fill the void in resource materials in the field of aging. To assist in this effort, each of the ten sections comprising the text is preceded by an extended introduction. The purpose of the introduction is to place the area in question in historical perspective. To this extent, three time periods have been selected as representative stages in gerontological development: (a) the 1930s through the early 1950s, (b) the late 1950s through the early 1960s, and (c) the late 1960s through the early 1970s. In addition to this organizational aid, a name and subject index is provided so that the reader can obtain maximum benefit from the text as a reference source.

In way of acknowledgements, I would like to thank Drs. Erdman Palmore, Perry L. Thompson, and Robert T. Sigler for their encouragement in the creation of this volume. In addition, I want to express my appreciation to the various contributors for their kindness in permitting the republication of these materials. And finally, special mention is due my wife Jacque for her patience and fortitude during the writing of the manuscript. More than any other individual, she provided the understanding and support necessary to offset initial discouragement, an abominable temper, and a sagging ego.

Omaha, Nebraska   BILL D. BELL

CONTENTS

Section III
Economics, Housing, and Health

Section IV
Work, Retirement, and Leisure

Section V
Attitudes Toward Age and Aging

Section X
Contemporary Research Strategies

CONTEMPORARY
SOCIAL
GERONTOLOGY

Section I

THE DEMOGRAPHY AND ECOLOGY OF AGE

THE SOCIAL GERONTOLOGISTS OF THE 1930s through the early 1950s concentrated much of their attention on the demographic aspects of aging. In general, the work of these scholars was descriptive in nature. Attempts were made not only to describe the extent of this population (Thompson and Whelpton, 1933) and where it was to be found (Kiser, 1950), but also how often the aged tended to move (Lee *et al.*, 1957) and the characteristics of their migratory patterns (Coale, 1955). In like manner, efforts were made to relate a number of social variables, such as age, sex, health, income, race, and social status to the demographic picture (Valaoras, 1950; Coale, 1955). For the most part, these early writings document in detail a significant increase in the absolute and proportionate numbers of elderly persons in the United States.

The late 1950s and early 1960s witnessed a continuation of a basically descriptive approach to the demography of age (Bowles and Traver, 1964). During this period of time, however, thought was also given to the various social outcomes of these demographic trends (Beattie, 1964; Beale, 1964; Sheldon, 1958). Accordingly, attention began to focus on the minority group status of the aged (Barron, 1961) as well as potential subcultures of aging (Rose, 1962). What followed was an attempt to harmonize a migratory picture of age with the problems engendered by a variety of social and geographical settings.

Gerontologists of the late 1960s and early 1970s have capitalized upon the descriptive and analytical work of these earlier generation demographers. It is recognized, for example, that large numbers of elderly persons are to be found in the urban areas of the nation (Atchley, 1972; Jackson, 1971). It is also evident that the urban environment presents the older person with a unique set of problems to be overcome. By the same token, however, large proportions of older persons still reside in the rural and semiurban areas of the midwest and midsouth (Goldscheider, 1966; Brotman, 1968).

In completing the picture, however, contemporary social gerontologists have cast considerable doubt upon a number of traditional understandings regarding the demography and ecology of the aged. It is now clear, for instance, that the majority of older persons are not migratory by nature (Birren, 1969). Many, perhaps most, prefer to remain in their familiar surroundings well into late life.

3

In this regard, the institutionalized view of the aged has been shown to be exaggerated as less than 5 percent reside in a supervised (i.e. institutionalized) environment (Atchley, 1972). In similar fashion, the mass migrations of the elderly to the sunshine areas of the nation have been overemphasized. Those individuals making this transition are frequently atypical of the general aged population. This fact is pointed up quite succinctly in the paper by Chevan and O'Rourke as well as in the work of Bultena and Wood in Section III.

The papers to follow give primary attention to the principal locations of today's elderly. The selections, however, do not focus on the social and psychological implications of these settings. On the other hand, these issues receive ample consideration in subsequent portions of the text. The present papers are, nevertheless, representative of the character of contemporary demographic research in that all stress the commonalities as well as emphasize the individual differences of the aged regardless of geographical setting. As each paper makes clear, the aged do not constitute a homogenous group in any real sense of the term. Indeed, age is suggested as only one of many factors useful in depicting the demographic character of the elderly.

The first of these papers focuses on the urban aged. Attention is given to the proportion of older persons in the nation's cities as well as to the problems unique to an urban environment. Birren invokes the Lewinian concept of *life space* to stress the point that cities are first and foremost social organizations and secondarily physical organizations. Threats to the life space of the elderly include redevelopment, relocation, and rehousing within the urban setting.

Accompanying various changes in the life space of the aged are significant alterations in physical and mental well-being. For Birren, "the proximal environment assumes an importance in the aged not often perceived by the mobile young adult." He argues that the urban life space should offer a sense of support in the presence of familiar persons and objects, as well as provide for a variety of individually selected patterns of social involvement.

The paper by Rose provides a number of valuable insights into the character of life in small town America. He points out, for example, that a much larger proportion of rural than urban residents are self-employed and that these self-employed persons are less likely than urban employees to retire completely and suddenly at a fixed age. Such gradual retirement suggests less anxiety over declining income in the later years in the rural areas of the United States than in urban areas.

The migration of the young from rural areas has meant a disproportionate increase in the numbers of the rural aged. As such, political power in these areas has fallen into aged hands. This is in sharp contrast with the youthful politics of the urban setting. Similarly, contrasts exist in the housing as well as interpersonal sectors. On the other hand, more opportunities for meaningful social relationships seem to characterize the rural domain.

The final paper in this section goes beyond the urban or rural character of the elderly and addresses a much broader question, the regional homogeneity of the aged. Chevan and O'Rourke report the findings of a study "in which techniques of multivariate analysis were used to describe the relationships which obtain between the distribution of the older population and some of its conditional characteristics." The issue at point concerns whether those older persons who are isolated, ill housed, in poor health, and with inadequate transportation facilities are concentrated in some areas and not in others.

The use of a Q analysis enables the authors to make a number of observations relative to the regionality and homogeneity of the aged. In general, this technique demonstrates that the older population is not distributed across the United States in a homogeneous fashion. On the other hand, different styles of aging are observed and can be associated with the Q groups (i.e. geographical regions) established in the analysis.

REFERENCES

Atchley, R. C. *The social forces in later life*. Belmont, California: Wadsworth Publishing Company, 1972.

Barron, M L. *The aging american*. New York: Thomas Y. Crowell, 1961.

Beale, C. L. Rural depopulation in the United States; some demographic consequences of agricultural adjustment. *Demography*, 1964, *1*, 264-272.

Beattie, W. M., Jr. The place of older people in different societies. In P. F. Hansen (Ed.), *Age with a future*. Copenhagen: Munksgaard, 1964.

Birren, J. E. The aged in cities. *Gerontologist*, 1969, *9*, 163-169.

Bowles, G. K., and Traver, J. D. The age-sex-color composition of net migration in the United States. *Population Index*, 1964, *30*, 307-308.

Brotman, H. B. *Who are the aged: a demographic view*. Ann Arbor, Michigan: University of Michigan-Wayne State University Institute of Gerontology, 1968.

Coale, A. J. The population of the United States in 1950 classified by age, sex, and color—a revision of census figures. *Journal of the American Statistical Association*, 1955, *50*, 16-54.

Goldscheider, C. Differential residential mobility of the older population. *Journal of Gerontology*, 1966, *21*, 103-108.

Jackson, J. J. The blacklands of gerontology. *Aging and Human Development*, 1971, *2*, 156-171.

Kiser, C. V. The demographic background of our aging population. In *The social and biological challenge of our aging population: proceedings of the Eastern States Health Education Conference, March 31-April 1, 1949*. New York: Columbia University Press, 1950.

Lee, E. S. Miller, A. R., Brainerd, C. P., and Easterlin, R. A. *Population redistribution and economic growth: United States, 1870-1950, Vol. 1: Methodological considerations and reference tables*. Philadelphia: American Philosophical Society, 1957.

Rose, A. M. The subculture of the aging: a framework for research in social gerontology. *Gerontologist*, 1962, *2*, 123-127.

Sheldon, H. D. *The older population of the United States*. New York: John Wiley & Sons, 1958.

Thompson, W. S., and Whelpton, P. K. *Population trends in the United States*. New York: McGraw-Hill Book Company, 1933.

Valaoras, V. G. Patterns of aging in human populations. In *The social and biological challenge of our aging population: proceedings of the Eastern States Health Education Conference, March 31-April 1, 1949*. New York: Columbia University Press, 1950.

Chapter 1

THE AGED IN CITIES

JAMES E. BIRREN

THE PROBLEMS of the aged in the city have to be looked at in broad scope so key ideas can be evolved that will lead to improvement of the city, the common place of residence of the aged. The aged have not joined, or have not been able to join, the flight of the young family to the dubious "high water level" of suburbia to avoid the noise, the smog, the dirt, the social tensions, and the poorer housing of the "older city." The aged especially should be considered when we try to improve our present cities and plan cities of the future. Not only do millions of aged persons live in cities but they live in sections of cities with least adequate housing.

A haunting overtone of America's monumental work of recreating a higher quality of life in cities is the question of whether the past has overcommitted the future to patterns of buildings, uses of land, and ways of living. Whether we will be free enough to make more than just minor changes in our cities is a different question than deciding upon the principles along which bold strides might be made in improving the quality of urban life. It is the second of these questions that we are concerned with here.

It should always be kept in mind that cities are primarily social organizations and secondarily physical organizations. The structure of cities in steel, bricks and mortar, wires and pipes has followed man's desire to gain the advantages of congregate living. If gains in congregate living and working in cities appear to be growing smaller in relation to increasing disadvantages, it is to matters of social organization that we should first turn our attention.

While considerable experience has been built up by business and industry in surveying sites and buildings for economic feasibility, little sophistication has been developed in surveying the social functions of proposed potential facilities. Even less experience has been developed to evaluate the outcomes of construction in meeting proposed social functions. Control of construction has been concentrated in persons who can best judge matters of material design and safety. Securing a building permit involves screening plans and construction inspection by experts in engineering and architecture.

It has not followed that the patterns of organization of cities which are good for young persons or efficient for commerce and industry are meeting the needs of the aged. By contrast, an urban way of life that is optimum for the aged may also provide the young with an environment with social and personal functions considered primary to physical design and construction. Old people live in unattractive, inexpensive housing in the centers of cities. If urban renewal is undertaken, new shopping areas, apartment buildings, restaurants, and hotels are too expensive for the elderly, and their housing is too unattractive to keep in the same area. Hence, the elderly as marginal residents of city center are displaced when renewal proceeds.

Reprinted by permission from the *Gerontologist*, 1969, *9*, 163-169.

Some Basic Issues

Fact gatherers in the government and universities are providing valuable statistical material for digestion and policy formation. That the nineteenth century city, blown up in size to cover twentieth century populations and functions, is breaking down hardly needs statistical support. Less often realized is that there are millions of the aged poor silently trying to cope with the inadequacies of the city and getting less than their share of its goods and services. The position of the aged in the cities is to a large extent an economic issue. There has been a downward trend in the number of aged persons living with relatives. However, rather than resulting from a decline in strength of family ties *per se,* it more likely reflects the fact that there has been a rise, however small, in the economic position of the aged. There is an inverse relation between income level and living with relatives, suggesting that an aged person lives with relatives as a compensation for poverty rather than as a choice of living arrangements. Given adequate income, the aged live near but independent of their children or other relatives.

Most elderly persons have resided a long time in their communities. The 1963 Social Security Survey of the Aged indicated that 80 percent of couples over the age of sixty-two had lived ten or more years in their community at the time of survey. The median number of years in the community was thirty-two, and the median residence in the current dwelling was sixteen years. Two thirds of the married couples had equity in a nonfarm home with a median equity of $10,100. The median assets of married couples was $11,180 (including their home). The data on assets should be considered along with income data. For married couples with at least one member over age sixty-five, 41 percent

were classified as poor or near poor on the basis of income, i.e. less than $2,500 per year. These data obscure the fact that there were large numbers with limited or no assets ($2/5$ of married couples had less than $500 in financial assets) and very small incomes (15% had less than $1,500 per year). If all the assets of individuals are prorated as annual income over expected life, the median incomes for married couples over sixty-five would be $3,795. This figure suggests a strong economic basis for the nonmoving of the aged. That is, even if the over sixty-five couple spent one third of their annual income (plus assets), they could spend only $1,265 a year for housing or about $105 a month. At least one half of the aged couples would appear to be "locked into" their housing arrangements because they have too little money for alternatives.

Of the nearly 19,000,000 persons over age sixty-five, about two-thirds live in urban areas. Many rural aged leave their farms and move into small towns or nonfarm rural areas where they are relieved of the heavy work of farming yet remain in contact with friends and the familiar landscape of the area. Some retired farmers do move to cities, as do miners from thinly settled areas. Such aged have diverse expectations and needs when they come to the city and may make several housing changes. While change of residence among the aged is somewhat less frequent than among the young-adult population, large numbers of the aged nevertheless do change their place of residence. Upward mobility with increased income and attempts to improve one's housing apparently is a constant process with the young. The aged often appear to be dissatisfied with their housing but do not attempt to move as frequently as the young. About one fifth of the national population change their residence in a year. A survey in Los Angeles indicated that about 90 percent of individuals fifty years and older were dissatisfied with their living arrangements, but only 13 percent actually did move during a one-year period. Two things stand out: higher dissatisfaction and lower mobility among the aged than among the young.

Discussions of the needs of the elderly in the modern city often degenerate into a narrow discussion of housing for the aged. This is not to deny the very great importance of housing. The principle is, however, that good or pleasant housing is not the most important aspect of urban life. Discussions of the position of the aged in the city should be organized around the concept of life space. The individual's life space is that part of the city he occupies physically, socially, and psychologically.

The urban life space of the aged individual involves not only the characteristic services available to the young but also the ease of access to these services. Young adults, because of their higher mobility, can adapt themselves more easily to the scattered nature of urban functions. Because they can drive, they can cope with considerable distances between schools, places of entertainment, housing, and work. In the suburban sprawl surrounding our cities, it is the active function of the mother to integrate the services needed to maintain a growing family. She drives one direction to the market, another direction to take a sick child to the pediatrician or dentist; still other scattered trips are needed to take the youngsters to sports events, special schools, and social functions. These functions are geographically organized in specialized buildings for the efficiency of the professional person.

The elderly person can hardly organize and cope with many professional specializations widely separated geographically.

The mere lower mobility of the aged, due in part to his not being able to drive an automobile, for example, markedly reduces the life space of the aged person in most American cities. Absent is an organizing or integrating force to deploy services for the benefit of the individual. Some compensation is possible if the individual moves into an older neighborhood or community with its clustering of small shops and narrow streets. Paradoxically, it is in the most deteriorated areas of cities that aged persons may lead their most independent existence and integrate for themselves combinations of needed services. The replacement of deteriorated areas with high-rise housing usually results in the shopping areas being placed a long way off in large specialized complexes. Many of these shopping centers are almost impossible to approach on foot.

The specialized nature of modern cities results in separation of many social sites and functions. Consider, for example, the cemetery. Older cities have within communities or neighborhoods cemeteries in which local residents are buried. Widows may visit graves on Sundays to place flowers, gossip with other widows, and share family information. In modern urban societies the social value of the cemetery has disappeared. To visit a grave of a member of a family by traveling a long way by car and caring for the grave among strangers in a complex of graves of unfamiliar persons is to crown the obvious anonymity of the large city. The community cemetery had a socializing role which cannot be served by physically more attractive but remote cemeteries.

Individual differences in the social, psychological, and physical needs are greater in an aged than in a young population. Marked individual differences in the aged occur in energy levels and desire for physical activities and in participation in cultural events. In comparison with the present young-adult population, the aged have a lower average level of educational attainment and a rather sizable proportion of functional illiterates. Thus, despite high motivation, many of their interests must necessarily be undeveloped as a consequence of the limited educational opportunity available when the older generation was young. In addition to the wide range of educational differences, the current population of retired persons has a high proportion of foreign-born individuals because of the large immigration waves of the early part of this century.

An optimum life space for the aged is one that offers support in the presence of familiar objects and persons, plus the opportunity for an individually selected pattern of privacy and involvement with social groups. Persons of all ages seem to like a relationship of detached involvement in which they can remove themselves to a private sanctuary yet alternately seek contact with others. The life space of the individual should be socializing in the sense that it surrounds him with a stream of information that is at times useful and at other times emotionally supportive. It does not follow, however, that a permanent place of residence remains for the aged individual supportive of an adequate life space. An aged individual may reside in the area where he settled as a young adult and yet live in a lonely and symbolic fashion the relationships of his early life. If in fact the number of daily personal contacts is counted and an estimate is made of the intimacy of these contacts, it may be found that he is poorly or tenuously related to the community of which he has been a long-time but increasingly marginal resident.

The dramatic growth of clubs for the aged is evidence of the considerable unmet affiliative needs of the elderly, needs which are commonly not met by place of residence alone. Mere residence in an age-diverse community is no indication that the aged person is integrated in a satisfying and supportive matrix of social relationships. The nonworking retired resident in an apartment building largely occupied by middle-aged adults can be a remarkably isolated person. The opportunities for friendship diminish once the worklife ceases since in urban life friendships tend to evolve from work relationships.

With the shrinking life space of advancing age, more and more psychological support derives from objects near at hand. The proximal environment assumes an importance in the aged not often perceived by the mobile young adult.

Mental Health and the Community of the Aged

The aged, like the young, most enjoy affiliating with those of nearly their own age. Most old friends of the aged tend to be elderly, and most likely new friends will also be elderly. It should come as no surprise, then, that the elderly are found in enclaves. To call such grouping *age segregated* is to miss the main point that they can be voluntary, hence are *age congregated*. The urban elderly seem to thrive best among similarly aged individuals in places adjacent to the life activities of other age groups. Mental health would thus seem to be promoted by a balance of independence and interdependence, independence being provided by a range of facilities close at hand and useful to all age groups, with dependence provided by peer-group relations. Evidence exists that not only are friends important in the enjoyment of life's activities but that they provide a shock-absorbing quality in crisis situations. The supportive environment for the aged should, therefore, provide the opportunity for friendships at three levels: casual, intimate, and confidante. The candid soul-searching permitted by a confidante relationship appears to be an important factor in mental health in crises. The emotional and informational exchanges between close friends is as sustaining for the aged as for the young; and if the environment does not provide opportunities for making and keeping close friendships, it is indeed impoverished. Quite possibly, if we were to look at the mental health of the aged in as much detail as we do that of the young we would find a considerably higher proportion of psychopathology than we now recognize.

Redevelopment, Relocation, and Rehousing

When areas of cities deteriorate and become economically unproductive, there is a desire to "clean it all up." Areas that need redevelopment commonly contain old people who are poor. In order to redevelop an area, the aged along with the poor young have to be relocated. Almost no relocation housing is available to the aged because they have so little money (over 50% of them have substandard incomes) and mobility. If redevelopment proceeds and the aged are dislocated, it is very unlikely that they will ever return to the original area from which they were displaced. Even if public housing were built in part of the redevelopment area, it is usually not possible for the displaced aged to qualify on income for rental in public housing. Furthermore, other functions of redeveloped land tend to be upgraded and do not serve one of our neediest groups in society, the aged urban poor.

Housing units themselves are relatively easily designed and constructed compared with a social design of the community that considers replacement of familiar people, objects, and places.

This all suggests that economic planners, physical planners, and social planners should get together early in redevelopment activities so that rehousing of the aged can result in an upgrading of their life space rather than displacement and permanent downgrading.

Specialized Approach for the Aged

As mentioned previously, the low mobility of the aged requires that services be brought closer to the individual. Decreases in the range of services used by the aged in cities may result from the fact that older persons become discouraged by a succession of obstacles that would not inhibit the young, e.g. high bus steps, the need to cross wide busy streets to catch a bus, the fast timing of traffic lights, high curbs, and the inadequate labeling of buildings.

Not only do many aged persons need rehabilitation, but also facilities need rehabilitation to increase their use in relation to needs. Banks, physicians, shops, lawyers, and parks, for example, may be underused by the aged because of the energy it takes to get to them. Older persons often go without replacing their broken eyeglasses, teeth, or other personal items until they find a less taxing way of getting them than by using public transportation, even if it exists.

Rarely do cities provide a centralized information service to the aged to tell them where they might find what they need, whether it be in the area of health, housing, or recreational pursuits.

Range of Options

The range of options in living arrangements available to older adults should be even greater than those available to the young-adult population to accommodate individual differences. A group of seventy-year-olds will contain at one extreme men who run a mile a day or surf and at the other extreme bed-ridden patients. It will contain women who play an instrument in a symphonic group or paint and women whose mental powers are seriously impaired. Research has shown that a variety of life styles can lead to life satisfaction. Both the energetic activist and the rocking-chair noninvolver can achieve adaptation with the issues of their lives with success and satisfaction. The environment must offer the opportunity of leading appropriately active roles, if desired, as spouse, parent, single person seeking a mate, work or part-time work, and community volunteer. Unless the older person can have easy access to options, we can hardly expect him to fashion a life space unique for his interests and needs.

Limitations of vision, hearing, and mobility restrict individuals from participating in events which interest them and which are highly appropriate to their backgrounds and experience. The extent to which various physical limitations of individuals can be overcome in public functions by appropriate engineering and architectural design is unknown since communication with designers and the relevant scientists is scant. Designers must share with behavioral, social, and medical scientists the planning of the environment. In addition, following up evaluations of construction and redevelopments should be made by a multidisciplinary group so that we can learn from mistakes. There is considerable need for involvement of architects and city planners with behavioral and social scientists in deciding upon the goals and patterns of living arrangements for the aged. It is only by such a joint exchange of information that we can begin to describe adequately the social system in which the older person functions and the design of the supporting environment with options.

It has been suggested that, since life satisfaction of elderly persons can go up when they live in housing projects with others of the same age, cities for the aged should be developed. It does not follow that if people will be better adjusted when they live in a building with people of similar ages, that adjacent buildings must also be occupied by the same age groups. In fact, individual differences among aged persons are probably so large that they do not lend themselves to congenial living in large areas of housing for the aged alone. While most daily contacts seem congenial with others of similar age and background, this is not the whole issue and need not in itself imply that large areas of cities should be lived in and used by narrow age groups. It seems highly desirable that age groups share the use of buildings and services, such as parks, beaches, cultural centers, and churches. In the interests of efficiency alone, it should be pointed out that working-age adults rarely use such services and places during the week workday. This suggests that congregate living arrangements for the aged can be distributed in communities so that the sharing of facilities and services can be carried out efficiently.

Summary of Key Issues

Cities are primarily social organizations and secondarily collections of concrete, steel, and wooden structures. That structure follows function can be lost sight of, and the social "creaking and cracking" now heard in cities suggests that planners thought that function was determined by structure. The concept of *life space* should be used in discussing the position of the aged in cities since it implies more of the functional relations of living than does the more limited structural term *housing*. The city should provide the largest possible life space for its residents, a life space that contains many options and the opportunity to express individual differences in needs and desires. More than one half of the population over sixty-five can exercise little or no choice of place of residence or other features of their life space because of their low incomes.

Almost one half of the aged are poor. Because of this, they are most unlikely to be able to buy or rent the facilities needed to provide adequate life space in the city. Representation of the special needs of the elderly seems to be weak in the city because they have no fixed relationship with industry, nor are they particularly good consumers. Planning for the position of the aged, even though there are nineteen million of them in the total population, is inadequate and often occurs merely as an afterthought. Representation of the aged in the administrative organizations of cities must be achieved so that the needs of the elderly are met in proportion to their numbers and individual requirements.

The urban environment must provide a plurality of facilities designed to meet a wide range of individual differences. While aged members of society tend to become more dependent upon others for their existence, they cannot be treated as a homogeneous group.

One of the strong embarrassments of the position of older persons in the city is their limited mobility. Many tendencies in urban renewal which otherwise improve the construction of the modern city tend to disturb the lives of older persons. Planning would seem best designed to encourage living arrangements of older persons adjacent to areas where they can share common facilities with other age groups. In addition, they should live in a community in which most of the common daily needs can be met within walking distances. Nothing is more at variance with the needs of the older person than the huge shopping complex with its wealth of goods and services when the aged do not have a way of reaching it or after arriving there do not have the income to purchase the available goods and services. Generally speaking, older persons seem to gain satisfaction and support from association with familiar objects and places and from association with persons of a similar age and background.

Planning the life space of the aged should become a joint responsibility of physical and social planners, of engineers, architects, and biological, behavioral, and social scientists. The training of such persons will anticipate the planning and construction needs of tomorrow.

REFERENCES

Goldschieder, C. Differential residential mobility of the older population. *Journal of Gerontology*, 1966, *21*, 103-108.

Rosow, I. *Social Integration of the Aged.* New York: The Free Press, 1967.

U.S. Department of Health, Education and Welfare. *Patterns of Living and Housing of Middle Aged and Older People.* Washington, D.C.: Public Health Service Publication No. 1496, 1967.

U.S. Department of Health, Education and Welfare. *1963 Social Security Survey.* Washington, D.C.: Government Printing Office.

Chapter 2

PERSPECTIVES ON THE RURAL AGED

ARNOLD M. ROSE

I N ANALYZING THE rural elderly, three sets of factors must be kept in mind: (a) factors associated with aging in American society, (b) characteristics of life today in small towns and the open country, and (c) characteristics of life in small towns and the open country some sixty years ago when the present generation of older people were in their formative years. The reason for distinguishing the third set of factors from the other two is that rural life, which was much different sixty years ago in the United States than it is today, has had a profound effect on the present generation of older people. This generational influence is to be sharply distinguished from the influence of aging as such since it is much more temporary. Rural life today is much less distinguishable from urban life. When the present generation of rural adults becomes old, their generational characteristics and problems will be little different from those of the urban elderly but much different from the generational characteristics and problems of present rural older people.

In separating out the influence of these three sets of factors, which we shall call, respectively, the factors of aging, of rural life, and of generation, it is to be understood

Reprinted by permission from *Older Rural Americans*, E. Grant Youmans (Ed.), Lexington, Kentucky: The University Press of Kentucky, 1967, 6-21.

that this is an analytic distinction. Their influence on the elderly is in fact inextricably intertwined.

AGING IN AMERICA

In distinguishing the factor of aging† from the generational influence, we did not intend to imply that the former was unchanging while the latter was changing. The condition of being an older person is not merely a function of relatively immutable biological characteristics but also of cultural characteristics, which happen to be changing at a rapid pace in contemporary American society. The limitations on the elderly, the opportunities before them, the attitudes of younger generations toward them, and their attitudes toward themselves or older people are, since the 1950s, undergoing changes of almost revolutionary proportions.

Before considering these changes, let us first examine the social psychology of the typical older person in present American society. There are two outstanding social psychological problems of older people in American society today, and they are related in part: one is the loss of social roles and the other is the development of negative attitudes toward the self.

Loss of Occupation

Most employed persons are obliged to retire from their jobs sometime during their sixties, and occupation is a chief life role for most men and for a significant

†The discussion of the aging factor is largely a revision of two earlier analyses by the author, adapted to the aging in rural society: "Mental Health of Normal Older Persons," *Geriatrics*, 16 (Sept. 1961), 459-64; and "The Subculture of the Elderly: A Framework for Research" in *Older People and Their Social World*, ed. A. M. Rose and W. A. Peterson (Philadelphia: F. A. Davis Company, 1965), Ch. 1.

proportion of women. The chief life role for most women is childbearing and child-rearing, and this has been accomplished for most American women in their fifties or, increasingly because of the younger age at which women now voluntarily stop having babies, in their forties. After they are no longer engaged in childbearing, many American women find new roles in employment or voluntary associations, but these also are greatly reduced by the mid-sixties.

The loss of the chief life function, occupation for a man and childrearing for a woman, may be damaging to the conception of the self, especially if all the individual's values have been concentrated on this function and if he has no other valued activities that can provide him with substitute goals and satisfying roles. On the other hand, if he has the latter and feels a growing strain between carrying on the chief life function and the physical ability or interest in doing so, retirement can be a relief and an avenue to a happier life. There is evidence that, for many males in our society, particularly in the lower- and middle-income classes, retiring from the job is looked forward to with pleasure and anticipation. Still, there is a great deal of individual variation.

Complete and sudden retirement is almost unique to industrial society. In most other societies, there is a gradual sloughing off of the primary occupation, and although the roll and the group participations associated with it change, the individual's conception of himself does not change rapidly. In agrarian areas many farmers are able to cut down on their work role gradually, thereby reducing the sense of loss which often accompanies abrupt retirement.

Attitudes Toward Aging

The problems of retirement are intimately connected with the problem of the reduced prestige of aging. In past centuries, wisdom was associated with age, but today the pace and complexity of events have prompted us to attribute wisdom only to the expert. Also, the elderly person was relatively rare in the past; today, the percentage of those over sixty-five years of age in the population has climbed to one in eleven. This inflation may have helped to reduce the popularly evaluated worth of the elderly person. Respect and praise in our society are generally accorded for achievement, and valued achievement is mainly a product of occupation, including childrearing for women. Loss of occupation in retirement removes the occasion for manifestations of praise and respect.

Changes in Family Roles

Old age often brings changes in family roles. Even before one reaches the age of sixty-five today, one has lost the childrearing role and assumed the grandparental role. The latter generally does not occupy as much time as the former and is frequently more pleasant, if the older couple and the younger families are in separate households. With retirement there is often a change in husband-wife roles; when he was employed full time there was a natural division of labor and power between them; upon retirement, he tends to intrude into her sphere. Either he wants some chores to keep himself busy or he feels he ought to help out when she is busy and he has nothing to do. He expects to take on these tasks as an equal (or sometimes, if he had a directive role in his occupation, unconsciously he expects to be a superior). Previously his wife has had little interference in running the house. Under the circumstances, either he meets rebuff, with some damage to his self-conception, or he starts a permanent conflict, or he threatens his wife's conception of herself, or they work out a new division of labor. This problem is less likely to occur if the man is a farmer and gradually retires from that occupation.

If either or both of the old couple move in with one of their married children's families, the required role adjustment is even more drastic. In other societies, and in our own society until about fifty years ago, the family included the older generation, but today in our society the older person is regarded as an extra member. The older couple living with their adult children in past centuries very often were regarded as the heads of the household, whereas today they are generally the subordinates. Either of the older folks intrudes on the functions of the younger wife, except when she needs a baby sitter. The young couple's interests are generally different from those of the older persons, and there is always a question whether the latter should be included in the young couple's or family's activities. Entertainment of friends is often difficult in someone else's home, and if the move into the younger couple's home has entailed a movement into another community, there are often no friends nearby for the elderly person to invite.

In most cases, movement into the home of a married child involves some depreciation in self-conception arising from the down-grading of a role from an independent to a dependent person. Even the role of grandparent is not a satisfying one in our society if the grandparent lives in the same home: the younger family tends to be child centered today, but older persons often regard children as subordinates or pets. To have to accommodate to a domi-

nating child is an annoyance to a grandparent who lives in his own home; it can be traumatic to the grandparent who lives in the child's home. The difficulties of elderly parents living with their adult offspring in our society generally have kept them from living together; today this living arrangement is the atypical rather than the typical one, although research literature shows that other kinds of intergenerational relationships are maintained today.

When one of an older couple dies, the remaining person is cut off from his major social relationship. Both a role change and a narrowing of the self-conception is involved. Whereas there always may have been psychologic dependency on the spouse, awareness of this does not always exist until the spouse is dead. If there are strong group memberships, the psychologic dependency of the surviving person can be transferred partly to them. But the groups to which the older person belongs, especially the informal ones, are likely to consist also of older persons who die at an increasingly rapid rate. With each friend's death, the older person loses another role, another source of prestige, another social support, and part of himself. No loss of prestige is involved in the status of widowhood itself. However, the widowed woman may experience a strong sense of loss if she depended heavily for her social relationships on friends of her deceased husband rather than on her own personal friends.

Decline in Physical Powers

With the inevitable decline in physical powers, most older persons recognize that the future will bring even more incapacities and eventually death. For some, physical decline is so gradual and the unwillingness to face old age so strong that the realization that one is old may come as a traumatic shock that may result in depression of some duration. This depression may take the form of a disorganization of one's roles and of a strongly negative self-conception. For the majority, evidences of physical decline intrude themselves in one's self-conception as early as the thirties, so that the traumas occur in numerous small bits over a quarter of a century and leave no sudden, shocking realization for the individual to cope with. Still, it is probable that no individual is pleased with or is fully adjusted to the thought that he may become permanently infirm. Whatever the general level of aspirations of the individual, he probably hopes to continue his freedom of movement, but when that seems to be disappearing, he probably feels there is little left to which he can aspire.

For many aging persons there is some awareness of declining mental powers, and this may be as painful an experience as that of declining physical powers. However, declining mental powers usually involve less awareness, with the result that their total impact on emotional health may be less.

Fear of Death

Whereas death may not be so terrifying as in the days when there was an active belief in hell and many individuals had private reasons for predicting that this was to be their residence in the afterlife, the fear of the permanent unknown probably is still strong in most persons. Generally, death is welcomed only by those who are suffering great physical or mental pain or who have reached such a condition of lassitude that one nothingness seems to be an inconsequential substitute for another. The fear of death is so powerful that individuals who have little to live for and whose life offers them nothing but misery still refuse the release of death. The perception of the world is a personal one, and few individuals can conceive of the world without themselves, except perhaps in an academic sense. Most older people probably reconcile themselves to the thought of death, but once the conception has been formulated, it casts a shadow over a person's thoughts and over his expectations for the future by which he lives.

Summary

Although old age may bring a release from a boring job and from striving for scarcely attainable goals, resulting in a mellowness that comes to some old people, for most persons it brings disturbances to one's roles and self-conceptions that tend to result in minor forms of ill health. There tends to be a movement from head of household to dependent, from lack of awareness of psychologic dependency to poignant awareness, from rise in prestige to decline, from having a meaningful life role to having to search for a new role, and from being an active person to being a partial invalid. Opportunities for developing negative self-conceptions multiply, and mild depressions or neuroses thereby are more likely to result. It is even conceivable that the high rate of psychosis among older people is at least partly stimulated by these conditions. All of these mental states create problems for all the younger people who have to cope with older persons or who have responsibility for them in any way.

THE RURAL SETTING

Rural areas include both the open country, where farming is the usual occupation, and small settlements, where chief occupations range from mining and forestry to trade, transport, and service. A much larger proportion of rural than of urban residents are self-employed, and self-employed people are less likely than employees to retire completely and suddenly at a fixed age. The more gradual retirement of the farmer or small-town merchant eases many of the problems mentioned below as characteristic of retirement from occupation. With gradual retirement there is also less strain on income, and there may be less anxiety over declining income in the later years in the rural areas of the United States than in the urban areas. There is one significant additional burden on the income of the aging rural person, however, and that is the necessity of journeying and living away from home to get medical care for the more serious chronic diseases. This can add a serious additional strain on economic resources and also tends to stimulate anxieties about living among strangers at a time of personal crisis. It is likely that the rural aged make less use of medical facilities for these reasons.

The Community Dominated by Older People

With a decrease in the number of persons engaged in certain rural occupations, especially in agriculture and mining, there has developed a population imbalance. Most of those leaving rural areas are young adults, and they leave behind a disporportionate number of older persons. The nation has become familiar with localities to which older people migrate, such as St. Petersburg, Asheville, Tucson, and San Diego, but much less attention has been paid to the rural counties in many other states which also may have large numbers of older people (Doerflinger and Marshall, 1962). Even when the older couple abandon the family farm (usually by selling it to a large-scale operator), they characteristically move into a nearby village or town. In some midwestern rural counties, one half of the adult population is over sixty years of age.

Although such communities may not be actually controlled by the aged, these communities often reveal the pervasive influence of older people. Political actions are geared to their interests. It is difficult to get school bond issues passed, there is strong opposition to the real property tax, a considerable share of local tax receipts are devoted to the county's share of Old Age Assistance payments, and the town is more likely to have a park than a playground. The general outlook of the community is marked by the large number of older inhabitants: the drug stores display items appealing to older people, merchants make benches available in front of their establishments, homes tend to be shabbier because their elderly inhabitants are neither physically nor financially able to paint them, and the aged are everywhere in evidence. Political representatives from declining rural areas in state legislatures are as likely to reflect the generally conservative attitudes of the disproportionate number of older constituents as they are the economic interests of the farmer and small-town merchant.

Housing

In many American cities new housing programs have been initiated to fill the special needs of older people. The building of these apartments, both publicly and privately owned, dates mainly from the mid-1950s. An apartment house designed for older inhabitants usually has several of the following features: entranceways without steps, all units on the ground floor or accessible by elevators, handrails in the corridors, handrails in the bathrooms, electric outlets that can be reached without bending, shelves that can be reached without standing on ladders or chairs, and small units supplemented by common rooms. Little of this kind of housing is yet available in rural areas, although government financing is equally available and presumably private contractors are available to build it.

Many small-town elderly hold on to the large old houses in which they reared their families, even though such houses are no longer suited to their needs. The lag is partly social psychological and partly economic. It is difficult to find a buyer for a large old house in an area of declining population. But there is also an attachment to the old home, despite its inadequacies. It is a place where the adult offspring, with their growing families, may visit. To move from it would require disposal of much furniture and other personal property to which there are personal attachments. If the old home happens to be located along a highway or in a tourist area, it is frequently turned into a tourist home as a means of supplementing income. This provides the older or widowed homeowner with a range of outside social contacts, although superficial ones.

Opportunities for Social Life

Because of the high proportion of older people in many rural areas of the United States, most of them have ready physical access to other persons of their own age. Of course, if they remain on the farm, they are often dependent on the automobile as a means of visiting their friends. If they are too physically handicapped to drive an automobile, the rural setting may isolate them. Unless they have the means and the inclination to travel, or unless they happen to live in a tourist area, both of which circumstances are rare, rural old people are largely cut off from broader social relationships. On the other hand, it is probable that rural old people are not so age graded and isolated by voluntary associations as are older people in the cities.

Just as rural areas have been laggard about accepting the modern forms of housing for older people, they have been slow about developing the modern forms of recreation for older people. Especially since 1950, the cities of the United States, through the initiative of social workers, churches, civic groups, or of older people themselves, have created a wide variety of recreational and social organizations. Many of these have names that reflect an optimistic view of old age: Golden Age Club, Live-Long and Like-it Club, Life Begins at Eighty Club. Any large northern city may boast of more than one hundred such clubs, although those familiar with them estimate informally that they attract no more than 5 to 10 percent of the population over sixty-five years. These clubs seem to do a great deal for the morale of those who participate in them.

But these clubs and organizations have been practically absent from rural areas, largely because local governments or private organizations have done little to create them.

THE GENERATIONAL FACTOR

Many of the attitudes of today's rural elderly population can be explained by the fact that they grew up in the years around 1900. Whether they grew up in rural areas of the United States or, less frequently, of Europe, their way of life was very different from that of the youngsters in rural areas today. Rural life is not greatly distinguishable from urban life today in most northern states: the farm is run like an industry, the stores offer the same range of merchandise, travel to cities is frequent, and radio and TV keep people in constant touch with the world. The farm and the small town of sixty years ago was much more closed, limited, and isolated. One could escape it only by migrating to the big city, as many did. But those who stayed retained much of the old-fashioned, almost frontier-like, mentality, even as changing technology and economic organization changed the way of rural life for their offspring. In the South, chronic economic depression and technological backwardness, coupled with the pervasiveness of the caste system and the extreme social isolation, made the rural white or Negro of the lower income group into a peasant.

Conservatism

The evident conservatism of today's elderly citizens has led many observers to conclude that aging brings conservatism. That may be, but it has not yet been demonstrated. A simpler explanation of the conservatism of most elderly people today, especially the rural ones, is that they always were conservative.

But the conservatism of the rural areas of the United States in 1900 went far deeper than politics. Modern technology had made little impact on the farms by then, and although some farmers were prosperous, they were not affluent, as many farmers are today. If they had migrated from Europe, many had been peasants, and theirs was essentially a medieval mentality. There was tight control of the children by the parents and even a good deal of patriarchal domination of the whole family. Fundamentalism in religion was probably stronger in rural areas then than it is today. Education seldom went beyond the primary grades and even then was usually provided in one-room school houses by poorly educated teachers. Rural life in the United States in 1900 did not often produce bold, open, inquiring minds in its

young people, and when it did, the young people migrated to the big cities.

Influence of Poverty

The tight control of the American economy after the Civil War by the big city bankers, industrialists, and railroad owners helped to prevent prosperity on the farm, except for the brief period of World War I. The fact that agriculture was so competitive and so risky, especially as an efficient technology was being adopted in the first four decades of the twentieth century, kept most farmers poor until 1940. Many of the rural aged today have experienced bankruptcy and mortgage foreclosure. Poverty and consequent lack of access to the advantage of modern household technology have helped to mold the attitudes of the contemporary rural aged.

As they perceive the affluence of the younger generation, on the farms as well as in the cities, many older persons who have been economically deprived through most of their lives must feel some resentment. Of course, they feel some compensation in their attachment to the old-fashioned virtues, but the envy is still there. Prosperity came to the farms too late (during the 1940s) to benefit most of the elderly of today, and they are still poor and deprived. The amenities of modern life, and even such necessities as good medical care, are still not theirs. A significant number among them are resentful and crabbed.

REFERENCES

Jon A. Doerflinger, and Douglas G. Marshall, *The Story of Price County, Wisconsin* (Madison: University of Wisconsin Agricultural Extension Service, 1962).

Chapter 3

AGING REGIONS OF THE UNITED STATES

ALBERT CHEVAN AND JOHN F. O'ROURKE

IT SEEMS OBVIOUS that the study of aging in American society must be heavily dependent on a consideration of the distribution and condition of the older population. Typically the distribution of the older population is indexed in terms of the percentage of older persons in the population of a given area (Hitt, 1956; Sheldon, 1960). The condition of the older population is frequently indexed in terms of income distribution, family status, housing conditions, or any of a number of other social, economic, health, or psychological variables (Riley and Foner, 1968; Sheldon, 1958). It is noteworthy, however, that most of the studies of the distribution of the older population are persented in terms of single variables related to geographic areas while most of the studies of the older population's condition make no observations on the basis of their geographic distribution. One is hard pressed to find studies which consider the distributional tendencies of the older population together with a consideration of the condition or status of the population as it is reflected in some of its characteristics. The report of The Council of State Governments is a notable exception (The Council of State Governments, 1955). Simply put, the question of how the various indicators of the well-being of the older population are distributed has not been thoroughly considered.

The tendency of investigators to compartmentalize their observations about the distribution and condition of the population may be too easily accepted. This paper reports the findings of a study in which techniques of multivariate analysis were used to describe the relationships which obtain between the distribution of the older population and some of its conditional characteristics. Thus, the purpose of this investigation was to examine the grounds on which assumptions about the homogeneity of the older population may be based and to test whether the assumptions are warranted.

Descriptions of the older population as, "financially deprived, isolated, poorly housed, immobile," imply a homogeneity which may or may not exist in fact. Riley and Foner (1968) have indicated the social and psychological consequences of taking the stereotype of the older person seriously. There are two processes at work, and both call for further analysis to avoid the pitfall of the assumption of homogeneity. Findings from the macroscopic level may be easily assumed to hold for all lower level areas, and there is the possibility of unwarranted generalization from specific findings in small areas to the macroscopic level. In either event it is important to observe the extent to which findings derived from one geographic level hold at another. For studies made at the national level, this reduces to asking what kinds of geographic variations are found in the characteristics of the older population at state and lower levels. For specific studies, this means establishing the range of variations which exists in other kinds of areas. The conclusions drawn on the assumption of homogeneity have important implications for

Reprinted by permission from the *Journal of Gerontology*, 1972, 27, 119-126.

the way in which one conceptualizes the old age status in American society.

In carrying out a test of the assumption of homogeneity, attention was focused on characteristics of the population aged sixty-five and over *exclusively* as these are reflected in data compiled at the state level. The choice of state data was prompted by a desire to find a unit intermediate between traditional geographic regions and units smaller than states, such as counties or Standard Metropolitan Statistical Areas. Selection of the latter areas for the units of analysis presents difficulties because of the large proportion of the population not in metropolitan areas and the great variability in the size of metropolitan areas. States have an additional merit as units of analysis in that they have well established regional associations, which counties or metropolitan areas do not have. Finally, the states have intrinsic political meaning which is significant to planners as well as to people who live in them.

In the present study, data for twenty variables were abstracted from the 1960 Census of Population for the population aged sixty-five years and older residing in the continental United States. Hawaii, Alaska, and the District of Columbia were excluded from this study. Their inclusion seriously affects the analysis because, when included among the states, they supply twenty-one of the extreme values for the variables in Table 3-I. Standard Bureau of the Census definitions were used for all variables (US Bureau of the Census, 1963). Several variables require further definition. *Inmigrants* were computed as the ratio of a reconstructed 1955 population sixty and over to the number migrating to a state between 1955 and 1960. *Outmigrants* were computed as the ratio of the same reconstructed 1955 population to the number migrating from that state between 1955

and 1960. The 1955 population was obtained by first subtracting from the 1960 population aged sixty-five and over those not reporting residence in 1955 and those migrating to a state between 1955 and 1960. Most older adults reported money income from some source in 1959. The percentage of those aged sixty-five and over receiving income is a measure of those receiving any money income. Gifts, money received from the sale of property, income "in kind," bank withdrawals, and loans are not considered money income, and presumably account for those not receiving an income. The variable list is presented in Table 3-I, which associates with each variable the state whose population has the highest or lowest value for the variable and the value for the total United States.

It is readily apparent that there is a wide range of differences between states in terms of these variables and that some variables are more widely dispersed than others. For example, the percentage of the population aged sixty-five and over living on rural farms ranges between a low of 0.6 percent in Rhode Island and a high of 24.2 percent in Mississippi. Wyoming and Kentucky represent the extremes of the older persons who, in 1960, were residing in the state in which they were born. Similar extremes of difference are demonstrated for most of the other variables.

Twenty-six states appear in these extreme positions. Of the possible forty mentioned, Florida and Mississippi account for ten extremes. This foreshadows some of the outcomes of the subsequent analyses. In the cases of some of the variables, the extreme value is startlingly different from the value for the total United States. Whereas 7.7 percent of the older population of the United States is nonwhite, the comparable value for the state of Mississippi is 39.1. On the face of it, Table 3-I dispels any easy

TABLE 3-I
HIGH AND LOW STATE VALUES AND TOTAL US VALUES OF SELECTED
CHARACTERISTICS OF THE OLDER POPULATION

Population Characteristic	High Value	Low Value	Total US Value
1. % of state population aged 65+	11.9 (Iowa)	5.4 (NM)	9.0
2. % 65+ in urban areas	89.0 (RI)	27.0 (Minn)	70.0
3. % 65+ in rural farm areas	24.2 (Miss)	0.6 (RI)	7.7
4. % 65+ living as primary individuals	28.3 (Nev)	13.5 (NC)	19.7
5. % 65+ married and living with spouse	58.7 (Fla)	42.9 (Cal)	49.3
6. % 65+ living in child's household	16.8 (Md)	6.7 (Utah)	11.7
7. % 65+ living in group quarters	7.6 (Mass)	2.1 (Miss)	4.8
8. % 65+ born in state of residence	83.9 (Ky)	8.9 (Wyo)	48.3
9. % 65+ foreign born	41.9 (Conn)	0.9 (Miss)	19.6
10. % 65+ nonwhite	39.1 (Miss)	0.1 (Me)	7.7
11. % 65+ inmigrants	36.0 (Fla)	1.4 (NY)	....[a]
12. % 65+ outmigrants	11.4 (Nev)	1.7 (La)	....[a]
13. % 65+ receiving income in 1959	88.6 (Colo)	79.1 (Va)	83.6
14. % 65+ receiving income with income under $3,000	91.7 (Ark)	72.4 (Mont)	81.7
15. % males 65+ in labor force	39.2 (Neb)	19.8 (Fla)	30.5
16. % employed males 65+ in white-collar occupations	45.6 (Fla)	23.8 (Miss)	36.6
17. % 65+ living in owner-occupied homes	84.2 (Kan)	50.3 (NY)	71.9
18. Median years of education completed by 65+	8.8 (Me)	6.3 (SC)	8.3
19. Males per 100 females in population 65+	117.2 (Nev)	71.4 (Mass)	82.1
20. Children ever born per female 65+	4.6 (ND)	2.6 (Fla)	3.2

[a]These statistics represent interstate migration only.

notion that the elderly population is distributed across the states in a homogeneous fashion. A more careful examination of the data upon which Table 3-I is based will also demonstrate that this apparent lack of homogeneous distribution in the elderly population applies not only to the forty-eight states considered as a whole but also to traditionally conceived regional subgroupings of states, such as the Midwest or the West.

The purpose of this investigation was to determine whether there are bases other than the traditional one of geographic contiguity upon which regions may be described. Several previous studies have addressed themselves to the problem of regionality by using multivariate techniques. Factor analytic methods were used to de-lineate regions and subregions of the United States (Hagood, 1941, 1943). Also, factor analytic methods were used to establish regions of sociocultural homogeneity among nations of the world (Russett, 1968). Factorial ecology is well established among urban sociologists as a means of delineating homogeneous urban areas (Abu-Lughod, 1969; Sweetser, 1965; Nicholson and Yeates, 1969). The study being presented here is a logical extension of these previous studies, but it differs from them in focusing attention on a particular age group, the elderly.

The strength of factor analytic treatment is that it allows the description of relationships among variables which are not obvious from casual inspection. Given the large number of possible sets of variables within a long variable list, factor analysis discriminates among the sets and indicates those which are of greatest importance. In the present investigation, the twenty variables for the forty-eight states were first subjected to a Q analysis in which the original data were transposed so that the states became variables and the variables became readings (Fishman, 1969; Rummel, 1970). It is at this point that the exclusion of Hawaii, Alaska, and the District of Columbia took on added importance. In this transposition each variable was transformed to a score between zero and one. The state with the smallest value supplied the lower or zero boundary and the state with the highest value supplied the upper or one boundary. All other states fell at some proportionate distance between these two extremes.

Changing the extreme or outlying values changes the values for all states in this transformation by increasing their variability. Therefore, Q analysis without Hawaii, Alaska, and the District of Columbia was favored on the grounds that it yielded groupings of states in which fewer states were excluded from membership in some group.

The transposed data were submitted to a principal components analysis, and the resulting factor loadings were subjected to a varimax orthogonal rotation. This step yielded groupings of states which are closely related to one another because of their similar configuration among the variables. In the next step the manner in which the groupings of states differ was investigated through a conventional factor analysis. The same data that were used for the Q analysis were used without transposition in this step. The factor scores that this principal components analysis and varimax rotation yielded were now available as indicators of the dimensions along which Q groups differ. These techniques provided a test of

the traditional assumptions about regionality.

RESULTS

The question of whether populations aged sixty-five and over are distributed over anything like conventionally conceived regions of the country is approached through a Q analysis. The outcome of the Q analysis of the twenty variables for forty-eight states is shown in Table 3-II. Three large and three small clearly distinguishable groups of states emerge when loadings of $\pm$ .60 and above are used. The three large groups include thirty-seven of the forty-eight areas considered in the study and the three small groups include nine areas. Thus, a total of forty-six of the forty-eight states have strong loadings in some Q group and only Maine and Maryland are not included in any Q group.

The Q groups shown in Table 3-II and Figure 3-1 are somewhat like traditional regions, but both include states which are important exceptions or exclude states that are normally considered part of the regional groupings. In the case of Q Group I, all the states in the west north central geographic division are included, as well as states from four other geographic divisions used by the Bureau of the Census. Vermont and Oregon, at opposite ends of the nation, belong to Q Group I. In the case of its first five states, Q Group II tends to take on the identity of the northeastern part of the United States. However, this impression is greatly modified when one considers the remainder of the list which includes Illinois, Delaware, Ohio, California, and Michigan, and excludes Maine and Vermont. A more plausible rationale for the internal consistency of this group of states, which on the surface appears associated with the urban-industrial complex of the United

TABLE 3-II

Q ANALYSIS OF THE FORTY-EIGHT CONTIGUOUS STATES BY SELECTED CHARACTERISTICS OF THE OLDER POPULATION: VARIMAX SOLUTION

									Q Group				
I		II		III		IV		V		VI			
State	Factor Loading	State	Factor Loading	State	Factor Loading	State	Factor Loading	State	Factor Loading	State	Factor Loading		
Neb	93	Conn	94	Ga	96	NM	92	Colo	75	Fla	—87		
Iowa	93	NJ	93	Ala	96	Wyo	69	Wash	68	Ariz	—67		
Kan	93	RI	92	SC	91	Nev	62	Okla	63				
SD	86	Mass	90	NC	88	Utah	62						
Ind	80	NY	90	Tenn	83								
Mo	75	Ill	89	La	83								
Wis	75	Pa	88	Miss	81								
Minn	73	Del	73	Ky	72								
Idaho	68	Ohio	73	Va	70								
Vt	67	NH	70	Ark	66								
Ore	66	Cal	66	Tex	64								
Mont	63	Mich	66	WVa	63								
ND	61												

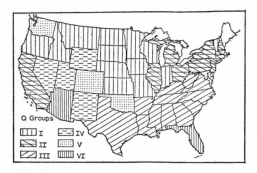

Figure 3-1.

States, will be supplied by the factor analysis.

Q Group III bears the strongest regional identity and is easily labeled southern. If the Bureau of the Census definition of the South were followed, then the inclusion of Florida, Maryland, Delaware, and Oklahoma would complete this list. Once again, it seems more reasonable to conceptualize this list in social and economic terms rather than on traditional geographic bases.

The four states in Q Group IV are all located in the Mountain Geographic Division of the Western region. Three other Q groups account for the other four states in the Mountain Division. Thus, states which would be expected to be included on the basis of geographic contiguity are excluded on other grounds, as yet undefined. Similarly, no geographic rationale exists for the configuration of states in Q Groups V and VI. The diversity of the population aged sixty-five and over in the Western Region of the United States is emphasized in Figure 3-1. Only Q Group II states are not found in this region of eleven states and no two states in the Pacific Division belong to the same Q group.

There remain two states, Maine and Maryland, which failed to achieve factor loadings of ± .60 or higher in any Q

group. Both of these states achieved loadings of .50 in two Q groups. This indicates their marginality when considered as regional members, since the decision to include them in any Q group would be arbitrary. Two other states, Kentucky and North Dakota, achieved acceptable factor loadings in Q groups other than those in which they were placed, indicating dual membership. Kentucky was placed in Q Group III because of the higher loading on that Q group. North Dakota was placed in Q Group I because it would have formed a seventh Q group with but a single member if the second, and slightly higher loading, were given precedence.

The Q analysis allows the observation that the criterion of geographic contiguity does not afford a reasonable foundation for grouping the older population of the continental United States. The usual reasoning behind employing the contiguity criterion is that, compared with noncontiguous groupings, states which border are most likely to have populations with similar characteristics. The Q analysis dispels that notion, but by itself, provides no alternative explanations for groupings of states achieved. Rather than speculate on what is common among geographically separate states, the technique of factor analysis will be enlisted as an aid in the interpretation of Q groups.

The factor loadings from the varimax solution of the principal components analysis of the twenty selected characteristics for the older population are shown in Table 3-III. Five factors were extracted in the factor analysis using eigenvalues greater than 1.0. These factors account for 82.3 percent of the variance which occurs among the forty-eight states.

When items with factor loadings of ± .60 and above are examined, it is apparent that the five factor structures represent

TABLE 3-III

FACTOR ANALYSIS OF SELECTED CHARACTERISTICS OF THE OLDER POPULATION: VARIMAX SOLUTION

Population Characteristic	Factor					h^2
	I	II	III	IV	V	
1. % of state population aged 65+	-70	-38	-06	-29	31	81.2
2. % 65+ in urban areas	-30	17	60	42	11	66.5
3. % 65+ in rural farm areas	48	-11	-68	-41	03	86.7
4. % 65+ living as primary individuals	-24	62	03	-02	68	90.5
5. % 65+ married and living with spouse	15	14	07	-85	19	80.0
6. % 65+ living in child's household	34	-38	12	46	-66	91.7
7. % 65+ living in group quarters	-89	-03	-16	23	-04	88.2
8. % 65+ born in state of residence	40	-68	-36	-04	-29	83.5
9. % 65+ foreign born	-71	16	23	42	-10	76.5
10. % 65+ nonwhite	84	-33	-08	13	-01	84.7
11. % 65+ inmigrants	10	43	70	-31	-08	78.9
12. % 65+ outmigrants	-16	89	-02	-08	-08	83.1
13. % 65+ receiving income in 1959	16	-11	08	-05	91	86.9
14. % 65+ receiving income with income under $3,000	59	-61	-18	-26	24	87.7
15. % males 65+ in labor force	-23	38	-75	20	-12	81.8
16. % employed males 65+ in white-collar occupations	-17	01	82	33	-05	81.2
17. % 65+ living in owner-occupied homes	-03	13	-24	-83	02	75.9
18. Median years of education completed by 65+	-78	46	11	-18	14	87.9
19. Males per 100 females in population 65+	08	77	-06	-40	18	80.3
20. Children ever born per female 65+	72	-07	-42	-18	-01	73.4
% variance accounted for	23.9	18.3	15.4	14.2	10.5	

clearly differentiated population structures. Factor I, which accounts for 24 percent of all variance, consists of a population with a high proportion of nonwhites combined with a low proportion of foreign born, a low proportion of older persons in the total population, high fertility in the past, low education, and a low proportion in group quarters. Although doing so anticipates the next step, these characteristics are customarily associated with a southern population, and this factor may be so labeled. The characteristic of low income, also associated with a southern population, barely fails inclusion in this factor. Moreover, rural farm residence, which is usually included in traditional lay conceptions for the South, loads only moderately on this factor.

Factor II is a mobility factor and characterizes a highly mobile population, both currently and probably in the past. There is a high outmigration coupled with a low proportion of residents born in the current state of residence, a high sex ratio, and a high proportion of the elderly living as primary individuals. There is a high degree of consistency among these four items, but the fifth item, low proportion with income under $3,000 in 1959, is not one commonly associated with the previous four items.

Factor III is an occupational factor and contains the two variables dealing with work status and occupation. These variables are represented by a high proportion of the employed in white collar occupations and a low proportion of males in the labor force. A third variable, low proportion residing in rural farm areas, coupled with a high proportion residing in urban areas, indicates an urban setting for this factor, such as the states in Q Group II. However, one characteristic loading heavily on this factor, a high proportion of inmigrants, does not fit the image of these states. Other variables which might be expected to appear in this factor if it were associated with Q Group II also do not appear.

Factors IV and V characterize different sets of living arrangements of the older population. Factor IV, on which only two items load strongly, stresses living without a spouse and living in rental units. Factor V places emphasis on a high proportion living as primary individuals and a low proportion living with a child. A high proportion reporting income in 1959 accompanies these two variables as part of Factor V, and would seem to facilitate the living arrangements implied by them. Such conceptual neatness must be tempered with the knowledge that populations rather than individuals are being described and generalization to the individual level is neither easy nor warranted. Thus, the five factors are clearly different from one another and have apparently rational internal structure.

The communalities for each variable shown in Table 3-III reveal that some variables are more strongly represented in the factors than others. The percentage in urban areas carries the lowest communality, 66.5. Urban residence is least related to the other variables, and knowledge of this variable contributes least to distinctions between the older populations of states. Location of residence within the state is not without importance, for the communality of rural farm residence is much greater than that of urban residence. This may be the result of the great diversity in the urban population, which includes persons in urbanized areas and places of 2,500 inhabitants or more outside urbanized areas.

The Q analysis and the factor analysis operate on basically the same data. It remains to establish the relationships between the two outcomes. The mean varimax factor scores for the six Q groups serve

TABLE 3-IV
MEAN FACTOR SCORES AND FACTOR SCORE STANDARD
DEVIATIONS FOR Q GROUPS

| Factor | | Q GROUP | | | | | |
		I	II	III	IV	V	VI
I	Mean	—.61	—.82	*1.36*	*.59*	—.22	.44
	S.D.	.37	.40	.63	.39	.37	.46
II	Mean	.14	—.26	—.70	*2.26*	.03	*.87*
	S.D.	.84	.39	.34	1.07	.26	.70
III	Mean	—.79	.43	—.24	—.09	*.56*	*3.45*
	S.D.	.59	.38	.61	.29	.15	.66
IV	Mean	—.67	*.92*	.02	.19	.02	*—1.82*
	S.D.	.37	.81	.89	.77	.47	.98
V	Mean	.31	—.41	—.13	—.07	*1.93*	—.37
	S.D.	.48	.79	1.08	.74	.03	.03

this purpose and are shown in Table 3-IV. This table was obtained by computing five varimax factor scores for each state, summing the factor scores for the states within each Q group, and dividing the sum by the number of states in a Q group. Mean factor scores of ± .50 or greater are italicized to stress the configurational pattern of each Q group. The standard deviation of each mean factor score is included in Table 3-IV.

The overall impression from Table 3-IV is that the grounds for establishing Q groups differ greatly from one group to another. The sets of variables associated with each factor are given different weightings within each Q group, and the cast of each Q group varies as a result. Furthermore, only two or three factors are of importance in any Q group, and Q groups take their imprint from these two or three factors. The Q groups remain more or less neutral in other factors.

Q Group III, as expected, has the highest mean for Factor I and the lowest mean for Factor II. In contrast with the southern states, the states in Q Group II score low on Factor I and high on Factor IV and are more or less neutral on other factors, including Factor III where a high loading was expected because of the urban nature of these states. On this basis, it is possible to say that the older populations of Q Groups II and III are the most dissimilar of any groups on the characteristics of Factor I. A parallel logic applies to comparisons between other Q groups. The basis for the unusual combinations of states in Q Groups IV, V, and VI is apparent in Table 3-IV. Florida and Arizona are the states which are most positive on Factor III and most negative on Factor IV. The populations of Q Groups IV and V are strikingly different on four of the five factors, albeit the states which comprise these groups are all west of the Mississippi River. The thirteen states in Q Group I, in the aggregate, score somewhat negative on Factors I, III, and IV.

Summary

The Q analysis establishes several major points about regionality. First, it produced six distinct groups of states whose older populations have characteristics which exhibit high degrees of internal consistency.

Three of these groupings consist of twelve states or more and these may be called the main aging regions in the United States. The three smaller groupings have such uniqueness as to constitute regions in themselves. Two states, Maine and Maryland, have marginal characteristics and so defy placement in any particular region. It should be emphasized that the aging regions which emerge in the Q analysis do not conform to traditional geographic conceptions of regionality in the United States, although Q Groups I and III do have some of the geographic bloc characteristics of regions. The analysis demonstrates conclusively that the older population is not distributed across the United States in a homogeneous fashion. It suggests that there are different styles of aging which may be geographically associated with the Q groups established in the analysis.

REFERENCES

Abu-Lughod, J. Testing the theory of social area analysis: The ecology of Cairo, Egypt. *American Sociological Review,* 1969, *34,* 198-212.

Fishman, J. A sociological census of a bilingual neighborhood. *American Journal of Sociology,* 1969, *75,* 323-339.

Hagood, M. Statistical methods for delineation of regions applied to data on agriculture and population. *Social Forces,* 1943, *21,* 287-297.

Hagood, M., Danilevsky, N., and Beum, C. O. An examination of the use of factor analysis in the problem of sub-regional delineation. *Rural Sociology,* 1941, *6,* 216-234.

Hitt, H. The demography of America's aged: A critical appraisal. In I. L. Webber (Ed.), *Aging: A current appraisal.* Gainesville: Press, University of Florida, 1956.

Nicholson, T. G., and Yeates, M. H. The ecological and spatial structure of the socio-economic characteristics of Winnipeg, 1961. *Canadian Review of Sociology & Anthropology,* 1969, *6,* 162-178.

Riley, M., and Foner, A. *Aging and society.* New York: Russell Sage Foundation, 1968.

Rummel, R. J. *Applied factor analysis.* Evanston, Ill.: Northwestern University Press, 1970.

Russett, B. M. International regions and the international system. In C. L. Taylor (Ed.), *Aggregate data analysis.* Paris: Mouton & Company, 1968.

Sheldon, H. D. *The older population of the United States.* New York: John Wiley & Sons, 1958.

Sheldon, H. D. The changing demographic profile. In C. Tibbitts (Ed.), *Handbook of social gerontology.* Chicago: University of Chicago Press, 1960.

Sweetser, F. Factorial ecology: Helsinki, 1960. *Demography,* 1965, *2,* 372-386.

United States Bureau of the Census. *Census of the population: 1960. Volume I, Characteristics of the population, parts 1-51.* Washington: Government Printing Office, 1963.

Section II

THEORIES OF AGING: SCIENTIFIC AND APPLIED

THE GERONTOLOGICAL WORK OF THE 1930s through much of the early 1950s was largely atheoretical in nature. By and large, scholars of this era were content to sketch the dimensions of the problems and concerns of an aged population. The theoretical frameworks utilized were usually implicit and often impressionistic in nature. As a consequence of this basically descriptive approach to aging, large quantities of frequently contradictory data began to accumulate.

Perhaps the first attempts to impose a semblance of order on the chaos of this "theory free" era were made in the late 1940s and early 1950s. Largely through the efforts of Havighurst and Albrecht (1953) and Cavan *et al.* (1949), the activity theory began to emerge as an attempt not only to integrate much previously accumulated knowledge, but also to explain a number of empirically based findings. In essence, this orientation suggested the health and well-being of the aged to be closely related to the physiological, psychological, and social activity levels of the aging adult. Such dimensions were considered in a state of dynamic tension. Reduction in activity levels in one area inevitably meant decrements in others. Although descriptive rather than explanatory in character, the activity theory stands as the first serious theoretical juncture in the history of contemporary social gerontology.

The impetus to theory building provided by Havighurst and Cavan was to bear fruit in the late 1950s and early 1960s. This proved to be the "golden age" of theory construction in gerontology. Although activity theory remained alive in a modified format, developmental (Anderson, 1958), role (Phillips, 1957), and identity-based (Miller, 1965) theories were emerging. Nevertheless, it was a theory quite opposed to these which stirred the imagination and engendered the criticism of scholars. The orientation in question was the disengagement theory.

The disengagement theory evolved in the late 1950s following the now famous Kansas City Study of Adult Life. As a result of this endeavor, Cumming and Henry (1961) set forth a formal exposition of this framework. By and large, the theory posits a functional relationship between the individual and society. The fact that individuals age and die and that society needs a continual replacement of "parts" is a fundamental tenet of the theory. In this view, both the person and society comprehend the necessity of the situation. As a consequence, the individual who can no longer produce effectively is expected to withdraw (i.e. disengage) from the on-going social life about him. This withdrawal encompasses not only a physical dimension by a psychological aspect as well. The disengagement processes which eventuate in a self-oriented personality are held to contribute to the maintenance of psychological well-being in late life. This process also makes possible a smooth transition of new "replacements" into the warp and woof of society.

The fact that Cumming and Henry regarded the above process as both inevitable and universal engendered a storm of criticism (Kutner, 1962; Maddox, 1963, 1964; Rose, 1964; Tobin and Neugarten, 1961). A positive result of such controversy, however, was a renewed attempt to link empirical research with a theoretical base. So successful was this new effort that the original authors were called upon to rethink their initial formulation (Cumming, 1964; Henry, 1964).

A final outcome of this period was an emphasis upon the differential qualities of age and aging. Expressed within the framework of continuity theory, gerontologists now viewed the processes of aging from an individualistic perspective. Instead of an inevitable process of disengagement or a continual pattern of activity being the case, individuals were acknowledged to represent a variety of "patterns" of aging (Cumming, 1964; Kutner, 1962; Maddox, 1963, 1964; Tibbitts, 1960; Rose, 1964; Tobin and Neugarten, 1961). The pattern of behavior one established in early life was now felt to be carried over relatively unchanged into late life. The continuity theory, therefore, was an attempt to account for many of the empirical inconsistencies discovered in this period.

If the previous era be regarded as one of theoretical development in gerontology, the period of the late 1960s and early 1970s can be seen as one of theoretical refinement (Atchley, 1972; Bengston, 1973). The activity theory, for example, was expanded to consider not only the type of activities engaged in by the older person, but also his phenomenal understanding of the meaning of these activities (Bengston *et al.,* 1969; Mercer, 1967; Lemon *et al.,* 1972). The disengagement theory, likewise, was forced to consider the individualistic character of the disengagement process. Cognitive and motivational factors were deemed essential to any explanation of disengagement phenomena (Back and McKinney, 1966; Seltzer and Atchley, 1971; Tissue, 1971). In the case of continuity theory, the life style or pattern notion of aging continued to be emphasized (Neugarten, 1965; Maddox, 1970; Havighurst *et al.,* 1968; Bultena, 1969; Palmore, 1968).

One final development continues to characterize contemporary theory in gerontology. By and large, the scholars of today are beginning to draw upon the rich theoretical resources of their respective disciplines. Sociologists, for example, are realizing the wealth of ideas provided by role and labeling as well as resocialization theories. Psychologists, too, have begun to place more stress on developmental models and have come to realize the usefulness of cognitive and exchange orientations. In addition, biologists have moved from an essentially deterministic course to one which recognizes individual and group potential. All in all, these shifts in perspective suggest a bright future for theoretical development in social gerontology.

The following papers are among the most recent explorations of the above-mentioned orientations. In addition to these "standard" frameworks, however, Gubrium, and Kuypers and Bengston present two fresh theoretical arrangements. True to the spirit of contemporary research, these authors draw insights from a variety of perspectives. Gubrium's theory, for example, is built around the interrelationship of two conceptual components: (1) environmental effects, such as social homogeneity, residential proximity, and local protectiveness; and (2) personal resources influencing behavior flexibility, such as health, solvency, and education. Kuypers and Bengston, on the other hand, borrow insights from labeling theory to argue the elderly susceptible to, and dependent on, social labeling because of their unique social reorganizations in late life.

The paper by Carp represents an attempt to clarify some of the components implicit in the disengagement framework. The author formulates and tests two disengagement-related hypotheses. First of all, it is hypothesized that, "disengagement from interpersonal relationships with family members and from those with friends are not coincident." In essence, the question addressed relates to the inevitability assumption of this formulation. Secondly, Carp hypothesizes that, "disengagement is not limited to immediate interpersonal involvement." Disengagement, it is argued, may be a personality trait and as such, may apply differentially to cathexes with objects, activities, and mental stimulations, as well as to those with persons.

The results of 295 interviews with residents of public and private housing indicate that disengagement from possessions, mental stimulation, and activities have much in common with each other and with disengagement from people. Nevertheless, the correlation between disengagement from family and from other people is observed to be negative. Disengagement from family is also negatively correlated with that from activities. "The results suggest that disengagement from the parental role is inversely related to disengagement from other people and that the concept of disengagement should be expanded to include withdrawal of investment from possessions, ideas, and activities."

The paper by Tallmer and Kutner addresses still another dimension of the disengagement perspective. These authors suggest that factors other than aging *per se* (e.g. stress-inducing environmental and circumstantial disturbances) may account for the social consequences previously attributed to disengagement. For Tallmer and Kutner, time does not merely pass nor does an individual merely age. Instead, "what transpires as time elapses . . . forces the individual to alter his life style leading to social disengagement." The issue, then, concerns whether disengagement may be viewed as an extrinsic or an intrinsic process.

Utilizing the technique of partial correlation, the authors conclude that, "disengagement among the aged can be predicted to occur as a concomitant of physical or social stresses which profoundly affect the manner in which the life pattern of the person is redirected." In other words, disengagement tends to be primarily the result of extrinsic rather than intrinsic factors. It is the correlates of old age (i.e. failing health, loss of peers, death of relatives, etc.) which appear to account for the social phenomenon known as disengagement.

The paper by Lemon *et al.* makes explicit a long implicit perspective in gerontology, the activity theory. As the authors point out, a formal test of this orientation is lacking in recent literature. While data exist which link activity levels to life satisfaction, these findings often prove a function of time limitations or research design. What is needed, and what the authors pursue, is a formal axiomatic statement of activity theory. In addition, utilizing secondary data derived from a study of inmovers to a retirement community, they subject the activity orientation to empirical test.

It is observed that, "only social activity with friends was in any way related to life satisfaction. No significant relationship was found between activity with neighbors, relatives, formal organization, or solitary activity." The utilization of such specification variables as age, sex, marital status, and employment status, fail to alter these initial findings. By and large, "the data lend only limited support to some of the propositions of activity theory."

The continuity theory is the subject of the paper by Maddox and Douglass. These authors contend that the reduction of variance in functioning with age has not been adequately demonstrated. They suggest such reported reductions may be artifactual of methodological design, sampling bias, and selective survival. As a consequence, they hypothesize individual differences to remain relatively constant over time once these factors are accounted for. Similarly, they hypothesize the maintenance of social differentiation in late life.

Data from a continuing longitudinal study form the basis for the authors' analysis. The authors conclude that, by and large, individual differences do not decrease with age in late life. In some instances they report marked increases in individual differences. The range of observed individual differences they find also to be maintained. That is, the individuals in the sample tend to maintain the same rank on a variety of social, psychological, and physiological indicators in relation to their age peers well into the later years of life.

The paper by Gubrium represents a fresh attempt at theory construction. The author's model is derived from a series of intensive interviews with 210 persons, age sixty to ninety-four, in a variety of residential settings. Basically a socioenvironmental typology, Gubrium's formulation recognizes the interrelationship of two conceptual components: (1) environmental effects, such as social homogeneity, residential proximity, and local protectiveness; and (2) personal resources influencing behavior flexibility such as health, solvency, and education. Although still in the developmental stages, the socioenvironmental orientation has both predictive and explanatory import to the gerontologist.

Finally, the paper by Kuypers and Bengston suggests a creative alternative to the theories previously presented. Borrowing insights from labeling theory, the authors argue the elderly susceptible to, and dependent on, social labeling because of their unique social reorganizations in late life. Such dependency leads to what is termed the *social breakdown syndrome,* characterized by the loss of coping abilities and the development of an internalized sense of incompetence.

After specifying the conditions under which this syndrome is most pernicious, the authors suggest an alternative formulation, the *social reconstruction syn-*

drome. This orientation calls for intervention at a number of critical points. Among the inputs suggested are (1) a new definition of social competence with age; (2) liberation from the functional ethic and the evolution of alternative ethical standards for older persons; and (3) the provision of various social and physical resources to lessen the debilitating environmental conditions facing the elderly.

REFERENCES

Anderson, J. E. A development model for aging. *Vita Humana*, 1958, *1*, 5-18.

Atchley, R. C. *The social forces in later life: an introduction to social gerontology*. Belmont, California: Wadsworth, 1972.

Back, K. W., and Gergen, K. J. Cognitive and motivational factors in aging and disengagement. In I. H. Simpson and J. C. McKinney (Eds.), *Social aspects of aging*. Durham, North Carolina: Duke University Press, 1966.

Bengston, V. L. *The social psychology of aging*. Indianapolis-New York: Bobbs-Merrill Company, Inc., 1973.

Bengston, V. L., Chriboga, D. C., and Keller, A. C. Occupational differences in retirement: patterns of role activity and life outlook among Chicago retired teachers and steelworkers. In R. J. Havighurst, M. Thomae, B. L. Neugarten, and J. K. A. Munnichs (Eds.), *Adjustment to retirement: a cross-national study*. Assen, The Netherlands: Van Gorkum, 1969.

Bultena, G. L. Life continuity and morale in old age. *Gerontologist*, 1969, *9* (4, part I), 251-253.

Cavan, R. S., Burgess, E. W., Havighurst, R. J., and Goldhammer, H. *Personal adjustment in old age*. Chicago: Science Research Associates, 1949.

Cumming, E. New thoughts on the theory of disengagement. In R. Kastenbaum (Ed.), *New thoughts on old age*. New York: Springer, 1964.

Cumming, E., and Henry, W. *Growing old: the process of disengagement*. New York: Basic Books, 1961.

Havighurst, R. J., and Albrecht, R. *Older people*. New York: Longmans, Green, 1953.

Havighurst, R. J., Neugarten, B. L., and Tobin, S. S. Disengagement and patterns of aging. In B. L. Neugarten (Ed.), *Middle age and aging*. Chicago: University of Chicago Press, 1968.

Henry, W. E. The theory of intrinsic disengagement. In P. F. Hansen (Ed.), *Age with a future*. Copenhagen: Munksgaard, 1964.

Kutner, B. The social nature of aging. *Gerontologist*, 1962, *2*, 5-9.

Kuypers, J. A., and Bengston, V. L. Social breakdown and competence: a model of normal aging. *Human Development*, 1973, *16*, 181-201.

Lemon, B. W., Bengston, V. L., and Peterson, J. A. Activity types and life satisfaction in a retirement community. *Journal of Gerontology*, 1972, *27*, 511-523.

Maddox, G. L. Activity and morale: a longitudinal study of selected elderly subjects. *Social Forces*, 1963, *42*, 195-204.

Maddox, G. L. Disengagement theory: a critical evaluation. *Gerontologist*, 1964, *4*, 80-82.

Maddox, G. L. Persistence of life style among the elderly. In E. Palmore (Ed.), *Normal aging*. Durham, North Carolina: Duke University Press, 1970.

Mercer, J. R., and Butler, E. W. Disengagement of the aged population and response differentials in survey research. *Social Forces*, 1967, *46*, 89-96.

Miller, S. J. The social dilemma of the aging leisure participant. In A. Rose and W. Peterson (Eds.), *Older people and their social world*. Philadelphia: F. A. Davis, 1965.

Neugarten, B. L. Personality and patterns of aging. *Gawein,* 1965, *13,* 249-256.

Palmore, E. The effects of aging on activities and attitudes. *Gerontologist,* 1968, *8,* 259-263.

Phillips, B. S. A role theory approach to adjustment in old age. *American Sociological Review,* 1957, *22,* 212-217.

Rose, A. M. A current theoretical issue in social gerontology. *Gerontologist,* 1964, *4,* 25-29.

Seltzer, M. M., and Atchley, R. C. The impact of structural integration into the profession on work commitment, potential for disengagement, and leisure preferences among social workers. *Sociological Focus,* 1971, *5,* 9-17.

Tibbitts, C. *Handbook of social gerontology.* Chicago: University of Chicago Press, 1960.

Tissue, T. L. Disengagement potential: replication and use as an explanatory variable. *Journal of Gerontology,* 1971, *26,* 76-80.

Tobin, S. S., and Neugarten, B. L. Life satisfaction and social interaction in the aging. *Journal of Gerontology,* 1961, *16,* 344-346.

Chapter 4

SOME COMPONENTS OF DISENGAGEMENT

FRANCES M. CARP

CUMMING AND HENRY (1961) presented disengagement as an inevitable mutual withdrawal which results in decreased interaction between the aging person and other people in the social system to which he belongs. Subsequently, disengagement theory and research have been concerned primarily with immediate personal interactions, and these personal interactions have been treated as relatively homogeneous.

It is recognized that various approaches to measurement yield different scores on disengagement. For example, Tobin, Havighurst, and Neugarten speak of the "various components of engagement-disengagement" (1962). However, the components to which they refer are "activity level, ego involvement, degree of positive affect, change in level of activities since age 60, and affect concerning the change in activity." Tobin et al. (1962) developed rating scales to measure these variables for each of eleven roles. While they recognize that activity and affect regarding activity may vary from role to role, Tobin et al. have been interested in the relationships between activity and affect rather than in relationships among roles. These and other investigators recognize that disengagement is not a unitary phenomenon in the sense that number of hours spent in interaction with family and friends is one measure,

Reprinted by permission from the *Journal of Gerontology*, 1968, *23*, 282-286.

while investment in the relationships is another.

This may still be a simplistic view. Disengagement may operate differently in various relationships. Treating family and friends together may obscure the process. The general developmental literature indicates that the relative importance of family members and of friends changes from one life stage to another (Gesell and Ilg, 1949; Hurlock, 1964). In regard to old age, the matter remains equivocal. Rosow (1964, 1966, 1967) stresses the socialization advantage of age-homogeneity and points to the greater interaction and mutual assistance among old persons in neighborhoods with high density of old people. Shanas and Streib (1965) conclude that, "in a rapidly changing world, the family becomes more important, not less important." This suggests that, as friends are lost in old age, relationships with kin become increasingly important. Carp (1966a) found that, while old people took advantage of an opportunity to form new acquaintanceships and enjoyed the increased sociability with friends and neighbors, these relationships did not replace ties with family members. Satisfaction with family improved as friendships expanded. Contact with family did not change.

Disengagement may operate in aspects of life other than the immediately interpersonal. The "social system" of an adult is not completely defined by his immediate interpersonal contacts. Libido normally is invested not only in other persons but also in possessions, activities, and cognitive pursuits. Perhaps disengagement can be more competently measured and understood if some of these additional aspects can be identified and included.

This study is an effort to clarify some components of disengagement. It has two hypotheses: (1) disengagement from interpersonal relationships with family members and from those with friends are not coincident, and (2) disengagement is not limited to immediate interpersonal involvement.

THE GENERALITY-SPECIFICITY OF DISENGAGEMENT ACROSS INTERPERSONAL INTERACTIONS: Previous measures of disengagement imply that interpersonal involvements are summative across all available role relationships. For example, Tobin and Neugarten (1961) used "number-of-persons-interacted-with-per-month," "number of hours per day spent in interaction with others, and intensity and quality of interpersonal relations." Tobin *et al.* (1962) used a total role-activity score which was based on ratings of activity level in eleven life roles: worker, spouse, parent, grandparent, kin-group member, homemaker, friend, neighbor, citizen, club member, and church member. The implication is that all role activities are involved in engagement-disengagement, and that units from the various role relationships are additive. To put it another way: while, obviously, the interpersonal behavior of old persons is conditioned by role availability, and the old person can express involvement only within those roles still available to him, the extent of his disengagement can be gauged by adding score units across roles. This inevitably implies that disengagement affects all role activities in the same direction at the same time. On the other hand, Shanas and Streib (1965) suggest that, as relationships with friends diminish, those within the kin group assume greater importance. Rosow (1964, 1966, 1967) finds that involvement with neighbors is largely determined by age composition of the neighborhood. Carp's (1966a, 1966b, 1967) findings are similar, and add that the quality of relationship with family is improved by increase in contact with neighbors and satisfaction with nonkin relationships.

For this study, interpersonal relationships were divided into two categories: those with family and those with other persons. If disengagement is a general trait, scores on engagement-disengagement with family should correlate positively and significantly with those on engagement-disengagment with other people. If disengagement does not affect similarly the relationships with family and with friends, correlations should be insignificant. If the process affects these relationships differentially, as suggested by Rosow (1964, 1966, 1967), Shanas and Streib (1965), and Carp (1966a, 1966b, 1967), correlations should be negative.

APPLICABILITY OF DISENGAGEMENT TO NONPERSONAL ROLES: It seems possible that engagement-disengagement is a personality trait or a process of aging which applies to cathexes with objects, activities, and mental stimulation, as well as to those with persons. Life roles are not limited to those which are patently interpersonal. Libido is invested in transactions with the external world through activities, and through involvement with society by keeping up with the news, reading new books, listening to controversial radio and television broadcasts, etc. The ego may be heavily invested in objects.

If disengagement is the normal preparation for death, disengagement must be accomplished not only with ties to persons, but also with those to material possessions and to worldly activities and ideas. Therefore, the index of disengagement used in this study included an item in each of these areas. If disengagement occurs in relation to the by-products of experience in the social system, as well as to immediately interpersonal aspects of that system, scores on the nonpersonal items should correlate with those on the immediately personal ones.

Materials and Methods

SUBJECTS: *Ss* for the study were 295 old people in San Antonio, Texas. They were old (range 54 years to 93 years, median 74) and poor (median income $94.40 per month, modal income $70.00) residents of a metropolitan area. One hundred ninety lived in apartments in Victoria Plaza, a public housing facility for the elderly; 105 lived in private homes, apartments, or rooms.

DATA COLLECTION: The data were provided by the interviewer who, on two occasions at an interval of approximately eighteen months, had spent several hours (typically 6) with the *S* to obtain extensive interview and test data on his history, current status and attitudes in regard to health, finances, family, and self, and his plans and anticipations of the future. In the interim, the interviewer had collected sociometric data three times. Following the last interview and test session, the interviewer recorded a number of judgments about the respondent. The items on which the interviewer evaluated the *S*'s disengagement were as follows:

1. More willing to let family (children) run own lives
   ..... 1) no
   ..... 2) don't know
   ..... 3) yes
2. Less interested in material things
   ..... 1) no
   ..... 2) don't know
   ..... 3) yes
3. Less interested in mental stimulation (news, books, discussion, etc.)
   ..... 1) no
   ..... 2) don't know
   ..... 3) yes
4. Less interested in taking part in activities
   ..... 1) no
   ..... 2) don't know

..... 3) yes
5. Less interested in people (other than kin)
   ..... 1) no
   ..... 2) don't know
   ..... 3) yes

The Disengagement Index required the interviewer's estimates regarding change in the *S* over the approximately eighteen-month period between intensive interview sessions. It involved ipsative rating rather than a normative rating (Kelly and Lingoes, 1962). The person was compared to himself at another time rather than to a reference group of other people. For example, the interviewer would check "Yes" to Item 2, "Is less interested in material things," for a person who gave the impression of being less concerned with the way his house looked, the kinds of furniture it had, etc. than he had been previously. People who continued to mention during the interview that they wanted good clothes, to have their hair fixed every week, to buy new furniture, or in other ways to "keep up with the Joneses," would be checked "No." The items focus on the presence or absence of change, on disengagement as a process, and, therefore, the index is less likely to confound an age change with a stable personality behavior trait (Rosow, 1963).

Also, these are estimates of interest or willingness, not necessarily of performance. For example, in some instances the person seemed extremely interested in people but the circumstances of his life made it impossible for him to enjoy much social participation. His rating sheet would be checked "No" in Item 5.

The format of the family item in the Disengagement Index seems preferable to a more traditional and less specific wording. The element of control or influence is central to the early parent-child relationship. Therefore, the dissolution of control must be intrinsic to disengagement. Frequency of contact occurs when an aged parent is fed, bathed, and otherwise treated like an infant. In such a situation of role reversal, high frequency of contact does not mean absence of disengagement. Similarly, intensity or closeness of relationship may vary quite independently of basic role quality. Identification of the variables of parent-child interactions during maturity and life, and explication of the relationships among them, remain fragmentary. Hence, the focus is on one basic factor, the locus of control or influence. The release of this directive role seems intrinsic to disengagement as it related to the aging process. Therefore, the family item of the index was directed at the element of control.

TREATMENT OF DATA: On a random sample of 100 *Ss,* a different interviewer read the interview and test responses and then filled out the Disengagement Index. Interjudge agreement on "Yes" responses was 96 percent. For the analysis reported here, the scores of the interviewer who had been in contact with the *S* were used.

To assess the commonality of disengagement from parental role and from the role of friend and acquaintance, zero-order correlations between judgments on Item 1 and Item 5 were calculated. To determine whether there is commonality among disengagement from persons and from objects, activities, and mental stimulation,

zero-order correlations between Item 1 and Items 2, 3, and 4, and between Item 5 and Items 2, 3, and 4 were calculated. For this purpose, responses were categorized: "Yes" vs. "No" and "Don't know." Point biserial correlation coefficients were computed, and the significance of the difference of each correlation coefficient from zero was assessed in terms of the standard error (McNemar, 1955).

Results

The results are reported in Table 4-I. Inspection of the table shows that disengagement from possessions, mental stimulation, and activities have a fair amount in common with each other and with disengagement from people. However, loss of interest in playing an influential role within the family shows no commonality with any of the other four. The rating on disengagement from this parental role showed no relationship to ratings on interest in material things and mental stimulation. It showed statistically significant negative correlations with interest in activities and in other people.

Discussion

These findings suggest that the concept and the measurement of disengagement could well be broadened to include release of attachment to possessions, to activities,

TABLE 4-I
INTERCORRELATIONS OF DISENGAGEMENT INDEX ITEMS

	Possessions	Stimulation	Activities	Other People
Family	—.06	—.05	—.19[a]	—.21[a]
Possessions		.30[a]	.30[a]	.26[a]
Stimulation			.27[a]	.28[a]
Activities				.52[a]
N = 295				

[a]Indicates significant difference from 0 at $P < 0.01$.

and to ideas which impinge upon the person from his environment. This is not surprising. The "social system" in which an adult lives is not limited to, or adequately defined by, the direct interpersonal contacts he makes.

The results also suggest that care must be taken in identifying the component parts of disengagement. Disengagement from family and from friends seems to have different meanings and timings. Among this group of people, those who appeared to be loosening the directive bonds of parenthood were not simultaneously loosening friendship ties or showing reduced interest in worldly affairs. The difference between the two aspects of disengagement is supported by the relationships between other data on these Ss which have to do with family and friends. For example, there was no relationship between frequency of visiting friends and frequency of visiting children ($r = -.06$). Nor was there one between frequency of seeing children and number of friends ($r = -.07$). Frequency of visits with children was inversely related to number of leisure pastimes in the company of others ($r = -.11$, $P<0.05$) and to membership in organizations ($r = -.12$, $P<0.05$). These correlations support the dissimilarity of engagement with family and with friends. This dissimilarity may have particular relevance to traditional measures of engagement-disengagement which summate measures of activity or involvement for these role relationships, as well as to understanding the nature of disengagement.

In regard to disengagement from family and from friends, this study indicates only that the two are not simultaneous and identical. Other studies must clarify the nature of variables and their relationships with each other and with other variables. The results are consistent with the view

that, as involvement in activities and with friends and acquaintances diminishes, the parental role becomes relatively more important to the aging person. This may reflect the investment of diminished energy in the most valuable domain, or it may result from situational thwarting of other outlets.

It may be relevant to further studies to note that disengagement from the directive parental role was associated with more positive self-image, while continued engagement in it was related to signs of maladjustment. Persons who were disengaging from the family role selected a larger number of favorable adjectives for self-description ($r = .27$, $P<0.01$). They reported fewer ailments which were of a neurotic type ($r = -.12$, $P<0.05$), and they showed fewer signs of maladjustment on the Senility Index of Cavan, Burgess, Havighurst, and Goldhamer (1949) ($r = -.16$, $P<0.01$).

It may be useful also to mention that there was no relationship between frequency of contact with children and satisfaction with family ($r = .05$). Frequency of visits with children was inversely related to satisfaction with friends ($r = -.13$, $P<0.05$). In general, the Ss who moved into Victoria Plaza, where opportunities for peer relationships were many, made new friends and indulged in more social activities. This increased peer engagement was accompanied by increased satisfaction with family as well as increased satisfaction with friends, though there was no consistent change in frequency of contact with family. Life satisfaction and self-esteem improved (Carp, 1966a). Disengagement from the controlling role of parenthood may be facilitated by opportunities for continued engagement among peers. On the contrary, environmentally determined disengagement from peers may increase dependency upon the parental role and retard the development task of disengaging from an earlier parent-child relationship or lead to regressive behavior in relation to adult children.

Summary

Two-hundred ninety-five old people were rated on an Index of Disengagement which includes items on own children, other people, activities, ideas, and material possessions. The correlation between disengagement from family and from other people was negative. Disengagement from family also correlated negatively with that from activities. Correlations were positive among disengagement from possessions, ideas, activities, and people other than family. The results suggest that disengagement from the parental role is inversely related to disengagement from other people and that the concept of disengagement should be expanded to include withdrawal of investment from possessions, ideas, and activities. Corollary data suggest that disengagement from the parental role which was appropriate at an earlier life stage may be facilitated by relationships with other people and that limitation of peer contact may increase dependency upon the family and retard the developmental task of disengaging from the parental role.

REFERENCES

Carp, F. M.: *A future for the aged.* Univ. Texas Press, Austin, 1966, 287 pp. (a)

Carp, F. M.: Effects of improved housing on the lives of older people. Chap. 12 in: F. M. Carp (Editor), *Patterns of living and housing of middle-aged and older people.* U.S. Govt. Print. Office, Washington, D. C., 1966, pp. 147-159. (b)

Carp, F. M.: The impact of environment on old people. *Gerontologist, 7:*106-109, 1967.

Cavan, R. S., Burgess, E. W., Havighurst, R. J., and Goldhamer, H.: *Personal adjustment in old age.* Science Research Associates, Inc., Chicago, 1949, 199 pp.

Cumming, E. and Henry, W. E.: *Growing old: the process of disengagement.* Basic Books, New York, 1961, 293 pp.

Gesell, A. and Ilg, F. L.: *Child development: an introduction to the study of human growth.* Harper & Brothers, New York, 1949, 475 pp.

Hurlock, E. B.: *Child development.* McGraw-Hill, Inc., New York, 1964, 4th Ed., 776 pp.

Kelly, E. W., and Lingoes, J. C.: Data processing in psychological research. Chap. 9 in: H. Borko (Editor), *Computer applications in the behavioral sciences.* Prentice-Hall, Inc., Englewood Cliffs, N. J., 1962, pp. 173-203.

McNemar, Q.: *Psychological statistics.* John Wiley & Sons, Inc., New York, 1955, 2nd Ed., 408 pp.

Rosow, I.: Adjustment of the normal aged. Chap. 38 in: R. H. Williams, C. Tibbitts, and W. Donahue (Editors), *Processes of Aging: Social and Psychological Perspectives.* Atherton Press, New York, 1963, pp. 195-223.

Rosow, I.: Local concentrations of aged and *intergenerational friendships. In:* P. F. Hansen (Editor), Age with a Future. *Proceedings of the Sixth International Congress of Gerontology, Copenhagen,* 1963. Munksgaard, Copenhagen, 1964, pp. 478-483.

Rosow, I.: Housing and local ties of the aged. Chap. 5 in: F. M. Carp (Editor), *Patterns of Living and Housing of Middle-Aged and Older People.* U.S. Govt. Print. Office, Washington, D. C., 1966, pp. 47-64.

Rosow, I.: *Social integration of the aged.* The Free Press, New York, 1967, 354 pp.

Shanas, E. and Streib, G. F.: An introduction. Chap. 1 in: E. Shanas and G. F. Streib (Editors), *Social Structure and the Family: Generational Relations.* Prentice-Hall, Inc., Englewood Cliffs, N. J., 1965, pp. 2-8.

Tobin, S. S., Havighurst, R. J., and B. L. Neugarten: An empirical investigation of the disengagement theory. *J. Geront., 17:*475, 1962. (Abstract)

Tobin, S. S. and Neugarten, B. L.: Life satisfaction and social interaction in the aging. *J. Geront., 16:*344-346, 1961.

Chapter 5

DISENGAGEMENT AND THE STRESSES OF AGING

Margot Tallmer and Bernard Kutner

Disengagement theory by all odds is widely acknowledged to be one of the most inventive of conceptions about the nature of the human aging process. Although it has been accorded some rough treatment since it was proposed by Cumming and Henry (1961), it has certainly provided scientific investigators of aging and their counterparts in social gerontology much to gnaw upon. Both the theory itself and the implications that may be drawn from it for social planning, public policy, and program development in the field of aging have made deep impressions, aroused serious thought, and sparked off new research endeavors. This paper is but another manifestation of the thunder that has followed the appearance of the disengagement theory in the sociological firmament.

A provisional theory of the process of aging, disengagement theory attempted to explain, within a functional framework, the patent observation that people become increasingly more withdrawn as they advance into old age. The theory questioned an implicit assumption of the activity theory of aging. It suggested, contrariwise, that social and psychological withdrawal

Reprinted by permission from the *Journal of Gerontology*, 1969, *24*, 70-75.

may be a necessary component of successful aging. According to the original promulgation of the theory, disengagement is an inevitable, universal, self-perpetuating, gradual, and mutually satisfying process prepared for in advance by society and the individual. During the process, the degree and variety of social interactions lessen with advancing years. These alterations are accompanied by concomitant changes in the perception of the life space and by an increasing self-absorption and lessening of ego energy. In a later article (1964), Cumming modified the theory but generally held to its main themes. She suggested possible variations in the pattern of withdrawal. Henry (1963) had in the meantime retreated somewhat from his original theoretical position and had introduced both the possibilities of reengagement and the need for considering life style patterns of response. He acknowledged that neither the disengagement nor activity theory could explain much of the empirical evidence nor could either handle questions raised by the effects of intentional external activation.

Although disengagement is a characteristic process of the elderly, according to many sociologists (Havighurst, Neugarten, and Tobin, 1963; Parsons, 1942; Rose, 1964; Williams and Wirths, 1965), they differ in their explanations and assessments of the data. When parts of the disengagement theory are tested empirically, there are various findings that cannot be adequately explained by the unmodified theory (Desroches and Kaiman, 1964; Prasad, 1964; Zborowski, 1962). Investigations of the activity/morale relationship fail to provide conclusive evidence either for the activity or the disengagement theories. Data suggested as upholding the former theory (Havighurst, Neugarten and Tobin,

1964; Kutner, Fanshel, Togo, and Langner, 1956; Reichard, Livson, and Petersen, 1962) also partly substantiate the latter. Groups appear either low in activity but high in morale (Lowenthal, 1946b; Maddox, 1962; Maddox and Eisdorfer, 1962) or show a decrease in activity but no concomitant morale decrement (Maddox, 1962).

In regard to personality differences with age, some studies show consistent changes between the years of forty and sixty (Bortner, 1962; Guttmann, Henry, and Neugarten, 1959; Neugarten and Guttmann, 1958; Shaw and Henry, 1956), but such research is usually based on cross-sectional data and does not necessarily reflect developmental changes. Investigations based on Rorschach findings reveal that with advancing years there is a tendency toward constriction of the life space and a diminution of response to external stimulation due to increased inner personal concerns. Without the establishment of norms for this age group, the Rorschach's sensitivity as an instrument may be questioned (Caldwell, 1954).

Both theories deal with chronological age as an entity when in fact it comprises many factors. Other possible explanations of the aging process include life patterns (Reichard *et al.*, 1962) and personality (Havighurst and Albrecht, 1953; Havighurst, Neugarten, and Tobin, 1963; Williams and Wirths, 1965; Zborowski, 1962) as the deciding factor. Aging then would not mirror a sharp change but rather a continuing consistent process of development (Cavan, Burgess, Havighurst, and Goldhamer, 1949; Lowenthal, 1964a; Maddox, 1965). Associations between class status and successful aging have been amply demonstrated (Kutner *et al.*, 1956; Lowenthal, 1964a; Maddox, 1964; Mead, 1962; Tobin, Havighurst, and Neugarten, 1962).

Prevalence of the aged in the community has been related to morale (Blau, 1961; Talmon, 1963), and health as a factor has been investigated repeatedly (Britton and Britton, 1951; Havighurst and Albrecht, 1953; Jeffers and Nichols, 1961; Kleemeier, 1951; Kutner *et al.*, 1956; Landis, 1942; Lebo, 1953; Maddox, 1962; Schmidt, 1951; Taves and Hansen, 1962) as has marital status (Burgess, 1954; Cavan *et al.*, 1949; Kutner *et al.*, 1956; Pressey and Simcoe, 1950; Taves and Hansen, 1962). Other factors related to adjustment in old age include sex differences (Lebo, 1953; Tobin, Havighurst, and Neugarten, 1962) and retirement status (Blau, 1961; Cumming and Henry, 1961; Goodstein, 1962; Kleemeier, 1951; Leveen and Priver, 1963; Parsons, 1942; Reichard *et al.*, 1962; Taves and Hansen, 1962).

Although Cumming and Henry speak of disengagement as a process of sociopsychological withdrawal, they do not draw a fine distinction between these processes. It is possible for psychological withdrawal or disengagement to occur prior to or concomitantly with social disengagement. The present study, however, deals particularly with the process of social disengagement.

We have attempted in this study to limit ourselves to some of the aforementioned factors while replicating as much as possible the methodology of Cumming and Henry. While we do not attempt to deal with the full range of problems raised by their study, we have concerned ourselves with the issue that certain factors other than aging, namely, stress-inducing environmental and circumstantial disturbances, have social consequences previously attributed to disengagement. These environmental stresses were only superficially treated by Cumming and Henry.

Materials and Methods

SUBJECTS: A sample of 181 Ss, 101 women and 80 men, was drawn from the New York City area. They were deliberately selected to encompass a wide range of possible health statuses, extending from the physically active and employed to the institutionalized disabled. Table 5-I describes the age, sex, and marital status of the sample. In Table 5-II are found the sources from which the Ss were drawn. They may be broadly classified as those living at home and ambulatory (interviewed at a local Senior Citizen Center), those who are currently employed (seen at Union headquarters), those chronically ill aged domiciled at a hospital, and those temporarily ill and recuperating at a special wing of a local hospital. Socioeconomic status, computed by the Bureau of Census standards, showed a mean score slightly above the national average. This index did not reflect current income but rather mirrored economic status prior to retirement. While the sample in this study was not randomly

selected from the general population, it was felt that the group encompassed a wide spectrum of the aged population and moreover included the chronically ill, a group not considered by Cumming and Henry.

Each interview was of approximately ninety minute duration and followed a prepared schedule of questions.

Instruments

In this study we utilized the same measures of social engagement used by Cumming and Henry in formulating their theory. These included the following.

ROLE COUNT: An index of the number of roles in which an individual is involved. Cumming and Henry regard a high role count as six or more roles.

INTERACTION INDEX: a measurement of the density of interactions based on a subjective rating determined by the amount of each day spent in normatively governed interaction with others. Scores can vary from one to five and Cumming and Henry considered scores of three, four, or five to

TABLE 5-1
AGE, MARITAL STATUS, SEX, AND AGE DISTRIBUTION

	50–59 Yrs.	%	60–69 Yrs.	%	70–79 Yrs.	%	80–89 Yrs.	%
Married	19	50	26	40	25	41	6	38
Widowed	6	16	22	33	25	41	10	62
Single or divorced	13	34	18	27	11	18	0	—
	38		66		61		16	

Age (Yrs.)	Male	%	Female	%
50–59	17	21	21	21
60–69	29	36	37	36
70–79	28	35	33	33
80–89	6	8	10	10
Total	80		101	

Note.—The sample is white, lower-middle class in general, with about two-fifths native-born.

TABLE 5-II
NUMBER OF SUBJECTS IN EACH MAIN
CATEGORY

	N	%
Working people	46	26
Ambulatory living at home	80	44
Convalescent temporarily ill	26	14
Institutionalized chronically ill	29	16
Total	181	100

be evidence of high interaction.

SOCIAL LIFE SPACE MEASURE: a composite of the density and variety of interactions and an estimated numerical average of the separate contacts one has with other people within a monthly period. Because the length of each interaction is not reflected in this composite, lives with a great variety of interactions and contacts score highest.

HEALTH INDEX: a list of seven questions adopted from the study on aging by Kutner *et al.* (1956). This index consisted of a summary of scores based on the questions concerned with the respondents' current health status. The highest score attainable was thirty-four, which indicated that the respondent had continued in good health and presented no physical complaints. Low scores indicated current relatively severe health problems. Information on the duration of illness was not obtained. Actual scores ranging from four to thirty-two were used in the analysis.

COMBINED "ENGAGEMENT" SCORE—STATISTICAL TREATMENT: For purposes of analysis illness, widowhood, and retirement are treated as possible factors or stresses. Each S was scored zero, one, two, three, depending upon the number of stresses suffered, and the resulting stress index was then correlated with each of the engagement measures. Correlations and partial correlations between all the variables were obtained both for the total group of Ss and for the chronically ill as a separate entity. The latter were dealt with independently as the engagement measures appeared to have different meanings in this setting.

Results

The means of each of the stress groups as well as results of the correlation analyses are reported in Table 5-III.

TABLE 5-III
ANALYSIS OF EFFECTS OF STRESSES ON ENGAGEMENT MEASURES

Number of Stresses	N	Age	Life Space Mean Scores	Role Count Mean Scores	Inter-action Index Mean Scores
0	(42)	62.1	29.0	8.19	4.61
1	(56)	67.3	18.14	6.16	4.03
2	(66)	68.0	12.30	2.57	3.20
3	(15)	72.4	11.47	5.47	3.33
r stresses			—.46*	—.42*	—.45*
r stresses partialling out age			—.44*	—.38*	—.44*
r Age, partialling out stresses			.00	—.02	—.07

Note — All correlational analyses were carried out using product-moment correlations and are therefore to be interpreted with appropriate statistical constraints.

*$p < 0.01$

Inspection of the means in this table for each of the stress groups reveals a decline in engagement as stresses rise from zero to one and again from one to two. Beyond this point, as the number of stresses increase, no further decrease in engagement is noted. It may be noted that the one-stress and two-stress groups are nearly the same in age, although their engagement levels are quite different. The three stresses occurred in approximately the same proportions as first, second, and third stresses. Therefore, the finding of the greatest change between the zero- and one-stress groups must be attributed to the fact that a stress, *per se,* has occurred rather than being caused by any particular type of stress.

In order to test the hypothesis that these stresses are causally related to disengagement, previously associated with age, we have computed partial correlations between the engagement measures, stresses, and age. The correlations between the number of stresses and the engagement measures are notably high, even when age is partialled out, and accounted for approximately 20 percent of the variance in the engagement measures. The correlation between stresses and age was .44. When this association is partialled out of the correlation between age and engagement, the association between these variables drops to zero or becomes slightly positive. Recency of widowhood and retirement were associated with the age of the respondent, as might be expected. The size of the age samples did not permit independent exploration of the effects of recency of retirement or widowhood on disengagement at different age levels.

The combined engagement score yields essentially similar findings to those produced by the separate measures.

CORRELATIONAL ANALYSIS OF THE EF-FECTS OF SEPARATE VARIABLES ON ENGAGEMENT: Table 5-IV presents the correlations between the three engagement measures and individual variables which might be expected to affect these measures. Correlations between age and the engagement measures have been included to facilitate comparisons.

We note that all but two measures of the fifteen analyzed are affected to a greater extent by the five factors other than age. Marital status, residence, and working status all show as high or higher r's with the engagement measures as does age. These variables, however, yield scores which are somewhat confounded with the dependent variables, for, by definition, they are involved in the engagement scores themselves.

However, income status is a variable the scoring of which is completely independent of the engagement measures. Income status has a slightly larger effect on engagement than does age. As might be anticipated, welfare clients had lower engagement scores than those not dependent upon such means of support.

Health appears to have a much more powerful effect on engagement than does any other factor including age. This relatively high correlation is probably an underestimate of the influence of health, since our two most physically ill groups were domicilliary residents in constant social interaction, some of which may well have been involuntary. One may assume that a similarly ill group, sequestered in their own homes, would evidence much lower engagement scores.

Since the incidence of poor health, widowhood, and retirement can be expected to increase with age, it became necessary to evaluate the independent effect of each of these variables by partialling them out (Table 5-V).

TABLE 5-IV

INTERCORRELATIONS BETWEEN
ENGAGEMENT MEASURES AND SELECTED
VARIABLES FOR THE ENTIRE SAMPLE
(N = 181)

| | Engagement Scores | | |
	Life Space	Role Count	Interaction Index
Age	—.22*	—.20*	—.14*
Marital status	.23*	.36*	.39*
Living alone	.10	—.22*	—.21*
Working status	.46*	.45*	.27*
Welfare	.30*	.14*	.20*
Health	.38*	.39*	.40*

*$p < 0.05$.

TABLE 5-V

PARTIAL CORRELATIONS BETWEEN
MARITAL STATUS, WORKING STATUS,
HEALTH, AND AGE WITH
ENGAGEMENT MEASURES

| | Engagement Scores | | |
	Life Space	Role Count	Interaction Index
Age, partialling out marital status	—.20*	—.18*	—.11
Marital status, partialling out age	.21*	.35*	.38*
Age, Partialling out working status	.00	.02	—.01
Working status, partialling out age	.41*	.41*	.23*
Age, partialling out health	—.20	—.18*	—.10
Health, partialling out age	.37*	.38*	.39*

*$p < 0.05$.

We note that when marital status or health is partialled out from the correlations between age and the engagement measures, there is a relatively small reduction in the size of the correlations. When working status is partialled out, however, the correlations are reduced literally to zero.

This finding indicates that all of the association between age and the engagement measures can be accounted for by the correlation between working status and engagement and the tendency for fewer older people to be employed. When we inspect the correlations of marital status, working status, and health with engagement we find that they are not substantially lower than were the original correlations. Thus, the independent effect of these variables when age is held constant is still larger than the effect of age itself on engagement, and, in fact, entirely accounts for the correlations between age and engagement.

The correlation between marital status and life space (partialling out age) is significantly less than the correlation between role count and the interaction index and marital status, probably because life space measures a variety of separate social contacts, rather than duration. Similarly, the interaction index correlates significantly less high with working status than either other index.

Summary

The study was designed to evaluate a portion of the disengagement theory of aging. It deals with the proposition that the social withdrawal suggested by Cumming and Henry as being a normal consequence of aging obscures the fact that certain concomitant stresses associated with aging could produce the effects termed disengagement. Three stresses were selected as independent variables, namely, ill health, widowhood, and retirement. The dependent variables and the general methodology employed were similar to that utilized by Cumming and Henry in the Kansas City Study of Aging. Using the technique of partial correlation, there appears to be substantial evidence for our hypothesis that disengagement among the aged can be predicted to occur as a concomitant of physical or social stresses which profoundly affect the manner in which the life pattern of the person is redirected. Because they have ignored the apparently definitive effect of such factors on disengagement, Cumming and Henry were led to the conclusion that advancing age was a sufficient explanation of the facts obtained in their study. It is not age which produces disengagement in our investigation but the impact of physical and social stress which may be expected to increase with age.

REFERENCES

Blau, Z. S. Structural constraints on friendship in old age. *American Sociological Review,* 1961, *16,* 429-439.

Bortner, R. Test differences attributable to age, selection processes and institutional effects. *Journal of Gerontology,* 1962, *17,* 58-60.

Britton, J. O., and Britton, J. H. Factors relating to the adjustment of retired YMCA secretaries. *Journal of Gerontology,* 1951, *6,* 34-38.

Burgess, E. W. Social relations, activities, and personal adjustment. *American Journal of Sociology,* 1954, *59,* 352-360.

Caldwell, B. McD. The use of Rorschach in personality research with the aged. *Journal of Gerontology,* 1954, *9,* 316-323.

Cavan, R. S., Burgess, E. W., Havighurst, R. J., and Goldhamer, H. *Personal adjustment in old age.* Chicago: Science Research Associates, 1949.

Cumming, E. M. New thoughts on the theory of disengagement. In R. Kastenbaum (Ed.), *New thoughts on old age.* New York: Springer, 1964.

Cumming, E. M., and Henry, W. *Growing old.* New York: Basic Books, 1961.

Desroches, H. F., and Kaiman, B. D. Stability of activity participation in an aged population. *Journal of Gerontology,* 1964, *19,* 211-214.

Goodstein, L. D. Personal adjustment factors and retirement. *Geriatrics,* 1962, *17,* 41-45.

Guttmann, D. L., Henry, W., and Neugarten, B. L. Personality development in the middle-aged man. Paper presented at the meeting of the American Psychological Association, Cincinnati, 1959.

Havighurst, R. J., and Albrecht, R. *Older people.* New York: Longmans, Green, 1953.

Havighurst, R. J., Neugarten, B. L., and Tobin, S. Disengagement and patterns of aging. Paper presented at the International Social Science Seminar on Social Gerontology, Markaryd, Sweden, 1963.

Havighurst, R. J., Neugarten, B. L., and Tobin, S. S. Disengagement, personality and life satisfaction in the later years. In P. From Hansen (Ed.), *Age with a future.* Copenhagen: Munksgaard, 1964.

Henry, W. The theory of intrinsic disengagement. Paper presented at the International Gerontological Research Seminar, Markaryd, Sweden, 1963.

Jeffers, F., and Nichols, C. Relationship of activities and attitudes to physical well-being in older people. *Journal of Gerontology,* 1961, *16,* 66-70.

Kleemeier, R. W. Effects of a work program on adjustment attitudes in an aged population. *Journal of Gerontology,* 1951, *6,* 372-379.

Kutner, B., Fanshel, D., Togo, A., and Langner, T. S. *Five hundred over sixty.* New York: Russell Sage Foundation, 1956.

Landis, J. T. Social-psychological factors of aging. *Social Forces,* 1942, *20,* 468-470.

Lebo, D. Some factors said to make for happiness in old age. *Journal of Clinical Psychology,* 1953, *9,* 384-390.

Leveen, L., and Priver, D. Significance of role playing in the aged person. *Geriatrics,* 1963, *18,* 57-63.

Lowenthal, M. F. Social isolation and mental illness in old age. *American Sociological Review,* 1964, *29,* 54-70. (a)

Lowenthal, M. F. Some shortcomings of isolation theory. Paper presented at the 17th Annual Meeting of the Gerontology Society, Minneapolis, 1964. (b)

Maddox, G. Some correlates of differences in self-assessment of health among the elderly. *Journal of Gerontology,* 1962, *17,* 180-185.

Maddox, G. Some correlates of differences in self-asssessment of health status among the elderly. *Journal of Gerontology*, 1962, *17*, 180-185.

Maddox, G. Activity and morale: A longitudinal study of selected elderly subjects. *Social Forces*, 1964, *42*, 195-204.

Maddox, G. Fact and artifact: Evidence bearing on disengagement theory from the Duke Geriatrics Project. *Human Development*, 1965, *8*, 117-130.

Maddox, G., and Eisdorfer, C. Some correlates of activity and morale among the elderly. *Social Forces*, 1962, *40*, 254-260.

Mead, B. T. Emotional struggles in adjusting to old age. *Postgraduate Medicine*, 1962, *31*, 156-160.

Neugarten, B. L., and Guttmann, D. L., Age-sex roles and personality in middle age: A thematic apperception study *Psychological Monographs*, 1958, *72*, 1-33.

Parsons, T. Age and sex in the social structure of the United States. *American Sociological Review*, 1942, *7*, 604-616.

Prasad, S. B. The retirement postulate of the disengagement theory. *Gerontologist*, 1964, *4*, 20-23.

Pressey, S. L., and Simcoe, E. Case study comparisons of successful and problem old people. *Journal of Gerontology*, 1950, *5*, 168-175.

Reichard, S., Livson, F., and Peterson, P. G.

Aging and personality. New York: John Wiley, 1962.

Rose, A. A current issue in social gerontology. *Gerontologist*, 1964, *4*, 45-50.

Schmidt, J. F. Patterns of poor adjustment in old age. *American Journal of Sociology*, 1951, *57*, 33-42.

Shaw, L. C., and Henry, W. A method for the comparison of groups: A study in thematic apperception. *Genetic Psychology Monographs*, 1956, *54*, 207-223.

Talmon, Y. Dimensions of disengagement—aging in collective settlements. Paper presented at the International Social Science Seminar on Social Gerontology, Markaryd, Sweden, 1963.

Taves, M. J., and Hansen, G. D. Explorations in personal adjustment after age 65. *Geriatrics*, 1962, *17*, 309-316.

Tobin, S., Havighurst, R. J., and Neugarten, B. L. An empirical investigation of disengagement theory. Paper presented at the meeting of the Gerontological Society, Miami, 1962.

Williams, R. H., and Wirths, C. G. *Lives through the years.* New York: Atherton Press, 1965.

Zborowski, M. Aging and recreation. *Journal of Gerontology*, 1962, *17*, 302-309.

Chapter 6

AN EXPLORATION OF THE ACTIVITY THEORY OF AGING: ACTIVITY TYPES AND LIFE SATISFACTION AMONG IN-MOVERS TO A RETIREMENT COMMUNITY

Bruce W. Lemon, Vern L. Bengtson, and James A. Peterson

This research examines the relationship between types of social activity and life satisfaction among a sample of individuals in a retirement community. The principal intent in the paper is the statement, formal and explicit, of a theory which has long been implicit in gerontological literature, the so-called activity theory of aging. The essence of this theory is that there is a positive relationship between activity and life satisfaction and that the greater the role loss, the lower the life satisfaction. A second goal of the paper is to empirically test hypotheses derived from the theory thus constructed, using secondary data, as a means of illustrating theory-development applied to a common proposition in gerontology.

The Problem

Many researchers in gerontology have been concerned with the association between social activity and life satisfaction. Over two decades ago, Havighurst and Al-

Reprinted by permission from the *Journal of Gerontology*, 1972, *27*, 511-523.

brecht (1953) made the first explicit statement concerning the importance of social role participation in positive adjustment to old age. Since that time, several investigators have affirmed the general validity of this statement in varied contexts (Burgess, 1954; Kutner, 1956; Lebo, 1953; Reichard, Livson, and Peterson, 1962; Tallmer and Kutner, 1970; Tobin and Neugarten, 1961). A few have challenged the position (for example, Cumming and Henry, 1961; Neugarten and Havighurst, 1969). Maddox (1963) observes that most previous research supports the importance of social role participation in adjustment to old age and that implied in the theoretical orientation of most of the research is the assumption that

> . . . the social self emerges and is sustained in a most basic way through interaction with others . . . (conversely) structural constraints which limit or deny contacts with the environment tend to be demoralizing and alienating.

It seems clear, however, that adequate theoretical formulation built upon these and related concepts is still lacking. The deficiency of adequately formalized, let alone articulated, theory has been noted by several scholars in the field. Maddox (1963) for example, observes wryly that, "relevant gerontological literature is not distinguished by explicit statements of theoretical orientation."

It is the purpose of the present research to partly fill this void by presenting a formal axiomatic statement of activity theory and to test a small subset of hypotheses derived from the theory using secondary data.

Previous Research

On the basis of past investigations one is led to the conclusion that activity in general, and interpersonal activity in particular, seem to be consistently important for predicting an individual's sense of well-being in later years. Burgess (1954) and Lebo (1953) reported a greater amount of time in social and voluntary organizations to be characteristic of subjects with high personal adjustment. Kutner *et al.* (1956), as well as Reichard *et al.* (1962) have presented data to indicate a direct relationship between high levels of activity and high degrees of morale. Other studies published during the 1960s continued to give empirical support to this general relationship. For example, Tobin and Neugarten (1961) found that, with advancing age, activity becomes increasingly important for predicting life satisfaction. Tallmer and Kutner (1970) find no confirmation for Cumming and Henry's prediction that high morale is found among the highly disengaged (i.e. withdrawn from social participation).

A longitudinal investigation by Maddox (1963) revealed that both interpersonal activity and noninterpersonal activity were significantly related to morale. Lowenthal and Haven (1968) found relationships with a close confidant to be positively associated with mental health and morale. That is, the maintenance of a stable, intimate relationship appeared to be more important for predicting high morale than was sheer frequent social interaction or the maintenance of present social roles. In a cross-cultural study, Havighurst, Neugarten, Munnichs, and Thomae (1969) report a substantial positive correlation between total activity in twelve social roles and general life satisfaction. Data from subjects of six different nation-cultures were analyzed. The relationship holds up in retirees from two very different occupational styles (Bengtson, Chiriboga, and Keller, 1969).

Certain demographic variables and social conditions have been specified by a number of researchers as factors which increase or decrease the general relationship between activity and life satisfaction. These conditions are usually referred to as role losses or role changes; they include phenomena such as widowhood, retirement, and failing health. Rosow (1967) found high morale to characterize 72 percent of the subjects who had lost no major role; only 30 percent of those with three or four major role losses had high morale. Phillips (1957) found all differences in the proportion of maladjusted respondents among those who have and have not undergone role changes to be statistically significant.

An issue related to the amount and type of interpersonal activity is the extent of change in activity. In general, the literature suggests that the presence of a role change is inversely related to morale, and usually serves to decrease the strength of the relationship between activity and life satisfaction (see Cavan, 1962; Phillips, 1957). It appears that a change in roles may involve a disturbance of interaction patterns and social rewards.

Axiomatic Statement of Activity Theory

Of the many priorities for research effort in the field of aging, perhaps few are as crucial as the development of formalized, explicit theory. The reasons for this are summarized in the conclusion section of this paper. Kerlinger (1964) defines theory as:

> . . . a set of interrelated constructs (concepts), definitions, and propositions that present a systematic view of phenomena by specifying relations among variables, with the purpose of explaining and predicting phenomena.

There are many types, strategies, and purposes of theory in social research. Each has its advantages and limitations. The specific form of theory construction that will be utilized here, axiomatic, has been elaborated by Zetterberg (1965). The axiomatic theory presented below is in part constructed on the basis of findings reported in previous research and in part based on what might be called the activity model implicit in many studies used to explain these findings.

In addition to choosing the method of theory construction, it is necessary to define the substantive frame of reference that is appropriate to the constructs and concepts under investigation. This allows the research to be placed within the context of a much broader frame of discourse in the discipline. Concepts and issues from the general theoretical orientation are applied to the specific phenomena under investigation. Often researchers do not make explicit the substantive theory within which they are working. In this research, an interactionist framework is utilized, drawing primarily from the statement of the theory found in McCall and Simmons (1966) and in Rose (1962).

Definition of Concepts

Activity is defined as any regularized or patterned action or pursuit which is regarded as beyond routine physical or personal maintenance. The present study involves three separate types of activity: (1) informal activity includes social interaction with relatives, friends, and neighbors; (2) formal activity includes social participation in formal voluntary organizations; and (3) solitary activity includes such pursuits as watching television, reading, and hobbies of a solitary nature. Note that there is an ordering in terms of interpersonal intimacy or intensity; this should be kept in mind

throughout the discussion to follow. Note also that there is an implied gradient of frequency of activity in each type. Thus, some activities are more intimate than others; some activities occur more frequently than others.

Role support is defined as, "the expressed support accorded to an individual by his audience for his claims concerning his role-identity" (McCall and Simmons, 1966). Role-identity, the central concept of the interactionist framework, may be considered as the character and the role that an individual devises for himself as an occupant of a particular social position. Put differently, it is his imaginative view of himself, as he thinks of being and acting as an occupant of a social position (McCall and Simmons, 1966).

Self-concept is defined as, "that organization of qualities (i.e. role identities) that the individual attributes to himself" (Kinch, 1963).

Role loss is defined as an alteration in the set of behavior patterns expected of an individual by virtue of the loss of some status position within a given social structure. For example, a major role loss occurs when a male has his status of worker changed to the status of retiree.

Life satisfaction is defined as the degree to which one is presently content or pleased with his general life situation.

Interrelation of Concepts

THE SELF-CONCEPT AND ROLE-SUPPORT: One's self-concept can be viewed as a variety of role-identities acquired during one's lifetime. When we interact with strangers, only general social roles are taken into account; but as we come to know others more intimately we "act toward them not merely in terms of their social roles but also in terms of their role-identities" (McCall and Simmons, 1966). The more personal in nature the activity, the more specific and effective the responses of others are for reaffirming one's role-identities and thus one's general self-concept.

Individuals form their self-concepts or social selves through interpreting the reactions of others toward them. Throughout the course of the life cycle, interaction with others is what sustains one's social self (Maddox, 1963; McCall and Simmons, 1966). Although self-conceptions are relatively stable by adulthood, they must still be "reaffirmed from time to time by the confirming responses of other people" (Shibutani, 1961). Thus, the more one interacts with others or is exposed to the responses of others, even in adulthood, the greater the opportunity for reaffirming specific role-identities.

TYPES OF ACTIVITY AS SOURCES OF ROLE SUPPORTS: Activity in general, and interpersonal activity in particular, offer channels for acquiring role supports or reinforcements which sustain one's self-concept. The more intimate the nature of the activity, the more role supports one receives because specific role identities are being taken into account by the audience. Both types of interpersonal activity (formal and informal) offer greater potential for developing role supports than does activity of a solitary nature. Solitary activity cannot offer as much role support since it can only involve symbolic or mentally constructed audiences. In solitary activity the confirming responses of others are not actually present; this serves to make this type of activity less important as a source of role supports.

Informal activity is frequently on a personal or intimate level and is thus the most important type of activity for reinforcing the self-concept. The greater intimacy of informal activity usually involves more primary group relationships and spontane-

ity, which, in effect, makes the role supports more specific for confirming one's role-identities. In formal activity, role supports are usually geared toward more generalized social roles.

In sum, activity of an interpersonal nature holds the greatest potential for offering role supports, with informal activity being more effective than formal activity (i.e. participation in voluntary organizations). Solitary activity is the least effective of the three activity types for offering role supports; however, a minimum of role support is possible because the actor is imagining the confirming responses of others.

In addition to the intimacy of activity, the frequency of activity is also obviously related to potential role supports. The greater the frequency of activity, the greater the opportunity and probability that role supports will result from the interaction. Both the intimacy or nature of the activity and the frequency of activity relate to differential role supports.

ROLE SUPPORTS AND LIFE SATISFACTION: In complex societies, such as the United States of America, many sets of differential norms exist and are imposed upon a given individual simultaneously. Hence, each individual has a variety of role supports for sustaining the self-concept. One's general satisfaction with life is contingent upon adequately satisfying a number of different role identities.

The more intimate and the most frequent one's total array of activities, the more likely it is that one will receive sufficient role supports for reaffirming all of one's various role identities. This in turn results in a more positive self-conception (unless, perhaps, one's role is defined as deviant).

An individual's degree of contentment and pleasure with his life situation is dependent upon a positive self-concept. In order for the self-concept to be sufficiently reinforced, organization of role-identities must be validated by the audiences which react to the claims one has concerning specific role-identities. The more a person's specific role-identities (and thus his self-concept) are validated, the greater the probability of having high life satisfaction. On the other hand, a low degree of life satisfaction is encouraged by an individual's role-identities not being validated by his audiences.

ROLE LOSS, ROLE SUPPORTS, AND LIFE SATISFACTION: A role change causes a disruption in the equilibrium of role supports. When an individual is separated from his customary roles, either temporarily or permanently, he is likely to experience "an acute sense of hollowness and of being adrift" (McCall and Simmons, 1966).

The individual with a high frequency of intimate activity has a larger variety of mechanisms or channels for reestablishing an equilibrium in his role supports when a major role change occurs. From this reasoning, it follows that the person with high activity will not have as much of a decrease in life satisfaction as the person with low activity because his greater amount of role support acts as a cushioning mechanism or a source for shock absorption during the period of actual role change. The individual with high activity also has a larger repertoire of interactions and greater social life space which likewise facilitates the readjustment process; at the same time new role supports must be acquired. High activity may decrease frustration, anxiety, and the sense of hollowness likely to occur under such conditions.

It can be logically deduced from the fore-going that the frequency and intimacy of one's activity is directly associated with how one adapts to major role changes. If role changes were held constant, the individual with high activity would maintain greater life satisfaction than his counterpart with low activity.

Statement of Postulates and Theorems

On the basis of the foregoing interrelation of concepts, the following postulates and theorems relating activity to life satisfaction can be stated:

P 1. The greater the role loss, the less the activity one is likely to engage in.

P 2. The greater the activity, the more role support one is likely to receive.

P 3. The more role support one receives, the more positive one's self-concept is likely to be.

P 4. The more positive one's self-concept, the greater one's life satisfaction is likely to be.

There are three first-order theorems that can be deduced from these postulates:

T 1. The greater the role loss, the less role support one is likely to receive.

T 2. The greater the activity, the more positive one's self-concept is likely to be.

T 3. The greater the role support, the greater one's life satisfaction is likely to be.

Two second-order theorems can then be deduced from combining the above:

T 4. The greater the role loss, the less the positive self-concept.

T 5. The greater the activity the greater one's life satisfaction.

Finally, one third-order theorem can be deduced:

T 6. The greater the role loss, the lower the life satisfaction.

Hypotheses Tested in this Study

Because of the necessity of using a secondary data source in the present study, a complete testing of propositions resulting from the foregoing theory is impossible. It was decided, therefore, to concentrate on Theorem 5, since this is the most central part of the theory as it has been applied to problems of aging. The following hypotheses, then, are based on the proposition that the greater the frequency of activity, the greater one's life satisfaction is likely to be.

First, let us examine the case where activity is specified according to frequency within various categories. Since the types of activity are qualitatively distinguished in terms of intimacy (informal activity, formal activity, solitary activity) the frequency of activity cannot be summarized in additive fashion. Thus, specified hypotheses must be constructed for each type:

> *Ho 1:* Informal activity (with friends, relatives, and neighbors) is directly associated with life satisfaction.
>
> *Ho 2:* Formal activity (participation in voluntary organizations) is directly associated with life satisfaction.
>
> *Ho 3:* Solitary activity (leisure pursuits, maintenance of household) is directly associated with life satisfaction.

Second, in addition to the frequency of activity, the nature or type of activity is also hypothesized to be differentially related to life satisfaction. That is, the more intimate the type of activity (i.e. the degree to which one has close personal interaction with others) the higher one's life satisfaction is expected to be. The following hypotheses are based upon further specification of concepts in Theorem 5.

> *Ho 4:* Informal activity (with friends, relatives, and neighbors) is more highly associated with life satisfaction than formal activity.
>
> *Ho 5:* Formal activity is more highly associated with life satisfaction than is informal activity.

Finally, additional specification of the foregoing relationships is made by analyzing the conditions of role change. Role changes are hypothesized to decrease the magnitude of the relationships between various types of activity and life satisfaction. The role change involving retirement for the male, and widowhood for the female, are considered to be the two most salient role changes. The following hypotheses are based upon Theorems 5 and 6:

> *Ho 6:* The direct association between activity types and life satisfaction among females is less pronounced among widows and more pronounced among married women.
>
> *Ho 7:* The direct association between activity types and life satisfaction among males is less pronounced among retirees and more pronounced among employed men.

Sample Description and Data Collection

The sample used in this study was drawn from a larger population of persons who were potential in-movers to Laguna Hills Leisure World, a retirement community located in Southern California. Other publications (Hamovitch, Peterson, and Larson, 1969; Peterson, Hadwen, and Larson, 1968)) have described in detail the methods and procedures of this research; only a brief summary will be made here. A systematic sample was defined, consisting of every third dwelling unit (after purchase but before the construction was completed). A sample N of 411 subjects (182 males and 229 females) were interviewed for the present study prior to their anticipated move to Leisure World.

Subjects were highly homogeneous concerning variables such as social class, marital status, religion, and race. Approximately 81 percent of the sample were married, 83 percent were middle and upper middle class, 84 percent were Protestant, and 10(

percent were Caucasian. The age distribution of the sample was as follows: 39 percent between fifty-two and sixty-four years of age, 46 percent between sixty-five and seventy-five, and approximately 15 percent over seventy-five years. Seventy of the 182 males were fully retired; 52 of the 229 women were widowed.

Trained interviewers were employed to conduct structured interviews with respondents in their homes. Over 200 items were included in the interview schedule, which took an average of $1\frac{1}{2}$ hours to complete.

The major dependent variable of this study, life satisfaction, was operationalized by using the thirteen-item Life Satisfaction Scale B (LSR-B) devised by Neugarten, Havighurst, and Tobin (1961). The major independent variables of this study (informal, formal, and solitary activity types) were measured by computing the frequency of interaction with close friends, neighbors, relatives; number of membership and degree of participation in formal organizations; and frequency of involvement with solitary activities (for the exact items see Peterson *et al.,* 1968).

Goodman and Kruskal's (1954) coefficient of ordinal association (G or "gamma") was judged to be the most appropriate statistical test of significance. Calculations for level of significance of gamma were computed by transforming gamma values to Z scores (Somers, 1962). Levels of measurement for independent variables as well as the dependent variable are ordinal in nature.

Results

Tests of Hypotheses Concerning Frequency of Activity and Life Satisfaction

Hypotheses 1 through 3 state the greater the frequency of the various activity types, the greater one's life satisfaction is

likely to be. Table 6-I shows gamma values and significance levels for these five relationships using the entire sample. Three tests are made of Hypothesis 1 in this table, keeping activity level with friends, relatives, and neighbors separate.

TABLE 6-I
ACTIVITY TYPES RELATED TO
LIFE SATISFACTION: GAMMA VALUES
AND SIGNIFICANCE LEVELS FOR THE
TOTAL SAMPLE (N = 411)

	Gamma Values	Significance Level
Informal activity with friends	.21	.05
Informal activity with relatives	.04	NS[a]
Informal activity with neighbors	.01	NS
Formal activity	.08	NS
Solitary activity	.01	NS

[a]Gamma is statistically nonsignificant at the .05 level or greater.

Only the relationship between informal activity with friends and life satisfaction was statistically beyond the .05 level (G = .21). This is, it will be noted, a very low relationship in terms of substantive significance. Informal activity with relatives or neighbors, formal activity, or solitary activity were not significantly associated with life satisfaction in the present sample.

Because of the low levels of association considering the total sample, it was decided to specify conditions under which these relationships are more or less pronounced. Thus, three variables were used as control measures: sex, age, and perceived health status. When analyzing data for males and females separately, only the relationship between informal activity with friends and life satisfaction among females was statistically significant (G = .23).

Age was controlled by dichotomizing

58

Contemporary Social Gerontology

subjects into two categories, sixty-four and under and sixty-five and over. Only relationship between informal activity with friends and life satisfaction among persons over sixty-five (G = .22) was statistically significant beyond the .05 level.

Subjects were divided into good health and fair health categories to control for perceived health status. Again, only the association between informal activity with friends and life satisfaction was significant beyond the .05 level, and this only for subjects with fair health (G = .26).

In summary, none of the hypotheses relating frequency of activity to life satisfaction received consistent empirical support. Only informal activity with friends was associated with life satisfaction, regardless of specification variables, and this was at a substantively insignificant level.

Tests of Hypotheses Concerning Type of Activity and Life Satisfaction

The degree of intimacy of activity is hypothesized to be positively associated with life satisfaction in Hypotheses 4 through 6. The three indexes of informal activity are hypothesized to be more highly associated with life satisfaction than is formal activity. Activity of a formal nature is likewise hypothesized to have a stronger association with the dependent variable than is solitary activity.

When considering the total sample (Table 6-I) the most well-supported suggestion is that informal activity with friends is more highly associated with life satisfaction than is formal activity. Because of the low magnitudes of gamma values for many of the relationships, apparent trends may be a function of chance variations and thus do not warrant emphasis. Thus, the findings for this set of hypotheses lend little or no substantive support to the theoretical propositions.

Tests of Hypotheses Concerning Role Loss Specifications

Role loss is hypothesized to decrease the magnitude of relationships between various types of activity and life satisfaction. The major role loss for males (i.e. retirement) and the major role loss for females (i.e. widowhood) are both analyzed for purposes of specifying either increases or decreases in the magnitude of association between activity and satisfaction.

Table 6-II indicates gamma values for specifying relationships between various activity types and life satisfaction under the condition of widowhood among females. Theoretically, relationships are hypothesized to be more pronounced among married subjects and less pronounced among widowed subjects (Hypothesis 6). Data indicate very minor support concerning four of the five activity types, with the one exception of formal activity. The magnitude of increases and decreases comparing the gammas of widows (N = 52) with the total female sample are extremely small and thus have little theoretical relevance. The only statistically significant relationship involves activity with friends and life satisfaction among married subjects, which is expected from previous findings.

Specification of relationships involving retirement among males in relation to the total male sample (Hypothesis 7) is presented in Table 6-III. The magnitudes of relationships between the various activity types and life satisfaction are hypothesized to decrease for male subjects who have undergone the role change from employee to retiree. Males who are still employed are expected to exhibit more pronounced associations between activity types and life satisfaction. Data do not support this hypothesis, and again the magnitudes for gamma values are extremely small. Four of the five activity types have slightly greater, rather than reduced, levels of association with life satisfaction among retired males (N = 111). This finding may, in part, be explained by the fact that subjects have mostly white collar or professional occupations which represent the most successful persons in terms of adjustment to retirement.

In general, the magnitude of the differences in increases and decreases is so small in most cases that chance variation may account for many of the changes.

Discussion and Conclusions

Implications for Activity Theory from These Data

While some of the relationships found in the data supported the theory being tested, most did not. There are two sets of implications for activity theory that seem warranted from these results: the first implications specific, and the second general.

In the first place, the most specific suggestion from these data is that participa-

TABLE 6-II

ACTIVITY TYPES RELATED TO LIFE SATISFACTION: GAMMA VALUES AND SIGNIFICANCE LEVELS FOR WIDOWED FEMALES AND MARRIED FEMALES COMPARED WITH THE TOTAL FEMALE SAMPLE

	Widowed Females		Total Female Sample		Married Females	
	(N = 52)		(N = 229)		(N = 177)	
Activity Type	Gamma Value	Signif- icance Level	Gamma Value	Signif- icance Level	Gamma Value	Signif- icance Level
Informal activity with friends	.06	NS	.23	.05	.33	.05
Informal activity with relatives	—.12	NS	—.02	NS	.01	NS
Informal activity with neighbors	—.14	NS	—.02	NS	.01	NS
Formal activity	.10	NS	.09	NS	.07	NS
Solitary activity	—.09	NS	—.06	NS	—.03	NS

TABLE 6-III

ACTIVITY TYPES RELATED TO LIFE SATISFACTION: GAMMA VALUES AND SIGNIFICANCE LEVELS FOR RETIRED MALES AND EMPLOYED MALES COMPARED WITH THE TOTAL MALE SAMPLE

	Retired Males		Total Male Sample		Employed Males	
	(N = 70)		(N = 182)		(N = 112)	
Activity Type	Gamma Value	Signif- icance Level	Gamma Value	Signif- icance Level	Gamma Value	Signif- icance Level
Informal activity with friends	.20	NS	.19	NS	.14	NS
Informal activity with relatives	—.05	NS	—.07	NS	—.10	NS
Informal activity with neighbors	.09	NS	.07	NS	.01	NS
Formal activity	.03	NS	.07	NS	.11	NS
Solitary activity	.08	NS	.06	NS	.00	NS

tion in an informal friendship group appears to be an important correlate of life satisfaction, but not, contrary to what may be deduced from a formal activity theory, frequency of activity in general.

Friendship is perhaps the type of relationship most likely to involve specific role supports. Friendships are not only more voluntary than the other informal activities with relatives and neighbors, but are more intimate in nature, i.e., characterized by primary relationships. Rather than reacting to only general social roles, as might characterize neighboring or formal activities, friends react toward one another in terms of their specific, idiosyncratic role-identities. The whole person, or in the somewhat more precise terminology of interactionist theory, the totality of one's role-identities, is thus taken into account to a greater extent. The friendship may also provide a sense of continuity and depth for one's role identities; this is especially important for the high life satisfaction in a rapidly changing, complex society.

The findings of this study, although intended to measure frequency of activity rather than intimacy or depth of a single relationship, may be considered alongside the data reported by Lowenthal and Haven (1968). They suggest that the presence of a stable, intimate relationship with a single "confidante" is the strategic correlate of high morale. The quality or type of interaction, not the quantity, is to them the more important predictor of life satisfaction. The present data concerning intensity of interpersonal activity provide some corroboration of this line of thinking. Future research should add the "confidante" concept to specify aspects of this theory.

In the second place, the more general conclusion from this study is that the data provide surprisingly little support for the implicit activity theory of aging which has served as the theoretical base for practice as well as research in gerontology for decades. The propositions that the greater the frequency of activity, the greater one's life satisfaction and that the greater the role loss, and the lower the life satisfaction were in the main not substantiated by this research.

The linear model upon which this and most other investigations of the social-psychology of aging is based appear simply insufficient to capture the complex interplay between the individual and his changing social system. As suggested in another paper (Kuypers and Bengtson, 1972) a model employing the features of systems theory seem more realistic. It makes more sense to focus on the process involved in adaptation to aging, rather than the static relations among elements; to construct a paradigm reflective of the cyclical qualities implied in feedback loops, rather than linear combinations of terms. Finally, one should attempt to examine the multiple interdependent contingencies among variables rather than two-by-two relationships. This the common-sense, simplistic statement of activity theory is incapable of doing.

The process of growing old involves a complex interchange between the individual, who carries with him a set of experiences and expectations, and his social world; the interplay may best be seen as a system implying a trajectory of ever-changing elements, some common to most members of his cohort, some idiosyncratic. To assert that activity in general is predictive of life satisfaction in general is to obscure the nature of this complex system.

Summary

This paper has presented a formal axiomatic theory in an attempt to articulate more precisely the so-called activity theory of aging. This theory suggests a positive relationship between social activity and life satisfaction in old age and further specifies that salient role loss is inversely related to life satisfaction. Various hypotheses derived from the theory were tested with data from a study of inmovers to a retirement community. Because the data are secondary (not originally designed to test the theory advanced here) only a portion of the postulates could be directly tested.

We can conclude from the results that, for this sample at least, only social activity with friends was in any way related to life satisfaction. No significant relationship was found between activity with neighbors, relatives, formal organization, or solitary activity. The use of various specification variables (i.e. age, sex, marital status, and employment status) did not change the initial findings of the total sample. The data lend only limited support to some of the propositions of the theory. Overall it points out the need to both revise or enlarge the theory, including as concepts personality configurations and availability of intimates (confidants), and second to test it on a broader spectrum of the aged population than the present sample of in-movers to a retirement community.

It is our conclusion that explicit theory development must be given higher priority by researchers. If social gerontology is to advance beyond the perpetuation of *ad hoc* descriptive analyses, to the higher level of science involving logically related and empirically verified propositions of a truly general nature, we must attend more to theory development.

REFERENCES

Bengtson, V., Chiriboga, D., and Keller, A.W. Occupational differences in retirement: Patterns of life-outlook and role activity among Chicago teachers and steelworkers. In R. J. Havighurst *et al.* (Eds.), *Adjustment to re-tirement: a cross-national study.* Netherlands: Van Gorkum: 1969.

Burgess, E. W. Social relations, activities, and personal adjustment. *American Journal of Sociology*, 1954, *59*, 352-360.

Cavan, R. Self and role in adjustment during old age. In A. Rose (Ed.), *Human behavior and social processes.* Boston: Houghton-Mifflin, 1962.

Cumming, E. M. and Henry, W. *Growing old.* New York: Basic Books, 1961.

Goodman, L. A., and Kruskal, W. H., Measurement of association for cross classifications. *Journal of the American Satistical Association*, 1954, *49*, 732-764.

Hamovitch, M., Peterson, J., and Larson, A. Housing needs and satisfactions of the elderly. *Gerontologist*, 1969, *9*, 30-32.

Havighurst, R. J., and Albrecht, R. *Older people.* New York: Longmans, Green, 1953.

Havighurst, R. J., Neugarten, B. L. Munnichs, J. M. A., and Thomae, H. (Eds.), *Adjustment to retirement: A cross-national study.* Netherlands: Van Gorkum, 1969.

Kerlinger, F. *Foundations of behavioral research.* New York: Holt, Rinehart & Winston, 1964.

Kinch, J. W. A formalized theory of self-concept. *American Journal of Sociology*, 1963, *68*, 481-486.

Kutner, B., Fanshel, D., Togo, A., and Langner, S. W. *Five hundred over sixty.* New York: Russell Sage Foundation, 1956.

Kuypers, J. A., and Bengtson, V. L. Competence and social breakdown: a social-psychological model of aging. *Human Development*, 1973. (in press).

Lebo, D. Some factors said to make for happiness in old age. *Journal of Clinical Psychology*, 1953, *9*, 384-390.

Lowenthal, M. F., and Haven, C. Interaction and adaptation: Intimacy as a critical variable. *American Sociological Review*, 1968, *33*, 20-30.

Maddox, G. Activity and morale: A longitudinal study of selected elderly subjects. *Social Forces*, 1963, *42*, 195-204.

McCall, G. J., and Simmons, J. L. *Identities and interactions.* New York: Free Press, 1966.

Neugarten, B., Havighurst, R., and Tobin, S. S. The measurement of life satisfaction. *Journal of Gerontology*, 1961, *16*, 134-143.

Neugarten, B., and Havighurst, R. J. Disengagement reconsidered in a cross-national context. Ch. 9 in Havighurst *et al.*, (Eds.), *Adjustment to retirement: A cross-national study*. Netherlands: Van Gorkum, 1969.

Peterson, J., Hadwen, T., and Larson, A. *A time for work, a time for leisure: A study of retirement inmovers*. Los Angeles: Gerontology Ctr., USC, 1968.

Phillips, B. S. A role theory approach to adjustment in old age. *American Sociological Review*, 1957, *22*, 212-217.

Reichard, S., Livson, F., and Peterson, P. G. *Aging and personality*. New York: John Wiley, 1962.

Rose, A. (Ed) *Human behavior and social processes*. Boston: Houghton-Mifflin, 1962.

Rosow, I. *Social integration of the aged*. New York: Free Press, 1967.

Shibutani, T. *Society and personality*. Englewood Cliffs, NJ: Prentice-Hall, 1961.

Somers, R. H. A new assymetric measure of association for ordinal variables. *American Sociological Review*, 1962, *27*, 82-94.

Tallmer, M., and Kutner, B. Disengagement and morale. *Gerontologist*, 1970, *10*, 317-320.

Tobin, S. S., and Neugarten, B. L., Life satisfaction and social interaction in the aging. *Journal of Gerontology*, 1961, *16*, 344-346.

Zetterberg, H. *On theory and verification in sociology*. New York: Bedminister Press, 1965.

Chapter 7

AGING AND INDIVIDUAL DIFFERENCES: A LONGITUDINAL ANALYSIS OF SOCIAL, PSYCHOLOGICAL, AND PHYSIOLOGICAL INDICATORS

GEORGE L. MADDOX AND
ELIZABETH B. DOUGLASS

THIS PAPER EXPLORES the relationship between age and individual differences. The nature of this relationship is important for understanding the later years of life and for developing methodologies appropriate for investigation of the human life-span.

Differentiation increases with age. Literature on human development repeatedly suggests this is generally the case (Neugarten, 1973; Sarbin, 1954). But the applicability of this generalization to the middle and late years of life is debatable, and the literature reflects uncertainty on the issue. The uncertainty persists not only because of substantive differences in theory about human development and change but also because reliable data are not available to test adequately the competing hypotheses.

One encounters, on the one hand, the claim derived from a life-span perspective that individual differences in life style and

Reprinted by permission from the *Journal of Gerontology*, 1974, *29*, 555-563.

intellectual functioning observed in the middle years are accentuated in late life (Bromley, 1966; Havighurst, 1957; Riegel, 1971; Riegel, Riegel, and Meyer, 1967). As Neugarten (1964) has argued:

> Within the social and cultural realms, we can expect differences between individuals to be accentuated with time, as educational, vocational, and social events accumulate one after another to create more and more differentiated sets of experiences from one person to the next.

Disengagement theorists have reinforced the argument for social variability. They argue that in the later years of life, for a variety of reasons, social constraints weaken. The observed variability in social and psychological functioning can in fact be accentuated at least at the begining of old age, as the individual activates preferred but suppressed conceptions of the self (Cumming and Henry, 1961). The literature on physiological functioning in late life also suggests that individual differences increase (Botwinick and Thompson, 1968; Comfort, 1968; Obrist, 1953). Dispersion of scores on a variety of physiological indicators increases over time for a cohort of older individuals apparently because some persons have maintained their earlier performance level while others have declined because of decremental aging effects.

On the other hand, one also encounters arguments for dedifferentiation in the later years. Proponents of this view in the literature on social, psychological, and physiological functioning typically argue that mean performance on a variety of parameters decreases in the later years (Kelly, 1955; Malmo and Shagass, 1949; Riegel *et al.*, 1967). With death being the end point of life, it is implied, individuals become increasingly alike as they approach this common denominator. Mean performance among the elderly decreases, and there is an apparent regression toward a progressively lower mean. Such dedifferentiation would presumably result from both selective mortality, which removes individuals who function least well, and increased morbidity, which limits the physiological functioning of survivors. Increased morbidity, in turn, constrains social and psychological functioning. In fact, then, there is not a regression toward the mean, in the statistical meaning of that term, but rather a narrowing of the range, with the less able person dying from the population.

The available literature thus offers contradictory conclusions, and assessment of the comparative strengths of the competing arguments has been difficult because adequate data often have not been available. Whether heterogeneity in populations remains stable, or decreases in the later years of life, and whether the hypothesized differentiation applies equally to social, psychological, and physiological phenomena, remain unresolved issues in the absence of reliable data. This paper presents data relevant to resolving these issues.

Some Methodological Considerations

(1) CROSS-SECTIONAL DATA SETS: Most of the studies which have explicitly examined age and variability have used cross-sectional data and have not made a clear distinction between age *differences* and age *changes*. Sequential observations of individual differences in particular cohorts are optimal for definitive tests of hypotheses regarding variability in the later years of life.

(2) SELECTIVE SURVIVAL: Selective mortality confounds tests of variability over time. The effects of subject loss due to death on the composition of any panel must be taken into account in studies of the relationship between aging and individual differences.

(3) SAMPLING BIAS: Related to selective survival is the problem of sampling bias. Less able persons in a population tend to refuse retesting as well as initial testing, particularly among the elderly. Such bias can produce artifactual differences in observed variability (Riegel *et al.*, 1967).

(4) TERMINAL DROP: A terminal drop (i.e. rapid change) in social, psychological, and physiological functioning immediately prior to death has been suggested by several writers as a possible source of individual differences in late life (cf. Riegel and Riegel, 1972, for further citations). In studying elderly persons, it is argued, investigators are in fact studying samples which include both elite survivors and an undetermined proportion of individuals experiencing rapid decline in functional capacity prior to death. The proportion of individuals in this terminal phase presumably would affect observed variability, although the extent of the effect remains a matter of conjecture.

(5) INTRAINDIVIDUAL VS. INTERINDIVIDUAL VARIABILITY: The effect of intraindividual variability in functioning on observed interindividual variability among elderly persons remains speculative. For example, increased personal as well as group variability in auditory reaction time appears to be related to aging, although the data for this conclusion are largely cross-sectional (Botwinick and Thompson, 1968; Obrist, 1953). However, the precise effect of such intraindividual variability on the assessment of individual differences within a group is unknown since relevant data are scarce.

(6) SEX AND AGE DIFFERENCES: Whether differentiation by sex increases with age has been debated in social psychological literature (Cameron, 1968; Neugarten, 1964; Palmore, 1968). It is, therefore, im-

portant in any discussion of individual differences in relation to age to anticipate that males and females may exhibit dissimilar patterns. Moreover, research evidence suggests the utility of distinguishing between the "younger aged" and the "older aged" (Riegel *et al.*, 1967; Spieth, 1965). Perhaps it is the "very old" among whom individual differences disappear rather than among "the old" in general. In any case, research on human variability must consider possible sex differences and the special effects of advanced old age.

Among these six considerations, this paper addresses items 1, 2, and 5 most directly.

Hypotheses

In the balance, our reading of the inconclusive evidence on variability in individual differences in late life leads us to propose two hypotheses.

(1) Individual differences do not decrease with age. Variability on a variety of indicators is at least maintained, if not increased, in late life. We contend that reduction of variance in functioning with age has not been adequately demonstrated and that the opposite is more likely to be the case. Reported decreases in individual differences, we propose, are artifactual rather than substantive; they are due to selective survival and/or sampling bias rather than to decreases in the individual differences among persons who survive to old age.

(2) Individuals tend to maintain the same rank on a variety of indicators in relation to age peers throughout the later years of life. Maintenance of individual differences in late life is not due, we argue, to "dynamic equilibrium" within a specific population, whereby there is random individual crossover and movement throughout the range of relevant scores (cf. Kelly, 1955, for an opposing argument). We re-

affirm that maintenance of differentiation in late life is not artifactual but substantive. Even if social activities are curtailed in an aged group, for example, those who earlier in life were the most active of their cohorts remain, relatively speaking, the most active; less socially active old persons become the less socially active very old persons. This hypothesis is based on evidence of a persistence of life style throughout the late adult years.

A major implication of these hypotheses is that any generalization about "the aged" which implies increasing homogeneity with age should be viewed with the same skepticism as generalizations made about other highly diverse social categories i.e. adolescents, adults, females, blacks, and Americans. Selective mortality does create a social, psychological, physiological elite among the older cohorts; and less diversity among the aged than among younger age groups is possible, though not demonstrated. What we seek to demonstrate in this paper, however, is a different point: In an identified cohort, the range of individual differences among survivors is maintained. These persons continue to grow, develop, change, in short, to maintain individual differences in the face of the decrements of aging.

Research Design

We have employed data from a continuing longitudinal investigation of human functioning at the Duke University Center for the Study of Aging and Human Development. The scope of this research and its principal findings through 1973 have been published in two volumes (Palmore, 1970, 1974). From this broader study we have concentrated on specific indicators of variability in individual differences over time. Our sample is composed of 106 current survivors of an original panel of 271 persons initially ranging in age from sixty to ninety-four; the mean age initially was seventy. Panelists were drawn from the area in and around Durham, North Carolina, and their social and economic characteristics reflect those of the area. Repeated measures of functioning in terms of a wide range of social, psychological, and physiological parameters have enabled us to test the two hypotheses in a defined sample.

Six rounds of observation are available, spanning an average of thirteen years from observation 1 to observation 6. At each observation we have been able to measure and compare the variability observed among nonsurvivors as well as survivors in the original panel of 271.

We tested the first hypothesis through the use of Pitman's (1939) test for correlated variances. Hypothesis 2 is tested by the Spearman rank order correlation.

For convenience in presenting data we have concentrated primarily on comparisons of surviving panelists at the first and sixth observations, though some information is presented on observations at time 2 through time 5.

From a battery of hundreds of measures covering a wide range of interdisciplinary variables, we selected nineteen measures as illustrative for our purposes. Complete information on the nineteen variables is not uniformly available for all six observations, so at any particular observation there may be less than nineteen variables for comparison. Only at time six are all nineteen variables available. There are fifteen variables with observations both at times one and six. When times three and six are compared, on the other hand, there are eighteen variables available.

The number of subjects available for specific analysis varies. This is because any given individual in our study sample of 106 may have missed one or more rounds

of observation during the approximately thirteen years. Moreover, some of the very old subjects who are unable to come to the center are seen at home, and certain procedures and tests are omitted.

These particular nineteen variables were selected for the following reasons: they were either ordinal or interval; they gave a broad spectrum of fairly representative social, psychological, and physiological functioning; the physiological and psychological measures were generally objective measures relatively independent of subjective judgments of investigators.

We were also able to test variability of intra-individual differences with respect to one variable, visual reaction time. This is important because it enabled us to assess the effect of personal instability in response *vis-à-vis* interindividual differences. As noted below, an individual's *reaction time* score used for interindividual comparisons was the grand mean of four reaction time mean subscores. An individual's *reaction time variability* score was the standard deviation of these four reaction time means around the grand mean of that individual's RT scores. Individual reaction time variability scores were assessed by Pitman's test of correlated variances to determine whether the dispersion of the variability of scores changed significantly over time. A paired t test was made to test whether *mean* individual variability changed from time one to time six.

Description of Variables

LIFE SATISFACTION AND LEVEL OF SOCIAL ACTIVITY. Morale and activity are defined in terms of scores based on the activity and attitude inventories developed by Havighurst and associates (Cavan, Burgess, Havighurst, and Goldhamer, 1949). The activity inventory score cumulatively assesses differences in physical vitality, in intimate social contacts with family and friends, in use of leisure time, in organizational membership and participation, in work role maintenance.

The attitude inventory includes items which, cumulatively, assess what might be called an individual's master definition of self in relation to others and environment: items, such as feelings about health, friends, work, economic security, religion, personal usefulness, happiness, family relationships.

SELF-HEALTH ASSESSMENT: Classification of subjects by self-assessment of health status was based on answers to the questions, "How do you rate your health at the present time?" The basic response categories were excellent, good, fair, and poor. A subject could in fact qualify his response by selecting "excellent for my age," "good for my age," and so on.

CONCERN ABOUT HEALTH: Self-health concern was measured on a four-point scale in response to the question, "How concerned do you feel about your health troubles?"

DEPRESSION: Subjects were rated by a psychiatrist as to presence and degree of depressive affect (not according to diagnosis of depression) after an extensive psychiatric examination.

WAIS: The psychological measure included was the Wechsler Adult Intelligence Scale score. The WAIS weighted scores uncorrected for age were used rather than intelligence quotients.

REACTION TIME: At the beginning of a visual reaction time task the subject was instructed to keep his finger on a start button until a signal light came on, and then quickly as possible he was to lift his finger from the start button and press the response button under the appropriate right or left light. There were twenty practice trials, ten of which involved only the right signal; ten involving the left signal. Following the practice trials there were sixty-four trials interspersed with four "conflict" trials when both signal lights came on simultaneously. For our purposes we studied lift times, the amount of time it took for the subject to raise his finger from the start button in responding to the signal light. Furthermore, we studied only the first forty measures, before any conflict situations were presented. The first forty life-time scores were averaged into four mean scores: the first ten right signals; first ten left signals; second ten right signals; second ten left signals. For our purposes in this study we computed a *grand mean* of these four mean scores, which we call the individual's reaction time score. In order to obtain several Reaction Time scores for each person, we were forced, because of the coding procedures, to use both right and left, early and late mean scores. A multiple analysis of variance (MANOVA) test indicated that there were significant right and left effects ($p<.0001$) and significant early and late effects ($p<.0001$) in the 4 RT means. Therefore, in averaging these four mean scores we have a right/left, early/late confound. We cannot be sure the extent to which change in variability is partially a result of these confounds. Reaction time was measured in milliseconds.

PHYSICIAN'S FUNCTIONAL RATING: Objective health status was measured on a six-point scale of physical functioning following an extensive medical and psychiatric evaluation by a project physician. This rating was the physician's estimate of the subject's capacity to function effectively in daily living and was determined after comprehensive examinations, which included a medical history, physical and neurological examination, as well as ophthalmological and dermatological examinations. The tests also included an audiogram, chest X-ray, electroencephalogram, electrocardiogram, ballistocardiogram, and routine blood and urine studies.

PERFORMANCE STATUS: Performance status was measured by the subject's ability to carry on his normal activities, or alternatively, his degree of dependence on help and nursing care, as assessed by a project social worker. The score was expressed in terms of percentage disability (from Karnofsky, 1948). Subjects were rated on this scale beginning at the third observation.

WEIGHT: Weight was recorded in pounds and was coded in terms of the "nearest 10 pounds."

CARDIOVASCULAR STATE: The presence or absence of cardiovascular disease was clinically assessed from EKG interpretations, estimates of heart size, the extent of aortic calcification, and evidence of peripheral arteriosclerosis, hypertension, or cardiac decompensation.

VISUAL ACUITY, RIGHT AND LEFT EYES: Visual acuity for both eyes was assessed on a far distance vision test with correction.

HEARING LOSS, BINAURAL: Binaural hearing loss was measured in terms of percentage hearing loss by a pure tone (MAICO) audiometric study.

DIASTOLIC AND SYSTOLIC BLOOD PRESSURE: The blood pressure values were obtained by cuff measures with the subject in a recumbent position.

BLOOD CHOLESTEROL: Total serum cholesterol determinations were made on blood drawn between 8 and 9 A.M. Analyses were made according to Bloor's method adapted to photoelectric colorimeter. The Liebermann-Burchard reaction was used.

Findings

Table 7-I reports changes in variability of individual differences for the series of social, psychological, and physiological measures considered in this study. We will concentrate on comparing observations one and six in this summary of findings. Fifteen variables are available for comparison in testing the first hypothesis.

(1) For eight out of the fifteen variables there was no significant change in variances between times one and six. Existing differentiation was *maintained*.

(2) For five out of fifteen variables there was a statistically significant increase in variance from the first to the last observation. Differentiation in these cases *increased*.

(3) For two out of fifteen variables there was a significant *decrease* in variance. A brief discussion of these two deviant variables is appropriate. The first variable illustrating a decrease in variance through time was self-health assessment. We know from previous longitudinal research that elderly subjects tend to over-estimate their health as they age (Maddox and Douglass, 1973). While most subjects are realistic in self-evaluation of health, those who differ with a physician's assessment of their health are much more likely to deny than to assume the sick role inappropriately. In this sense, they become more alike as they age; regardless of their objective physical condition, they tend to report good health. This measure, therefore, does not support our initial hypothesis.

The only other variable which contradicts our hypothesis is diastolic blood pressure. We offer an explanation for this contradiction because it alerts us to a problem in longitudinal research on older subjects. The observed pattern of blood pressure is quite probably a treatment effect. No detailed data are available on prescribed drugs being taken by the subjects at the time of each observation. We do know, however, that if a subject was found to have high blood pressure in the early observations of the study, his personal physi-

TABLE 7-I

CHANGES IN VARIABILITY: OBSERVATIONS 1 AND 6, 3 AND 6, FOR SELECTED
PARAMETERS OF FUNCTIONING

Parameter	N^a	Test for Correlated Variances[b] 1 and 6	Test for Correlated Variances[b] 3 and 6
Social/Social Psychological			
Life satisfaction	69	—.26[d]	—.20
Level of social activity	71	—.07	.05
Self-health assessment	72	.23[d]	—.03
Concern about health	64	—.37[e]	.04
Depression	60	e	.02
Psychological			
WAIS, full scale	59	—.10	—.15
WAIS, verbal weighted	63	—.09	—.12
WAIS, performance weighted	59	—.02	—.12
Reaction time	56	e	—.15
Physiological			
Physician's functional rating	55	.12	.07
Performance status	80	e	—.38[e]
Weight	63	—.07	e
Cardiovascular state	51	—.31[d]	.01
Visual acuity, right	55	—.46[e]	—.03
Visual acuity, left	53	—.45[e]	.06
Hearing loss, binaural	59	—.14	—.30[d]
Diastolic blood pressure	62	.30[d]	.22
Systolic blood pressure	62	—.04	.04
Blood cholesterol	33	e	—.18

[a]The basic sample size for this study was 106. For specific analyses the number of subjects varies because there was missing data at various points of measurement for many subjects. For each measure of functioning only persons who had all completed data for that one measure were included. No systematic bias appeared to operate in the omission of particular items. Some subjects were not available for study at a particular time of observation. Others were housebound at the time of observation and some tests or observations were omitted.

[b]A negative correlation indicates an increase in variance through time.
A positive correlation indicates a decrease.

[c]No data were collected for this variable at the times indicated.

[d]$p<.05$.   [e]$p<.01$.

cian was notified and he would normally be treated for the reported condition. Consequently, blood pressure (a relatively simple problem for medical management) would tend to be brought into normal range over time. Such intervention would logically result in the observed decrease in variance.

(4) Table 7-II presents the group variances for all measures for all observations. For six out of fifteen variables, the Time 1 variance was the *smallest* of the six variances. For six out of the nineteen measures available at the last observation, the Time 6 variance was the *largest* of the six. However, there was no linear, monotonic change in variance (except for the 3 measures of weight) from Times 1 through 6.

Contemporary Social Gerontology

TABLE 7-II

GROUP VARIANCES: OBSERVATIONS 1 THROUGH 6 FOR SELECTED PARAMETERS OF FUNCTIONING

Parameter	N^a	Time 1[e]	Time 2	Time 3	Time 4	Time 5	Time 6
Social/Social Psychological							
Life satisfaction	69	20.5[c]	23.9	22.5	23.5	26.2	31.1[d]
Level of Social activity	71	37.3	38.5	44.8[d]	31.2[c]	32.3	41.7[d]
Self-health assessment	72	3.2[d]	2.3	1.9	1.6[c]	2.2	2.0
Concern about health	64	.3[c]	.6	.7[d]	.6	.6	.6
Depression	60	b	1.1[d]	1.0	.6[c]	.9	.9
Psychological							
WAIS, full scale	59	869.4	813.4[c]	844.4	876.8	967.8[d]	942.0
WAIS, verbal weighted	63	378.7	369.4[c]	369.9	393.5	426.7[d]	403.9
WAIS, performance weighted	59	138.1	123.9[c]	128.5	141.8[d]	141.8[d]	141.3
Reaction time	56	b	109.3[c]	247.1	131.7	160.2	305.2[d]
Physiological							
Physician's functional rating	55	1.0[d]	.8	.9	.5[c]	.8	.8
Performance status	80	b	b	118.8	95.4[c]	175.7	239.1[d]
Weight	63	8.6[c]	8.9	b	b	b	9.1[d]
Cardiovascular state	51	1.3[c]	1.6	2.4	2.5[d]	1.6	2.4
Visual acuity, right	55	1.5[c]	3.4	3.6	2.9	2.2	3.8[d]
Visual acuity, left	53	1.2[c]	1.5	3.1[d]	2.9	2.1	2.8
Hearing loss, binaural	59	139.3	128.1[c]	129.4	150.5	162.3	167.6[d]
Diastolic blood pressure	62	1.7	1.0[c]	1.5	1.5	2.3[d]	1.0
Systolic blood pressure	62	5.3	4.4*	6.1	5.7	6.8[d]	5.6
Blood cholesterol	33	b	b	16.2	16.1[c]	16.5	21.8[d]

[a] See Table 7-I for explanation of sample size. [b] No data were collected for this variable at times indicated. [c] Smallest variance in the 6 observations.
[d] Largest variance in the 6 observations.
[e] Years between times of observation vary. In the early years of the study subjects were interviewed every 4-5 years. Later observations have been made at two to three-year intervals as the sample decreased in size and subjects became very old.

(5) This lack of a linear, monotonic change in variance over time led us to test the difference in variance between Times 3 and 6 to insure that our earlier findings were not an artifact of the particular observations selected. When Times 3 and 6 were compared, there were eighteen variables available. Sixteen of the eighteen showed a *maintenance* of variability. Two variables showed a significant *increase* in variance; there were no significant decreases in variance. This led us to reaffirm the hypothesized maintenance of variability with age.

(6) Table 7-III presents average variances over adjacent time periods. These averages provide additional information about the pattern of variance over the six observations. In columns 1 and 2, for fifteen out of nineteen measures the average of Times 1, 2, 3 variance was *smaller* than the average of Times 4, 5, 6 variance, indicating a general trend toward increase in variance through time.

(7) Mortality was controlled in this study by concentrating on subjects known to have survived through the last time of observation. Therefore, in reporting observations from Times 1 through 5, subjects who were not to survive have been removed. When mortality is controlled in this way, the basic study sample numbers 106. However, in columns 3 and 4 of Table 7-III, one observes that when mortality is not controlled, variance does decrease in ten of nineteen instances. From this we infer that reported decrease in variance with age is in most cases an artifact of sampling.

(8) Intraindividual variability of Reaction Time showed no clear pattern of change through time. Personal variability was analyzed in two ways:

(a) For each subject a grand mean of his four RT mean scores was computed. The mean RT scores plotted in the first graph of Figure 7-1 (solid line) represent the group mean of these individual grand RT mean scores. The standard deviations are represented by the dotted lines. Neither the five RT mean scores nor the associated standard deviations show significant change over time.

(b) The standard deviation of the four RT means around the grand mean of each subject became his RT variability score. The second graph of Figure 7-1 presents the mean RT variability scores (solid line) for all subjects; the dotted lines represent the standard deviations from these mean scores.

The sample variability (of individual variability in subtests) was subjected to the Pitman test for correlated variances. There was a fluctuation of variation through time, though no clear trend. Time 3 variability was the largest of the six observations; Time 2 was the smallest. There was a significant increase in variance ($p<.01$) between Times 2 and 6, but no significant change between Times 3 and 6.

A paired t test, comparing mean intraindividual variability for Times 2 and 6 ($t=.05$) and for Times 3 and 6 ($t=.15$) showed no significant difference. We conclude that stability in intraindividual variability in RT measures characterizes these subjects in late life.

(9) Finally, Table 7-IV presents the rank order correlations for the fifteen variables at Times 1 and 6 and the eighteen variables at Times 3 and 6. Rank order is clearly maintained in most measures of functioning. The maintenance of group variability is not simply due to "dynamic equilibrium" of persons fluctuating within the group without disturbing the appearance of stability of group variability. Those who score high on a particular variable in earlier observations tend to score high

TABLE 7-III

CHANGES IN VARIABILITY: OBSERVATIONS 1—3 AND 4—6 FOR SELECTED PARAMETERS OF FUNCTIONING, MORTALITY CONTROLLED AND NOT CONTROLLED

Parameter	Mortality Controlled[b] Average Variances		Mortality Not Controlled[c] Average Variances	
	Times 1—3	Times 4—6	Times 1—3	Times 4—6
Social/Social Psychological				
Life satisfaction	22.3	26.9[a]	31.8[a]	31.2
Level of Social activity	40.2[a]	35.1	42.9[a]	42.6
Self-health assessment	2.5[a]	1.9	3.0[a]	2.4
Concern about health	.5	.6[a]	.7	.8[a]
Depression	1.0[a]	.8	1.1[a]	.8
Psychological				
WAIS, full scale	842.4	928.9[a]	1007.5	1054.5[a]
WAIS, verbal weighted	372.7	408.0[a]	416.5	434.3[a]
WAIS, performance weighted	130.2	137.9[a]	159.8	165.9[a]
Reaction time	178.2	199.0[a]	195.1	531.6[a]
Physiological				
Physician's functional rating	.9[a]	.7	1.2[a]	.8
Performance status	118.8	170.1[a]	194.7	203.7[a]
Weight	8.8	9.1[a]	9.2[a]	8.7
Cardiovascular state	1.8	2.2[a]	2.5[a]	2.1
Visual acuity, right	2.8	3.0[a]	3.3	3.3
Visual acuity, left	1.9	2.6[a]	3.0	3.0
Hearing loss, binaural	132.2	160.1[a]	231.3[a]	206.7
Diastolic blood pressure	1.4	1.6[a]	1.8[a]	1.6
Systolic blood pressure	5.2	6.0[a]	7.6[a]	6.0
Blood cholesterol	16.2	18.1[a]	16.4	18.0[a]

[a]Larger of the two variance averages.   [b]Basic sample N = 106.   [c]Basic sample N = 271.

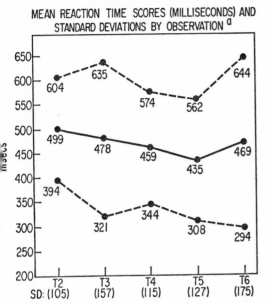

MEAN REACTION TIME SCORES (MILLISECONDS) AND STANDARD DEVIATIONS BY OBSERVATION [a]

[a] For each subject a grand mean of his 4 RT mean scores was computed. The above "Mean RT Scores" are the group means of these individual grand RT means.

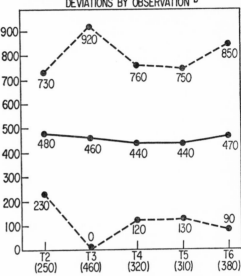

MEAN INTRA-INDIVIDUAL REACTION TIME VARIABILITY SCORES (MILLISECONDS) AND STANDARD DEVIATIONS BY OBSERVATION [b]

[b] The standard deviation of the 4 RT means around the grand mean for each subject became his RT variability score. The above mean RT variability scores are the group means of these individual RT variability scores.

Figure 7-1a, b.

later; low scorers tend to remain low scorers.

Conclusions

Our conclusions are straightforward. When the mortality and other losses within a defined sample are controlled, the observed variability of a number of social, psychological, and physiological measures tend to remain stable through time. In some instances there is a significant increase in individual differences. Increased variability of individual differences, moreover, is not due simply to increased personal variability or instability. On the contrary, there is stability through time in individual variability in at least the case of visual reaction time. Rarely is there a decrease in group time. Rarely is there a decrease in group

differentiation through time. Our first hypothesis is confirmed.

The range of observed individual differences is maintained, and within that range individual's rank ordering is relatively constant. The second hypothesis is also confirmed.

We have not in this paper dealt with the hypothesized terminal drop in scores prior to death. Insofar as terminal drop is a beginning of the death process, it is distinct from the gradual decrement of functioning within normal aging. Terminal drop would presumably be found prior to any disease-related death, regardless of age. The phenomenon warrants further longitudinal study.

This study challenges the generaliza-

TABLE 7-IV

PERSISTENCE OF RANK ORDER: OBSERVATIONS 1 AND 6, 3 AND 6 FOR
SELECTED PARAMETERS OF FUNCTIONING

Parameter	N^a	Spearman Rho, 1 and 6	Spearman Rho, 3 and 6
Social/Social psychological			
Life satisfaction	69	.65[d]	.60[d]
Level of Social Activity	71	.55[d]	.67[d]
Self-health assessment	72	—.02	.17
Concern about health	64	.35[d]	.29[c]
Depression	60	[b]	.02
Psychological			
WAIS, full scale	59	.92[d]	.94[d]
WAIS, verbal weighted	63	.93[d]	.93[d]
WAIS, performance weighted	59	.85[d]	.91[d]
Reaction time	60	[b]	.64[d]
Physiological			
Physician's functional rating	55	.12	.31[c]
Performance status	80	[b]	.48[d]
Weight	63	.89[d]	[b]
Cardiovascular state	51	.15	.44[d]
Visual acuity, right	55	.41[d]	.43[d]
Visual acuity, left	53	.36[d]	.53[d]
Hearing loss, binaural	59	.76[d]	.91[d]
Diastolic blood pressure	62	.45[d]	.44[d]
Systolic blood pressure	62	.51[d]	43[d]
Blood cholesterol	33	[b]	.57[d]

[a]See Table 7-I for explanation of sample size.
[b]Data were not collected for this variable at the times indicated.
[c]$p<.05$ [d]$p<.01$.

tion that, while children and adolescents become more differentiated through their development, adults become less differentiated in the later years of life. The data presented here provide evidence that development, change, and growth continue through the later years of the life-span in spite of the decrement of social, psychological, and physiological functioning which typically accompanies the aging process.

REFERENCES

Botwinick, J., and Thompson, L. W. Individual differences in reaction time in relation to age. *Journal of Genetic Psychology*, 1968, *112*, 73-75.

Bromley, D. B. *The psychology of human aging.* Penguin Books, Baltimore, 1966.

Cameron, P. Masculinity-feminity in the aged. *Journal of Gerontology*, 1968, *10*, 63-65.

Cavan, R. S., Burgess, E. W., Havighurst, R. J., and Goldhamer, H. *Personal adjustment in old age.* Science Research Associates, Chicago, 1949.

Comfort, A. Physiology, homeostasis and aging. *Gerontologia*, 1968, *14*, 224-234.

Cumming, E., and Henry, W. *Growing old: The process of disengagement.* Basic Books, New York, 1961.

Havighurst, R. J. The social competence of middleaged people. *Genetic Psychological Monographs*, 1957, *56*, 297-375.

Karnofsky, D. A. The use of nitrogen mustards in the palliative treatment of carcinoma.

Cancer, 1948, *1*, 634-656.

Kelly, E. L. Consistency of the adult personality. *American Psychologist*, 1955, *10*, 659-681.

Maddox, G. L., and Douglass, E. B. Self-assessment of health: A longitudinal study of elderly subjects. *Journal of Health & Social Behavior*, 1973, *14*, 87-93.

Malmo, R. B., and Shagass, C. Variability of heart rate in relation to age, sex, and stress. *Journal of Applied Physiology*, 1949, *2*, 181-184.

Neugarten, B. L. A developmental view of adult personality. In J. E. Birren (Ed.), *Relations of development and aging*. Charles C Thomas, Springfield, IL: 1964.

Neugarten, B. L. Personality change in late life: A developmental perspective. In E. Eisdorfer and M. P. Lawton (Eds.) *The psychology of adult development and aging*. American Psychological Assn., Washington, 1973.

Obrist, W. D. Simple auditory reaction time in aged adults. *Journal of Psychology*, 1953, *35*, 259-266.

Palmore, E. B. The effects of aging on activities and attitudes. *Gerontologist*, 1968, *8*, 259-263.

Palmore, E. B. (Ed.) *Normal aging*. Duke Univ. Press, Durham, NC, 1970.

Palmore, E. B. (Ed.) *Normal aging, II*. Duke Univ. Press, Durham, NC, 1974.

Pitman, E. J. G. Biometrika, 31:9, summarized in G. W. Snedecor and W. G. Cochran, *Statistical methods*. Iowa State Univ. Press, Ames, 1967, 195-197.

Riegel, K. F. The prediction of death and longevity in longitudinal research. In E. B. Palmore & F. C. Jeffers (Eds.), *Prediction of life span: Recent findings*. Health Lexington Books, Lexington, MA, 1971.

Riegel, K. F., and Riegel, R. M. Development, drop, and death. *Developmental Psychology*, 1972, *6*, 306-319.

Riegel, K. F., Riegel, R. M., and Meyer, G. Socio-psychological factors of aging: A cohort-sequential analysis. *Human Development*, 1967, *10*, 27-56.

Sarbin, T. R. Role theory. In G. Lindzey (Ed.), *Handbook of social psychology*, I. Addison-Wesley, Cambridge, MA, 1954.

Spieth, W. Slowness of task performance and cardiovascular disease. In A. T. Welford and J. E. Birren (Eds.), *Behavior, aging and the nervous system*. Charles C Thomas, Springfield, IL, 1965.

Chapter 8

TOWARD A SOCIOENVIRONMENTAL THEORY OF AGING

JABER F. GUBRIUM

I N THE LAST TWO decades, two competing approaches to the social interaction and morale of the "normal" aged have been fairly clearly delineated in gerontology. These two usually have been referred to as "activity" and "disengagement" theories. Both have suffered severe explanatory problems in that each has been unable to account for a significant number of documented instances of old people's behavior that contradict what might have been predicted from either of their viewpoints alone.

Instances of high morale or life satisfaction associated with isolation and/or inactivity (Gubrium, 1970; Messer, 1967; Townsend, 1957; Tunstall, 1966) are unaccounted for by activity theory, which would predict that only *moderate to high levels* of interaction or activity lead to high morale. Disengagement theory, on the other hand, remains unable to explain the felt despair or dissatisfaction with life expressed by some persons who are involuntarily "disengaged" or are socially isolated (Blau, 1956; Lowenthal and Boler, 1965, Tallmer and Kutner, 1970). This latter approach would predict a positive association between withdrawal and morale.

In view of the significant variations in

Reprinted by permission from the *Gerontologist*, 1972, *12*, 281-284.

existing data on the relationship between interaction and morale, it is obvious that both of these theories are limited as explanatory devices. Although there has been no absence of methodological criticisms of the theories (Carp, 1968; Cumming and Henry, 1961; Maddox, 1964; Prasad, 1964; Rose, 1964), there has been little or no systematic attempt to delineate dimensions of a perspective on interaction and morale that might account for more of the variation in available data than has either of them.

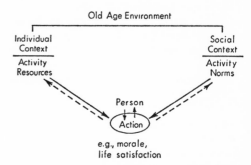

Figure 8-1. Schema of the socioenvironmental approach.

A socioenvironmental perspective would have the capacity to account for each of the anomalous cases cited above. This approach assumes that the environment of action for the aged is two-sided and consequently is built on the interrelationship of two contextual dimensions (Fig. 8-1). The first of these is social, referring to the normative outcomes of social homogeneity, residential proximity, and local protectiveness. The second dimension will be referred to as the "individual context" indicating those activity resources such as health, solvency, and social support that influence behavior flexibility.

The grounds from which this perspective on aging has developed are twofold. First, there has been a steady accumulation

of thinking and evidence in the gerontological literature directed at understanding the relationship between activity and
morale by combining environmental and
personal concepts (Blau, 1956, 1961; Bultena and Marshall, 1969; Carp, 1967, Messer, 1967; Rose, 1965; Rosow, 1967; Townsend, 1957). And second, our analysis of
data obtained from 210 old people, sixty
to ninety-four years, intensively interviewed
and observed in Detroit, corroborated the
utility of combining both social and individual contexts. Let us examine each context separately.

ENVIRONMENTAL EFFECTS

What is the meaning of the normative
effects of varied degrees of age-concentra-
tion on activity in old age? Taking leads
from Messer (1967) and Rose (1965), it
might be said that as the local environments of the aged become concentrated
with old people, it is likely that local activity norms become age-linked, i.e. persons'
expectations on each other's behavior become rooted in relatively common rather
than diverse experiences. If such age-concentrated environments are proximate as
well as age-homogeneous and exhibit relative continuity as such, then what Rose
calls a "subculture of aging" will probably
emerge. The behavioral implication of such
a subculture is that the activity that is expected of persons, sanctioned, or labeled
as deviant, is significantly different from
that in age-heterogeneous locales.

What differential burden does age-
heterogeneity as opposed to age-concentra-
tion place on personal variations in behavior flexibility? In highly heterogeneous
environments, the variety of situations that
persons are likely to encounter are maxi-
mal. This implies that any person must
have a sufficient command of himself to
"make-out," as Goffman states, from one

situation to the next. The resources he
possesses, then, must be sufficiently endow-
ed so as to allow him to fulfill a variety of
expectations. Now, what of homogeneous
environments? The variety of situations
with which persons are confronted here are
quite narrow in terms of demands on flexibility. Facility in one situation is likely to
mean facility in most.

The second context of old age environments refers to differences in persons'
capacities to engage in varied forms of activity. For the aged as a group, there are
at least three resources that specifically affect behavior flexibility. These are the behavior potential provided by good health,
solvency, and on-going social support (e.g.
having a living spouse).

How is it that personal resources affect
behavior with respect to the normative
demands of varied environments? Among
persons with good health and solvency,
normative burdens should be minimal in
the sense that these individuals possess
sufficient potential behavior flexibility to
eclipse local conditions and problems. In
contrast to them, those having relatively
minimal flexibility are most sensitive to
the conditions of and variations in local
norms. Those aged persons who can least
afford it are the most adversely affected by
normative demands.

If we dichotomize each of the two contextual dimensions of the socioenvironmental approach and think of the halves
of each as extremes, four types of resource-
norm situations emerge (Fig. 8-2.)

Before discussing these types and their
relative implications for morale among the
aged, let us assume that persons feel most
satisfied with themselves and their living
conditions when there is congruency between what is expected of them by others
of significance and what they may expect of
themselves (Secord and Backman, 1961,

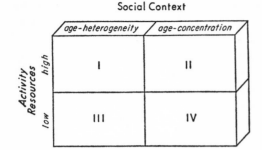

Figure 8-2. Types of resource-norm situations.

1965). Any inconsistency between these two bodies of expectations will be said to lead to life dissatisfaction among the aged.

It is safe to make such an assumption provided that the situation of self-regard is the same as the situation in which persons experience the expectations of others referring to self. If these situations are not the same, then the costs to self-conception of any changes in others' definitions of self may easily be nil. For an old person, what this infers is that if he commits his behavior and orients his mind to others in his locale, then how they conceive of him will influence his action. But, on the other hand, if "he's in it but not with it," then the mechanism of congruency may be inoperative.

Returning to our typology, then, we should expect persons to have comparatively high morale in types I and IV environments. The morale of persons in types II and III should be lower but for different reasons. In type III, dissatisfaction results from inability to perform as a "typically defined" member. In such age-heterogeneous locales, standard membership generally means possessing conduct typical of a variety of active and/or working adults. The low morale of type II environments was evident among several aged persons in the Detroit interviews mentioned above. These persons were in excellent health,

usually had high mobility resources, and were economically solvent. However, as long as they remained both geographically and psychologically oriented to their local age-homogeneous environments, they appeared to be bitter with immediate others and expressed rather sarcastic dissatisfaction with their living conditions, both physical and social aspects. Their dissatisfaction might best be described as humiliation.

The foregoing socioenvironmental approach to old age and its propositions are predictive of behavior contingent only on activity norms, activity resources, and the assumption of congruency. Several "intervening" factors may serve to alter empirically the behavior that would be expected based on the contingencies alone. Some of these are as follows:

1. Being part of a significant "circle" of age-homogeneous friends or having a confidante in an otherwise age-heterogeneous locale.

2. Not being behaviorally oriented to a local environment.

3. Having experienced life-cycle isolation.

4. Not possessing the psychological "coping" characteristics of the normal aged.

Any research testing socioenvironmental propositions would have to control, randomize, or analyze as deviant cases these potentially confounding influences.

REFERENCES

Blau, Z. S. Changes in status and age identification. *American Sociological Review*, 1956, *21*, 198-203.

Blau, Z. S. Structural constraints on friendship in old age. *American Sociological Review*, 1961, *26*, 429-439.

Bultena, G. L., and Marshall, D. G. Structural effects on the morale of the aged: A com parative analysis of age-segregated and age-integrated communities. Paper read at the annual meeting of the American Sociological Assn., San Francisco, 1969.

Carp, F. M. The impact of environment on old people *Gerontologist,* 1967, *7,* 106-108.

Carp, F. M. Some components of disengagement. *Journal of Gerontology,* 1968, *23,* 382-386.

Cumming, E., and Henry, W. E. *Growing old.* New York: Basic Books, 1961.

Gubrium, J. F. Environmental effects on morale in old age and the resources of health and solvency. *Gerontologist,* 1970, *10,* 294-297.

Lowenthal, M. F., and Boler, D. Voluntary vs. involuntary social withdrawal. *Journal of Gerontology,* 1965, *20,* 383-371.

Maddox, G. L. Disengagement theory: A critical evaluation. *Gerontologist,* 1964, *4,* 80-82.

Messer, M. The possibility of an age-concentrated environment becoming a normative system. *Gerontologist,* 1967, *7,* 247-250.

Prasad, S. B. The retirement postulate of the disengagement theory. *Gerontologist,* 1964, *4,* 20-23.

Rose, A. A current issue in gerontology. *Gerontologist,* 1964, *4,* 46-50.

Rose, A. Group consciousness among the aging. In A. Rose and W. A. Peterson (Eds.), *Older people and their social world.* Philadelphia: F. A. Davis, 1965.

Rosow, I. *Social integration of the aged.* New York: Free Press, 1967.

Secord, P. F. and Backman, C. W. Personality theory and the problem of stability and change in individual behavior: An interpersonal approach. *Psychological Review,* 1961, *68,* 21-23.

Secord, P. R., and Backman, C. W. An interpersonal approach to personality. In B. Maher (Ed), *Progress in experimental personality research.* New York: Academic Press, 1965.

Tallmer, M., and Kutner, B. Disengagement and morale. *Gerontologist,* 1970, *10,* 317-320.

Townsend, P. *The family life of old people.* London: Routledge & Kegan Paul,1957.

Tunstall, J. *Old and alone: A sociological study of old people.* London: Routledge & Kegan Paul, 1966.

Chapter 9

SOCIAL BREAKDOWN AND COMPETENCE: A MODEL OF NORMAL AGING

J. A. KUYPERS AND V. L. BENGTSON

THE ELDERLY INDIVIDUAL is faced with a variety of social reorganizations which pattern the nature of his personal functioning. Existing social-psychological models of aging have variously attempted to account for social reorganization by suggesting that changes may be stressful (stress theory), that they may be wrongly timed (disengagement theory), or that they must be compensated for (activity theory). These current perspectives on aging do not, however, adequately specify the mechanisms by which personal adaptive changes are contingent upon social-system changes.

In this paper, we shall propose a perspective new to the aging literature, the social-breakdown syndrome (SBS), which suggests that an individual's sense of self, his ability to mediate between self and society, and his orientation to personal mastery are functions of the kinds of *social labeling* and valuing that he experiences in aging. Further, we argue that the elderly are likely to be susceptible to, and dependent on, social labeling because of the nature of social reorganization in late life. That is, certain social conditions in the normal course of aging (role loss, vague or inappropriate normative information, and

Reprinted by permission from *Human Development*, 1973, *16*, 181-201.

lack of reference groups) deprive the individual of feedback concerning who he is, what roles and behavior he can perform, and, in general, what value he is to his social world. This feedback vacuum creates a *vulnerability to,* and *dependence on,* external sources of self-labeling, many of which communicate a stereotyped negative message of the elderly as useless and obsolete. The dynamic relationship between susceptibility, negative labeling, and the development of psychological weakness is detailed in the systems approach of social breakdown.

Unlike other major models of aging which attempt to define successful aging *within* the range of adaptation to environmental change, our argument is that aging, in general, assumes a pathological quality *because* of the nature of environmental changes. In other words, the relative sanity within an insane society and the general insanity created by that society are not the same. Our argument focuses on the latter i.e. expectable psychological consequences to certain noxious social reorganization in late life.

Social System Changes and the Passage into Old Age

From a sociological perspective, the most obvious characteristic of aging is change in social positions and social expectations with advancing years. The social system of an individual constantly changes as it reflects the new roles, the new norms, the new reference groups, and the new statuses which characterize different points of a life span. By now, a considerable body of research has shown that passage from middle age to old age is generally associated with a loss of norms, loss of roles, loss of reference groups, and a decrease in prestige. Other reviews have documented these generalizations (Bengtson, 1970; Cain, 1964; Riley *et al.*, 1968; Rosow, 1967; Rosenberg, 1972). We wish to briefly emphasize three aspects of social-system changes which result in increased vulnerability of the aged individual from the standpoint of social competence, and then to discuss the consequences of these changes from the perspectives of current theories of aging.

LOSS OF NORMATIVE GUIDANCE: Several studies have substantiated the common-sense observation that individuals are quite aware of the normative qualities associated with different points of the life-span. There are expectations, some quite diffuse and some role-specific, concerning appropriate behavior as one moves from one age-grade to another (Brim and Wheeler, 1966; Cain, 1964; Neugarten and Peterson, 1957; Neugarten *et al.*, 1965). However, several studies have suggested the notable absence, or inappropriateness, of norms specifically built around old age. For example, in their classic study of attitudes and aging, Havighurst and Albrecht (1953) found that most behaviors which were highly approved for older persons reflected the basic values of the local culture, applicable to all adults, not to the aged *per se*. Thus, the most approved activities included accepting minor civic responsibilities, voting regularly, keeping in touch with friends and relatives by visit or mail, maintaining an active special interest or hobby, being actively involved with the church and pursuing an active social life in the community, especially among persons of one's own age. Certain behaviors were strongly disapproved of in old age, ones which again focused on general rather than age-specific standards. The general prescriptions condemned life of isolation and inactivity, of solitude, of frequent violation of generational barriers, and of inattention to religion. Though

these data were gathered almost three decades ago, we suspect that much the same vacuum of norms appropriate to the later years would be true today. Thus, though age-grading systems in our society do define a period of 'old age' (Neugarten and Moore, 1968), and though older people in particular are conscious of the reality of age-appropriate behavior (Neugarten *et al.*, 1965), there is very little evidence of clearly-defined expectations concerning what the growing number of older people should do during this period of life.

SHRINKAGE OF ROLES: It has become commonplace in gerontological writings to note that the numbers and kinds of social contacts decrease with advancing years. Roles are literally lost as retirement, widowhood, death of friends, and decreasing physical mobility leave the individual less connected to his familiar personal world. Cumming and Henry (1961), Phillips (1957) and Blau (1956) all document reduction in social participation with age, though recent data from a longitudinal study (Palmore, 1968) questions the extent of a reduction in social activity within specifically defined roles. A cross-national study of aging (Bengtson, 1969), suggests that men in their seventies have very low activity in roles, such as club member, civic/political participant, and church member; slightly higher activity in the roles of friend, neighbor, and acquaintance; and the highest activity in family roles as parent and grandparent. The change-in-activity patterns, determined by comparisons with the subject's role activity at age sixty, as well as longitudinal studies carried out in Germany (Lehr, 1969), mirror this trend.

Thus, though the normative guidelines for behavior are borrowed from middle-age, and though activity is prescribed for roles outside the family, many of these roles of middle age are no longer available for older individuals. The decrease in the number of social positions traditionally open to the elderly further imperils 'competent' performance in social life by withdrawing the behavioral context for social activity.

LACK OF APPROPRIATE REFERENCE GROUPS: And finally, social-system changes in later life point to a decrease in appropriate reference groups (Rosow, 1967). While changes in the aggregate of individuals to whom a person looks in patterning his behavior occur throughout the life cycle, it is only in approaching old age that the very existence of such an aggregate becomes equivocal. Debate of this issue in the gerontological literature has focused on the possible emergence of a *subculture* of the aged, with its own group-consciousness (Rose, 1964). Several have argued that little evidence supports the existence of an elderly subculture (Streib, 1965; Rosow, 1967), and that the argument by Rose (1964) applies to only a limited number of persons involved in political action for the elderly. The reference group for the elderly seems to be more correctly people in their middle years (Rosow, 1967).

Indirect evidence of the lack of reference group is the almost complete absence of institutional provisions, i.e. the social structural aspects of socialization, to assist the individual in adapting to the marked changes in the social system. In the role-change termed *retirement,* for example, there are usually only formal ceremonies to mark leave-taking, the 'event' of retirement, but little meaningful attention to the nature of activity appropriate to the nonwork status itself (Maddox, 1966). Retirement ceremonies mark the end rather than the beginning. For the aging female who becomes *widowed,* there is also lack of any kind of institutional preparation and few

prescriptions for behavior (Lopata, 1972; Silverman, 1971). In the role-change represented by grown children leaving home, there is somewhat more evidence of socialization (Deutscher, 1964), simply because the focus of growing children's interaction is progressively and gradually less within the framework of the home. Even so, the *empty nest* (Spence and Lonner, 1971), may represent a dramatic change which the family undergoes with little or no social support.

SUMMARY: In this brief and selected review of research in the social psychology of aging, we have suggested that a person late in his life course is likely to experience, in an unprecedented way, the lack of defined behavioral guidelines specific to his age. Further, familiar roles of earlier periods of life are lost in various ways, not to be replaced with others of equal specificity. And finally, the person is left without a group of defined others with whom he can identify. The degree to which this argument realistically captures the universality of shifts in the social order of older persons is, of course, debatable. Individual variation must always be the counterpoint of any general statement of normal aging. However, we believe that insofar as role loss, normlessness, and lack of reference groups are likely and interrelated, they present the backdrop against which any theory of normal aging must be considered. The question of real import concerns the likely *consequences* to individual functioning and well-being that these changes portend.

THEORIES OF AGING—PERSONAL-SYSTEM CONSEQUENCES/SOCIAL SYSTEM CHANGES: In considering the state of existing theory on normal aging, we are concerned principally with the mechanisms or processes by which an individual is patterned by his social order. It is insufficient to say, for example, that the individual *adapts* to, or *copes* with, external changes. The researcher must characterize the process of adaptation, the points of influence, and possible consequences or side-effects of particular adaptations. In this light, we believe that the three principal social-psychological theories of aging have been inadequate in considering the ways in which an individual is dependent on feedback from his social order and the individual consequences if that feedback is absent or negatively toned.

The *multiple-stress theory* (Lowenthal, 1967) has been used to account for the antecedents of psychiatric disorder in the elderly. Briefly stated, impairment results from the accumulation of stress along the lifeline. Some persons' lives are more stressful than others. With repeated stress over time, adaptive strengths are taxed and breakdown may ensue. In our view, certain critical questions are left unanswered by stress theory. What constitutes stress? How does stress accumulate? Where is it stored? Are certain stressors common to the elderly? If so, are role loss and lack of reference groups considered stressors? If not, how does stress theory consider the experiential impact of role loss, normlessness, or loss of reference group? In short, stress theory as used in consideration of mental disorder in the elderly only posits and association but not the mechanisms of causality between stress and impairment; nor does it directly deal with the possibility of the stresses of social reorganizations.

The now laboriously researched, debated, and modified *disengagement theory* seems to account for social-system changes by proposing the 'intrinsic' necessity of social-system and personal-system disengagement (Cumming and Henry, 1961). In this model, one issue of concern is the *synchrony of timing* between social and individual changes. If changes of role loss

and decrease in normative regulation occur before the individual is ready, disequilibrium is created. Whatever the timing, however, this model suggests that what some may see as lack of normative guidance is really reduced normative *control,* a welcome change for the elderly person who psychologically is more highly invested in 'inner' personal concerns, termed the greater 'interiority' of old age. Subsequent analyses of the Kansas City data have suggested that certain personality types will experience the social-personal system severance with more equanimity than others (Neugarten *et al.,* 1968). In any case, these 'types' are apparently historically continuous and not centrally a product of recent social changes *per se.*

The *activity theory* (recently systematized by Lemon, 1972) seems to reify the continuity of life style into old age, for it suggests that psychological well-being is a function of the degree to which a person can maintain patterns of activity and involvement into late life. In this model, the relationship between the social system and the personal system does not or should not change as an individual passes from middle to old age. The norms impinging upon him do not markedly change; he is still *expected* to do much the same (keep busy) as he did in the middle years, with the exception that he is allowed not to work (whether he wants to or not) ; and he is *expected* to slow down a little (Havighurst and Albrecht, 1953). When roles are taken from him (e.g. retirement, loss of spouse, friends) successful adaptation is measured by his ability to compensate by increasing activity in other spheres. The sources of satisfaction, his self-concept, and his life style do not change much from what they were in the middle years; nor does his respect for productivity and conventional social norms.

SBS and Transition to Old Age

The *social breakdown* theory was initially developed to help explain the genesis of mental disorder in a general population. It is here offered as a sensitizing model, which explains something of the peculiar relationship between the elderly person whose social system is contracting and the broader social environment within which he lives. We shall argue that the probable consequence of social reorganization for the elderly is the creation of a basically negative cycle of events in which behaviors and attitudes toward the self develop; these the wider society, and ultimately the old person himself, defines negatively as incompetent. This is based on a further suggestion that the social-system changes outlined earlier in this paper create a general susceptibility to the syndrome and that the dominant societal view of assigning worth, *personal worth through social utility*, is a fulcrum in creating a negative spiral of breakdown. Note that we are here talking about *normal* aged individuals in a society that presents an environment conducive to negative labeling.

THE MALIGNANT CYCLE OF SBS: SBS, originally introduced by Gruenberg (1964) and Zusman (1966), offers a seven-stage formulation of the development of negative psychological functioning, specifically, mental illness. The seven steps of social breakdown are as follows:

(1) precondition of susceptibility;
(2) dependence on external labeling;
(3) social labeling as incompetent;
(4) induction into a sick, dependent role;
(5) learning of skills appropriate to the new dependent role;
(6) atrophy of previous skills;
(7) identification and self-labeling as sick or inadequate.

This formulation rests on the premise that mental health and illness are directly related to socialenvironmental conditions. The theroy thus offers considerable insight into the dynamic between the person's *sense of self*, the development of *skills* for dealing with self and environment, and the *feedback* given by the outside world. According to Zusman (1966):

> This concept (SBS) relates many symptoms of chronic mental illness to the attitudes and actions of those who are around the mentally ill person. The picture presented by the mentally ill person is felt to be a result of the interaction between a person suffering from an illness and his current environment. The concept emphasizes that an adequate description of a mentally ill person requires a statement of the conditions under which he has been observed.

As applied to the elderly, the parallel is clear. The symptoms of being old are associated with the negative attitudes and actions accorded the symbols of aging in today's society. In Zusman's (1966) formulation, the first stage involves the *precondition of susceptibility* (step 1) of the individual.

Insofar as the precondition is a product, as Zusman (1966) implies, of the confusion, vagueness, or lack of specificity of standards for appropriate behavior, a strong case can be made that the elderly are likely candidates of susceptibility. The crux of the question eventually will lie in the determination (empirically) of how these conditions relate to individual susceptibility.

According to Zusman (1966), the existence of "weakened or deficient inner standards" is critical for the development of social breakdown. While details of the genesis of "weakened standards" are unspecified, the implication throughout is that certain qualities of one's social world are the foundation for either strong or weak personal standards. We are suggesting, for the elderly, that the social reorganizations signaled by role loss, deficient or vague normative information, and lack of reference groups provide the beginning link between the kind of information society provides concerning what is expected and valued, and the personal guidelines established, which pattern action. While we underscore that research must critically examine the variations in development of susceptibility for the elderly, at this point we propose that the social changes experienced late in the adult life line are likely to create a vacuum of information concerning one's personal action and position in the wider society.

In the social-breakdown formulation, the initial step of susceptibility leads to an excessive dependence on current cues (step 2).

In other words, one's ability to employ previous ethics or guidelines, a necessary condition for aging according to activity theory, is reduced, forcing a heavy reliance on current (unvariable) cues. This dependence, in and of itself, does not lead to the genesis of social breakdown. The critical element is, rather, the nature and quality of the cues available to the individual. In Zusman's (1966) formulation, there occurs a *social labeling* (of the individual) as *incompetent* and in some contexts, as dangerous (step 3).

While the specific quality of social labeling of a mentally ill person and an elderly person are different, for both there is an emphasis on the negative quality of the cues. The elderly have the additional disadvantage of having vague or ill-defined labels. That is, negatively-toned stereotypes associated with loss of productive roles may become accepted by the individual in describing himself. From the dominant functionalistic perspective of Western society,

the elderly person is informed, directly and indirectly, of his uselessness, obsolescence, low value, inadequacy, and incompetence. To the degree that these specific messages are conveyed and to the degree that the elderly person, rendered susceptible, adopts them as true for the self, a cycle of events is established which leads to a generalized *self-view* of incompetence, uselessness, and worthlessness.

The remaining steps in SBS follow from this initial pattern of susceptibility, dependence, and negative social labeling. The individual is induced (step 4) into a sick role. He is involved in ceremonies which offer guidelines for behavior. This role induction is followed by the *learning of behaviors and skills* (step 5) appropriate to the negative role, and *by the atrophy of work and social skills* (step 6) which are not demanded in the new context. Finally, there occurs the psychological *identification* and self-labeling as useless, sick and inadequate (step 7).

The cycle of interaction is created in which a person, rendered susceptible, is ascribed negative value, is encouraged to develop skills and behavior in concert with this value, and finally incoporates the negative value as true for the self. This, in turn, leads to further susceptibility, dependence, low self-assessment, and the atrophy of coping skills.

In short, the system can be described as a vicious feedback loop with negative inputs (Fig. 9-1).

To what extent does this precondition of susceptibility exist in American society? We have argued that the major life commitments of the middle years, as well as the value bases of these commitments, are likely to persist into the late adult years. The elderly person bases his self-worth and looks to social acceptance in terms of these values; values which reflect a commitment

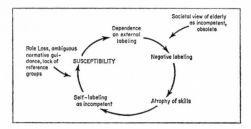

Figure 9-1. A systems representation of SBS as applied to old age with negative inputs from the external social system.

to the ethic of *personal-worth-through-social-utility* (i.e. productivity) prevalent in American society (Reich, 1970; Slater, 1970; Williams, 1970). Given this standard, the social utility of the elderly is negatively valued; hence the decreased status of the elderly and the development of susceptibility in an entire age-grade.

Intervention in the Vicious Cycle of Social Breakdown

Our analysis of the relevance of the SBS to understanding normal aging has underscored that the person is defined by, and eventually defines himself as, incompetent. Further, we suggest that competence can be variously viewed as (1) successful social-role performance, (2) adaptative capacity, and (3) personal feelings of mastery and inner control. According to the circular nature of the SBS, all of these aspects of competence are interrelated. On the one hand, they serve to define the nature of the developing incompetence of the elderly. On the other hand, they can also be interpreted as providing guidelines to break the vicious cycle of social breakdown. This is the implication of the system to which we now turn, for there are several possibilities of interventive effort suggested by each of the definitions of competence.

COMPETENCE AS DEFINED BY SUCCESSFUL

SOCIAL-ROLE PERFORMANCE: The major premise in this view is that a person's worth as ascribed by others is a function of his demonstrated ability to perform in defined social roles, particularly work and family roles. One must take, we feel, a relatively pessimistic view of society's ability and willingness to offer power and opportunity to the elderly in roles which are now being withdrawn. For example, we see little hope that forced retirement policies will be voluntarily decreased, affording greater flexibility for role performance. We also see little likelihood that alternative roles will be defined by the wider society which allow for greater social penetration by the elderly, despite lip service given to programs of volunteerism or foster grandparents programs by agencies.

Rather, we suggest that efforts must be made on an individual level to liberate the person from the dominant societal view that worth is contingent on his performance in economic, productive social roles. The distinction between social guidance and social control seems appropriate here. That is, to enable the elderly person to experience the lessened social expectation of role performance as a personal liberation would lie on the premise that there are alternative ways of assigning personal worth. We are suggesting that the development of freedom from a social-worth ethic would involve the development of personally defined bases for assigning worth, ones relying more on personal definitions of meaning and purpose, on expressive, creative, and introspective activities.

The accomplishment of this shift in values is by no means thought to be simple or straightforward. The elderly are, so to speak, prisoners of their own valuing past, and are likely to view expressive and nonfunctional activities as the wider society does, i.e. self-indulgent, useless, and nonpurposeful. On the other hand, there are several factors which suggest the possibility, inevitability, of such a shift in values where old age is concerned. First, with the emergent cultural forms of younger generations, with the greater public awareness of alternative life styles, and with the eventual historical and cultural infusion of more expressive, individuated ethics in society, one would expect that the ability and willingness of the elderly to experience reduced normative input as liberation from external control will increase. Second, with the demographic changes of the past decades, an unprecedented percentage of our population is continuing to live past sixty-five. The sheer numbers of these individuals for whom society traditionally has not assigned a positive social function are such as to imply a shift in positions as well as values.

COMPETENCE AS CAPACITY TO ADAPT TO ENVIRONMENTAL CHANGE: The premise in this view is that regardless of the specific nature of valuing and of social-ecological conditions, persons must possess the equipment to perceive their world realistically and must be able to cope with its demands. Most individual case work and clinical activities focus on this aspect of competence by aiding the person in his struggle to cope with his environment by building ego strengths, and by expanding awareness. While we would not minimize the importance of this individual approach to adaptation, it seems that, too often, this approach has ignored the importance of decreasing the noxious elements of one's environment, those aspects that often require extreme coping measures, and which severely strain existing adaptive strengths. In other words, while continual efforts must be made to enable the development of psychologically able individuals, substantial effort must also be directed toward lessening the variety of debilitating environmental conditions,

especially those of poor health, poverty, inadequate housing, dehumanizing institutional treatment, etc.

COMPETENCE AS PERSONAL FEELINGS OF MASTERY AND INTERNAL CONTROL: The premise of this view is that the experience a person has of himself as being causally important, as being in control of his destiny, and as being able to bring about desired effects is the foundation of an able, adaptable person. While it is true that eliminating the noxious conditions of existence will help create a benign environment, and while liberation from functional ethics will legitimize the creation of new options for action, the person must experience the source of his action, the locus of his control, as resting with himself. The externalization of control and decision-making power mitigates against the maintenance of personal strengths, for it places the responsibility for action outside the individual. Experientially, one is left with the rhetorical question: 'Why act, why initiate if it doesn't make any difference, if the real power to determine my fate lies outside myself?'

To enable the development of an internal locus of control, those who would envision themselves as serving the elderly must define as one of their major goals the systematic deinvestment of their power and control. They must, at all the subtle junctures of decision making, policy formation, and administration, acknowledge the experiential value to their clients of individual power and control. Self-government, resident directorship, political advocacy, and aging group consciousness are all part of the beginning vocabulary of practitioners which underscores this view, i.e. self-determination and individual control of policy and administration is the foundation for competent aging.

Can one imagine, for example, an old-age home whose personnel and decision-making bodies are exclusively comprised of the elderly themselves? While the nursing and social-service staff, for example, might be younger people, they are servants of the elderly board of directors, the elderly committee structure, and the elderly administrators. Imagine a program of continuing education entirely defined and run by the elderly, supported by society and government, but in no way controlled by the extension division of existing colleges and universities. Imagine a policy-forming committee in local government, staffed by the elderly whose charge is to define priorities, develop and administer programs which attempt to enhance the condition of their elderly constituency. Imagine a governmental agency with substantial funds (staffed by the elderly) which attempts to encourage the development of elderly foundations, elderly causes, and elderly advocates. We suggest that this approach would begin to transfer the locus of control to its rightful place, would enhance the effect of the elderly to define their own existence, and would provide society a source of exciting and relevant efforts to

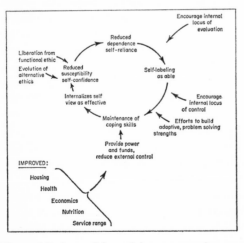

Figure 9-2. A possible social reconstruction syndrome.

improve the condition of the elderly. In short, it would allow elderly individuals to assume true competence in the sense of being their own locus of evaluation and control.

Summary

The purpose of this paper has been to present the SBS as a model which allows a sensitive explanation of three important issues in the social psychology of aging: (1) the interplay between the elderly person, whose social system is contracting, and the broader social environment within which he lives; (2) individual outcomes in terms of competence or well-being; (3) the processes of feedback by which this interplay becomes a vicious circle. Using the seven stages of the SBS, it was proposed that elderly individuals begin the cycle by being in a precondition of susceptibility, a vulnerable state created by the loss of historically familiar sources of feedback (roles, norms, and reference groups). As a second step, the individual becomes dependent on external evaluation and labeling. For the elderly, this labeling is systematically negative, being founded on a dominant ethic of personal worth through socioeconomic utility prevalent in our society. Eventual consequences to this social labeling as incompetent are the loss of psychological equipment to cope with the environment and the internalization of the negative self-view, thus completing a vicious cycle.

The cyclical nature of the SBS offers the prospect of intervention at various points of interaction. We suggested that efforts be made to liberate the person from the dominant societal view that worth is contingent on his performance in economic or productive social roles; further, we suggested that efforts be continued to enhance adaptive capacity by lessening the debilitating environmental conditions, poor health, poverty, and inadequate housing, and by facilitation of personal strengths. Finally, we suggest that, to enable the development of an internal locus of control, those who envision themselves as serving the elderly must deinvest their own power and control: self-determination by the elderly and individual control of policy and administration is the foundation of competent aging.

REFERENCES

Bengtson, V. L.: Cultural and occupational differences in social participation; in Havighurst *Adjustment to retirement: a cross-national study* (Van Gorkum, Amsterdam 1969).

Bengtson, V. L.: Adult socialization and personality differentiation: the social psychology of aging; in Birren *Contemporary gerontology: concepts and issues* (University of Southern California Press, Los Angeles 1970).

Blau, Z. S.: Changes in status and age identification. *Amer. Social. Rev. 21:*198-209 (1956).

Cain, L. E., Jr.: Life course and social structure; in Faris *Handbook of modern sociology.* (Rand McNally, Skokie 1964).

Cummings, E. and Henry, W.: *Growing old* (Basic Books, New York, 1961).

Deutscher, I.: The quality of postparental life: definitions of the situation. *J. Marriage Family. 26:*52-59 (1964).

Gruenberg, E. M. and Zusman, J.: The natural history of schizophrenia. *Int. Psychiat. Clin. 1:*699 (1964).

Havighurst, R. J. and Albrecht, R.: *Older people* (Longmans Green, London 1953).

Havighurst, R. J.; Neugarten, B.L., and Tobin, S. S.: Disengagement and patterns of aging; in Neugarten *Middle age and aging* (University of Chicago Press, Chicago 1968).

Lehr, U.: Consistency and change of social participation in old age; in Havighurst *Adjustment to retirement: a cross-national study* (Van Gorkum, Amsterdam 1969).

Lemon, B. W.: Bengtson, V. L., and Peterson, J. A.: Activity types and life satisfaction in a retirement community: an exploration of the activity theory of aging. *J. Geront.* (in press, 1972).

Lopata, H.: *Widowhood in American society* (Schenkman, Chicago 1972).

Lowenthal, M.F.: *Aging and mental disorder in San Francisco* (Jossey-Bass, San Francisco 1967).

Maddox, G.: Retirement as a social event in the United States; in McKinney and De-Vyver *Aging and social policy* (Appleton-Century-Crofts, New York 1966).

Neugarten, B. L. and Moore, J.: The changing age status system; in Neugarten *Middle age and aging* (University of Chicago Press, Chicago 1968).

Neugarten, B. L. and Peterson, W. A.: A study of the American age-grade system. *Proc. 4th Congr. Int. Ass. Geront., vol. 3,* pp. 497-502 (1957).

Neugarten, B. L.; Havighurst, R. J., and Tobin, S.S.: *Personality and Patterns of aging* (University of Chicago Press, Chicago 1968).

Neugarten, B. L.; Moore, J., and Lowe, J.: Age norms, age constraints, and adult socialization. *Amer. J. Sociol. 70:*710-717 (1965).

Phillips, B.: A role theory approach to adjustment in old age. *Amer. Sociol. Rev. 22:*212-217 (1957).

Palmore, E.: The effects of aging on activities and attitudes. *Gerontologist,* St. Louis *8:* 259-263 (1968).

Riley, M.W.; Finer, A. B., and Hess, A. H.: *Aging and society: an inventory of research findings, vol. 1* (Russell Sage Foundation, New York 1968).

Reich, C.: *The greening of American* (Random House, New York 1970).

Rose, A. M.: A current theoretical issue in social gerontology. *Gerontologist,* St. Louis *4:*25-29, (1964).

Rosenberg, S.S.: A sociological perspective on aging. *Sociol Focus* (1972).

Rosow, I.: *Social integration of the aged* (Free Press, New York 1967).

Silverman, P. R.: Widowhood and preventive intervention. *Family Coordinator 21:*95-102 (1971).

Slater, P.: *The pursuit of loneliness* (Beacon Press, Boston 1970).

Spence, D. and Lonner, T.: The empty nest: a

transition in motherhood. *Family Coordinator 20*:369-376 (1971).

Streib, G. F.: Are the aged a minority group? In Goulder and Miller *Applied sociology* (Macmillan, New York 1965).

Williams, R.: *American society* (Random House, New York 1970).

Zusman, J.: Some explanations of the changing appearance of psychotic patients: antecedents of the social breakdown syndrome concept. *Millbank Memorial Fund Quart. 64*: (1966).

Section III

ECONOMICS, HOUSING, AND HEALTH

D URING THE ERA OF THE 1930s through the early 1950s, considerable attention was devoted to the economic, housing, and health problems of the aged. Much of this research was sponsored and/or encouraged by agencies of the federal government in an effort to assess the extent of difficulties in these areas as well as to evaluate the effectiveness of programs directed toward alleviating these needs. Researchers, however, often tended to concentrate on specific problem areas. Housing, for example, drew a great deal of attention (Donahue, 1954; Chapin, 1951; Woodbury, 1950) as did medical (Felix, 1951; Monroe, 1951; Perrott, 1936; Woolsey, 1952) and financial matters (Woytinsky, 1943). Much of these efforts appear aimed at a comprehensive cataloguing of those difficulties facing the elderly.

Although this early research was mainly descriptive in nature, studies were not lacking which suggested the interrelatedness of these dimensions (Bond *et al.,* 1954; Chapin, 1951; Festinger *et al.,* 1950). Housing, for instance, was seen to influence the health and well-being of the older adult. Income, too, bore a strong relationship to both variables. As a consequence, there began to emerge the rudiments of what would shortly form the nucleus of some of the more far-reaching theories in social gerontology.

In summary, it must be said that these early research endeavors were limited in a number of ways. Most of the work was of a descriptive character and, therefore, guided by little theoretical insight. In addition, the survey design was used almost exclusively. Although recognition was given to the interrelated features of the various dimensions, little research was actually directed toward the multiple and interactional effects of all three. On the other hand, however, it should be acknowledged that such research did serve to delineate a number of problems facing the elderly in these areas, as well as provide some indication of the success of public and private support efforts. Finally, these findings provided valuable data for the framing of several theories of aging.

The late 1950s through the early 1960s saw a continuation and elaboration of the needs assessments and evaluations conducted earlier (Andrews, 1963; Burgess, 1960; Corson and McConnell, 1956; Epstein, 1959; Rothenberg, 1964;

91

Steiner, 1957). Although much of this research remained somewhat specialized in nature, its social and psychological character was becoming apparent. In general, the aging process was viewed against the backdrop of a number of critical variables. The influence of social attitudes and values, for example, was seen to affect not only the choice of housing arrangements (Beyer, 1962), but also the physical and emotional well-being of the elderly person (Busse, 1965; Donahue and Ashley, 1959; Richardson, 1963; WHO, 1959; Van Zonneveld, 1962). In addition, it was now considered unrealistic to examine the aspect of housing influence without an equal consideration of income and health (Kreps, 1963; Shanas, 1965; Turnbull *et al.,* 1957).

Besides stressing the interrelated character of the variables in question, the research of this era made use of more advanced techniques of data collection. Efforts were made to abandon single survey approaches to problem areas. In place of these, the longitudinal model was substituted. Although not to be fully utilized until the end of this period, these early longitudinal attempts succeeded in amassing significant quantities of data relative to the economic, physical, and locational problems of the elderly. Such data made possible not only a more realistic test of the theories generated during this time, but also provided the raw material for future theories. In addition, these findings enabled researchers to plan more appropriately for the future needs and requirements of a growing aged population. This era, then, can be generally characterized as a time of growth and expansion in the knowledge base regarding housing, income, and health.

The late 1960s and early 1970s again reflect a concern for assessing the economic, health, and housing needs of the elderly. This concern manifests itself as well in attempts to evaluate the success of remedial programs (Tissue, 1971; Hamovitch, 1969; McGuire, 1969; Travis, 1966; Brennen, 1967; Wendell, 1968; Williams, 1968). While fully recognizing the social and psychological character of each dimension, current research efforts are aimed at specifying the conditions and/or circumstances under which these factors constitute difficulties for the aged (Blenkner, 1967; Brinker, 1968; Chen, 1966; Goodstein, 1966; Krislov, 1968). In addition, considerable effort is made either to integrate the results of this research into presently existing theoretical formats, or to modify these structures in such a way as to better account for the observed results.

The desire for theoretical integration and formulation has gone hand in hand with improvements in methodology and research design. In general, the longitudinal framework has proven the most useful in terms of theory construction and verification (Palmore and Jeffers, 1971). In addition, contemporary gerontologists have made use of the field orientation of the social psychologist to explore the effects of housing and other programs on the health, attitudes, and behavior of the elderly. In this regard, a number of quasi-experimental designs have been employed (Carp, 1966; Sherman, 1968; White and Gordon, 1969). These formats have also proven useful in assessing the effectiveness of policy formulations.

Another focus of present-day research involves the aged's phenomenological understanding of their needs. The contemporary gerontologist has shown himself to be not only a social scientist but an enlightened social planner. That is, he is not only willing to pose questions, but he is also ready to provide solutions based on the aged's perceptions of their own problems. Proposals for national health insurance, guaranteed annual incomes, and greater variety in the housing of the elderly, for example, are evidence of this orientation. Furthermore, the effectiveness of these proposals has often been demonstrated by empirical research (Beckman, 1969; Beresford and Rivlin, 1966; Lawton and Lawton, 1968).

The focus of the early 1970s, then, is not upon research for research sake. Instead, it is directed toward the thorough exposition of problem areas utilizing sound theoretical frameworks. This use of sophisticated designs and statistical techniques has made possible the examination of facets of each area heretofore unexplored. Such efforts have brought an appreciation of the phenomenological as well as the objective dimensions of these areas. In turn, the proposals of contemporary gerontologists have reflected an approach to policy planning which acknowledges not only the aged as a group phenomena, but gives equal weight to the reality of individual differences.

The papers to follow have been selected as representative of contemporary research in the economics, housing, and health of the aged. These writings not only describe the dimensions of each problem area, but also discuss the various interrelated aspects of each. In addition, these authors reflect the modern concern for individual differences as well as illustrate the gerontologist's willingness to propose meaningful programatic solutions.

The paper by Schulz is an attempt to assess the economic impact of an aged population upon the industrialized countries of the world. The rising numbers of older persons as well as their increasingly earlier age at retirement are factors which dramatize the growing inequities in the transfer of income from a working to a nonworking population. In the author's estimation, the collective private or public mechanisms available to effect this transfer are closely related to two fundamental questions, the earnings-consumption pattern during worklife, and the retirement age decision. For Schulz, any decision to increase living standards in retirement must be bought by a decrease in someone's consumption potential before retirement. In addition, "equity dictates that there be some relationship between the gains achieved by the retired population and their sacrifices in terms of less consumption when they were young." The author feels that a partial solution to the social and financial cost problems arising from a sharply rising retirement population is to discourage movement out of the labor force.

Peterson is concerned more directly with the personal view of the economics of age. The author argues that the many indicators of economic adequacy presently available (e.g. the Social Security Poverty Index, the Bureau of Labor Statistics' "Retired Couple's Budget," and the BLS's "Three Budgets for a Retired Couple") provide little insight into the way older Americans feel about their financial condition. As a consequence, the author proposes a perceptual measure of income adequacy.

The measure in question was employed as a fixed-alternative questionnaire.

This instrument was administered to fifteen groups of retirees participating in multiservice senior centers or clubs in the Detroit metropolitan area. The findings indicate that 57 percent of the persons surveyed perceived their present finances to be inadequate. Thirty-five percent, on the other hand, saw their incomes as adequate, and another 8 percent viewed theirs as partially adequate. The non-married, females, blacks, those renting or buying a home, persons with low income, those living alone, and those with less education tend to be more likely to report their present finances to be inadequate. A comparison of the perceptual measure utilized with the more "objective" instruments mentioned above, indicates a reasonably similar pattern.

The paper by Lawton and Cohen looks at the issue of housing impact on the social and psychological well-being of older people. Utilizing a design incorporating a longitudinal dimension, the authors examine five housing sites in terms of the changes experienced by tenants during their first year of occupancy. These changes are then compared to change in groups of community residents who did not move into new housing during this period of time.

The authors report that following a year in the new housing, the rehoused were (1) "significantly poorer in Functional health than the community comparison subjects;" (2) "significantly higher in Morale, perceived more Change for the better, were more Satisfied with their housing, were more involved in External activities, and more Satisfied with the *status quo* than the community comparison subjects;" and (3) "not significantly different from the community comparison subjects in Loner status, Orientation to children or Continued breadth of activity."

Bultena and Wood focus attention on differences in the personal adjustment of older persons who have moved both to age-integrated and to age-segregated communities in a retirement state. They also examine a number of factors alledgedly related to differential adjustment. In addition, they present comparative data from a sample of males (N = 284) who have retired to their home towns in Wisconsin.

The findings indicate the migrants to retirement communities to have higher morale than those selecting regular age-integrated communities in Arizona. The authors feel this difference may be attributed in part to the differential characteristics of persons settling in these two types of communities. They point out that, "those in the retirement communities were drawn, to a greater extent than those in regular communities, from the higher socioeconomic segments of the aged population, and more often perceived themselves in good or very good health." By the same token, the structural features of these two types of communities are important to the morale of their residents. "The retirement community, with its greater opportunities for friendship interaction . . . and the functions it performs as a supportive reference group for leisure-oriented life styles, is found to provide an environment conducive to the adaptation of its residents to the retirement role."

The paper by Brody observes the major health needs of the aged to involve a number of chronic medical conditions. In surveying the various programs aimed at providing medical services to older people, the author notes the lack of a comprehensive philosophy of health care. Current modes of health care, for instance, are seen as primarily concerned with quantity rather than the quality of life. Health definitions, on the other hand, suggest a concern for not only the absence of disease, but also stress the physical, mental, and social well-being of the individual. For Brody, "the effectiveness of comprehensive health programs must be measured in terms both of the elderly person's response to the insults to which he is exposed and of the extent to which the health system enables him, or proposes to enable him, 'to rally,' respond, or function."

The final paper in this section presents and evaluates a newly-developed state-wide program of health care delivery to the elderly. The program in question focuses primary attention upon the rural aged. The writer describes the makeup of the MERCI project as well as the character of the screening and referral process. The initial phases of project utilization are then explored in depth. The writer concludes that such an adjunct medical system contributes significantly to the maintenance of the health and well-being of an aged population.

REFERENCES

Andrews, R. B. Housing for the elderly: aspects of its central problem. *Gerontologist*, 1963, *3*, 110-116.

Beckman, R. O. Acceptance of congregate life in a retirement village. *Gerontologist*, 1969, *9*, 281-285.

Beresford, J. C., and Rivlin, A. M. Privacy, poverty, and old age. *Demography*, 1966, *3*, 247-258.

Beyer, G. H. Living arrangements, attitudes, and preferences of older persons. In C. Tibbitts and W. Donahue (Eds.), *Social and psychological aspects of aging*. New York: Columbia University Press, 1962.

Blenkner, M. Environmental change and the aging individual. *Gerontologist*, 1967, *7*, 101-105.

Bond, F. A., Baber, R. E., Vieg, J. A., Perry, L. B., Scaff, A. H., and Lee, L. J., Jr. *Our needy aged: a California study of a national problem*. New York: Henry Holt & Co., 1954.

Brennan, H. J. *The economics of age*. New York: W. W. Norton, 1967.

Brinker, P. A. *Economic insecurity and social security*. New York: Appleton-Century-Crofts, 1968.

Burgess, E. W. (Ed.) *Housing the elderly in retirement communities*. Ann Arbor: University of Michigan Press, 1960.

Busse, E. W. The aging process and the health of the aged. In F. C. Jeffers (Ed.), *Duke University council on gerontology: proceedings of seminars 1961-1965*. Durham, North Carolina: Duke University Press, 1965.

Carp, F. M. Effects of improved housing on the lives of older people. In F. M. Carp and W. M. Burnett (Eds.), *Patterns of living and housing of middle-aged and older people*. Washington D. C.: United States Public Health Service, 1966.

Chapin, F. S. Some housing factors related to mental hygiene. In R. K. Merton, P. S. West, M. Jahoda, and H. C. Selvin (Eds.), *Social policy and social research in housing*. New York: Association Press, 1951.

Chen, Y. Economic poverty: the special case of the aged. *Gerontologist*, 1966, *6*, 39-45.

Corson, J. J., and McConnell, J. W. *Economic needs of older people.* New York: Twentieth Century Fund, 1956.

Donahue, W. (Ed.) *Housing the aging.* Ann Arbor: University of Michigan Press, 1954.

Donahue, W., and Ashley, E. E., III Housing and the social health of older people. In C. Tibbitts (Ed.), *Aging and social health in the United States and Europe.* Ann Arbor: University of Michigan Press, 1959.

Epstein, L. A. Money income of aged persons: a 10-year-review, 1948 to 1958. *Social Security Bulletin,* 1959, *22,* 3-11.

Felix, R. H. Mental health in an aging population. In W. Donahue and C. Tibbitts (Eds.), *Growing in the older years.* Ann Arbor: University of Michigan Press, 1951.

Festinger, L., Schacter, S., and Back, K. *Social pressures in informal groups: a study of human factors in housing.* New York: Harper & Bros., 1950.

Goodstein, S. Urban and rural differences in consumer patterns of the aged. *Rural Sociology,* 1966, *31,* 333-345.

Hamovitch, M. B., and Peterson, J. E. Housing needs and satisfactions of the elderly. *Gerontologist,* 1969, *9,* 30-32.

Kreps, J. M. (Ed.) *Employment, income, and retirement problems of the aged.* Durham, North Carolina: Duke University Press, 1963.

Krislov, J. Four issues in income maintenance for the aged during the 1970's. *Social Science Review,* 1968, *42,* 335-343.

Lawton, M. P., and Lawton, F. G. Social rehabilitation of the aged: some neglected aspects. *Journal of the American Geriatrics Society,* 1968, *16,* 1346-1363.

McGuire, M. C. The status of housing for the elderly. *Gerontologist,* 1969, *9,* 10-14.

Monroe, R. T. *Diseases in old age: a clinical and pathological study of 7941 individuals over 61 years of age.* Cambridge, Mass.: Harvard University Press, 1951.

Palmore, E., and Jeffers, F. C. Health care in a longitudinal panel before and after medicare. *Journal of Gerontology,* 1971, *26,* 532-536.

Perrott, G. St. J. The state of the nation's health. *Annals of the American Academy of Political and Social Sciences,* 1936, *188,* 131-143.

Richardson, I. M. Occupation and health. In R. H. Williams, C. Tibbitts, and W. Donahue (Eds.), *Processes of aging,* New York: Atherton Press, 1963.

Rothenberg, R. E. *Health in the later years.* New York: New American Library, 1964.

Shanas, E. Health care and health services for the aged. *Gerontologist,* 1965, *5,* 240; 276.

Sherman, S. R. Psychological effects of retirement housing. *Gerontologist,* 1968, *8,* 170-175.

Steiner, P. O., and Dorfman, R. *The economic status of the aged.* Berkeley: University of California Press, 1957.

Tissue, T. Old age, poverty, and the central city. *Aging and Human Development,* 1971, *2,* 235-248.

Travis, G. *Chronic disease and disability.* Berkeley: University of California Press, 1966.

Turnbull, J. C., Williams, C. A., Jr., and Cheit, E. F. *Economic and social security.* New York: Ronald Press Co., 1957.

Van Zonneveld, R. J. *The health of the aged.* Baltimore, Md.: Williams & Wilkins, 1962.

Wendell, R. F. The economic status of the aged. *Gerontologist,* 1968, *8,* 32-36.

White, E. L., and Gordon, T. Related aspects of health and aging in the United States. In M. F. Lowenthal and A. Zilli (Eds.), *Colloquium on health and aging of the population.* New York: S. Karger, 1969.

Williams, W., and Lyday, J. M. Income sufficiency and the aged poor. *Quarterly Review of Economics and Business,* 1968, *8,* 19-25.

Woodbury, C. Current housing development for older people. In W. Donahue and C.

Tibbitts (Eds.), *Planning the older years*. Ann Arbor: University of Michigan Press, 1950.

Woolsey, T. D. Estimates of disabling illness prevalence in the United States. *Public Health Service Bulletin 181,* Washington D. C.: Government Printing Office, 1952.

World Health Organization. Mental health problems of aging and the aged, sixth report. *World Health Organization Technical Report Series,* 1959, *171,* 3-51.

Woytinsky, W. S. Income cycle in the life of families and individuals. *Social Security Bulletin,* 1943, *6,* 8-17.

Chapter 10

THE ECONOMIC IMPACT OF AN AGING POPULATION

James H. Schulz

When persons speak about the aging of a population, they are generally describing a situation where the proportion of aged persons in the population is increasing. Such a definition is not completely unambiguous, however, since it neglects all other age structure shifts occurring, for example, as a result of changes in the relative proportion of the very young. But the numerous physical, social, and economic problems occurring among the older part of the population raise the question as to what impact demographic changes in the age structure of the population will have on these problems and their solutions.

Investigation (U.N. Dept. of Economics and Social Affairs, 1956) has shown that:

> ... in the greater part of the world, the age structure [since the earliest recorded censuses] has undergone little change. This is particularly true of the economically under-developed countries, or rather of all countries with a high fertility ... The reduction of mortality, as it has occurred historically, has had little effect on the age structure.

The reduction of fertility, however, in the more developed countries has had a considerable impact.

This phenomena of a population aging

is relatively recent and restricted to a small but growing group of countries. Using the classification scheme developed by Rosset (1964), we can classify nations with 8 percent or more of their population over the age of sixty-four as having aged populations. Currently, there are over twenty countries meeting this criteria, about one half of them with percentages greater than 12 percent.

As a result of past demographic history, the age patterns of these aged populations tend to have the shape of a barrel rather than a pyramid, as a result of the fact that there are relatively more middle-aged than young persons in the population. This middle-age bulge will grow older and result in increased aging of these nations, being relatively unaffected in the short run by changes in mortality or fertility levels.

As an example of these developments, Figure 10-1 shows for the United States the projected ratio of the over sixty-five population to the twenty to sixty-four population.

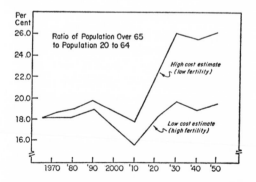

Figure 10-1. Source: United States Population Projections for OASDI Cost Estimates. Actuarial Study #62, 1966, p. 23. Reproduced in Reports of the 1971 Advisory Council on Social Security Communication from the Secretary of Health, Education, & Welfare, 82nd Congress, 1st session. Washington: GPO, 1971, p. 94.

Reprinted by permission from the *Gerontologist*, 1973, *13*, 111-118.

The Economic Problem Stated

Today, around the world, social security systems, typically covering old-age, survivors, disability and health insurance, are the principal institutional mechanism used to provide economic security to the retired aged. Such systems are viewed as devices for equitably (in greater or less degree) transferring income (hence output claims) to the aged from those persons in the active working population.

Thus, social security improvements often head the list of demands by the aged segment of the population, while being relatively unimportant to younger workers. But regardless of whether the mechanism for retirement income provision is social security, public assistance, private insurance, private charity, and/or self-help through the use of personal savings, the fundamental economic fact remains that the part of national output consumed in any particular year by the retired aged is produced by the working population.

Of course, old people are not the only population group claiming through public programs a share of the available goods and services. Education of the young, manpower programs, support for veterans, expanded preventive and treatment medical service for all ages, general poverty programs, and other general welfare programs in a sense compete with one another for shares of the gross national product. And to this competition might be added the competing claims of such nonwelfare programs as environmental protection, housing and urban development, and transportation, all of which, for example, have become so important as to now justify separate and powerful agencies in the United States government.

It is these (and other) alternative uses of our output that cause people to talk about the competition between the young and the old (US Senate Special Committee on Aging, 1970). Given the prospects for rising retirement income expectations in the future and a rising proportion of aged, together with rising perceived needs of other age groups, it is often suggested that a country will never be able to develop income transfer programs for the aged which will be adequate. The substance of the problem or question at issue, however, should be stated differently. The major economic issue is not whether, in the face of other problems, such as general poverty, urban blight, and increased demand for education, a nation can have new and better economic support for the aged. Rather the issue is better posed as to whether the people of the nation want a higher standard of living in their retirement years at the expense of a lower standard during the active working years.

While the economic status of the aged is dependent on the extent to which the society at any particular time is willing to transfer income from workers to the retired, the financing systems of all existing individual or collective private or public mechanisms available to carry out this transfer are intimately bound-up with two fundamental questions.

1. The earnings-consumption pattern during worklife and the extent to which people are willing and able to postpone consumption until the retirement period.

2. The retirement age decision which, together with age of entry, determines the relative size of the working versus nonworking years (taking birth and mortality rates as given).

Thus, to better provide for old age, people must save more during their working years, and/or they must develop institutions which will transfer the income they desire from the population which is working during the period they are retired. In creased saving for retirement means less income in the working years for consumption purposes. Alternatively, the transferring of adequate income in old age, if it is to be done equitably, must be based upon appropriate amounts of payments or tax contributions during the working years to support the then aged.

There is a growing debate in the United States (Projector, 1969) as to the intragenerational equity of both current private and public pension systems. For example, the Nobel prize-winning economist Paul Samuelson (1967) argues that because of population growth and continued economic growth, windfall gains will continue for future generations:

> The beauty about social insurance is that it is actuarially unsound. Everyone who reaches retirement age is given benefit privileges that far exceed anything he has paid in. And exceed his payments by more than 10 times as much (or 5 times, counting in employer payments)!

In contrast to the Samuelson view is one held by a number of economists including the noted American economist, Friedman (1971):

> [Social security] combines a highly regressive tax with largely indiscriminate benefits and, on the average, probably redistributes income from lower to higher income persons . . .
>
> What . . . working people are now doing is paying taxes to finance payments to persons who are not working. The individual worker is in no sense building protection for himself and his family—as a person who contributes to a private vested pension system is building his own protection. Persons who are now receiving payments are receiving much more than the actuarial value of the taxes that were paid on their behalf. Young persons who are now paying social security taxes are being promised much less than the actuarial value that the taxes paid on their behalf could buy in private plans.

The problem of intragenerational equity arises not only as a result of paying benefits to people who have a relatively few years of participation in the pay-in part of the system. It is created also by the numerous and frequent changes in pension formulas, benefit levels, benefit calculation procedures, and numerous other aspects of the pension system, changes which occur so frequently in almost all countries. All these changes make it difficult to analyze the relationship between the taxes paid and the benefits received by the current generation of retired people and make it almost impossible to make accurate predictions about future generations. Yet given the large number of social security systems in the world today whose benefits are fundamentally related to contributions (taxes) based upon earnings, it is mandatory that serious consideration and study be given to both intragenerational and also intergenerational equity matters. With regard to intragenerational equity, a considerable body of literature has been developed and testifies to the complexity of the subject (Atkinson, 1970, Brittain, 1967; Campbell, 1969; Chen, 1967; Goldin, 1971; Samuelson, 1958). Much work remains to be done.

Thus, to summarize, the economic impact of an aging population should be looked at in relation to two major questions.

1. What effect does the aging of a population have on the ability and willingness of that population to provide for themselves (and prior and succeeding generations) adequate income (and health, disability, and survivorship) protection in retirement?

2. As a population and its pension systems react and adjust to the changing demographic structure in response to question one—how should the burden or costs of retirement income be allocated among

groups within a particular generation and among various generations?

Let us look now at some of the key factors connected with adequate retirement income and intragenerational equity. First, is the demographic factor. Are nations aging and how rapidly?

Demographic Structure

A look at the United States experience illustrates current demographic developments. The US Bureau of the Census makes four different projections which differ in their assumptions for fertility.

The latest population projections of the census forecast a rising proportion of persons age sixty-five or older in the total population, rising from 10 percent in 1970 to 13 percent in the year 2020. If one looks at the proportion of persons age sixty or older, the proportion increases from 17 percent in 1970 to 19 percent in 2020.

In Western Europe there was a well-known drop in the birthrate from 1875 to 1935 which, at the time, created great concern; this trend reversed itself in the late 1930s, and birthrates went up (even during World War II) throughout the 1940s and 1950s. After 1965, however, the trend resumed its downward trend (Sauvy, 1970).

Data published by the United Nations (1971) show that there are two countries (Austria and the German Democratic Republic) with 15 to 16 percent of the population over age sixty-four, five countries (Belgium, France, Norway, Sweden, and England/Wales) with 13 percent, and seven countries (Denmark, the Federal Republic of Germany, Greece, Italy, the Netherlands, Switzerland, and the USA) with 10 to 12 percent.

Benefit Levels

The level of living which older people desire or expect when they retire is a key variable in determining the magnitude of the economic task faced by the working population in supporting the nonworking population. As stated above, a decision to increase living standards in retirement must be bought by a decrease in someone's consumption potential before retirement. Furthermore, equity dictates that there be some relationship between the gains achieved by the retired population and their sacrifices in terms of less consumption when they were young.

Historically, the great bulk of older people in most countries have enjoyed very low living standards, often sharply reduced from their preretirement years. It seems clear that this situation resulted not so much from an explicit decision of these people to live in poverty. Rather, it resulted from (a) frequent national economic fluctuations with recurring depressions and inflations, (b) individual difficulties in retirement preparation arising from (a) and from the generally low levels of income available during the working years, and (c) the lack of national retirement planning.

With the development of collective means of retirement security through pension systems, the economic situation of the retired has changed significantly. But still it is generally agreed that in almost all countries improvements must be made in pension systems. Thus, it is that the direction and magnitude of these improvements will influence and be influenced by the aging of a nation's population. Specification of any level of retirement income *adequacy* can be translated into its cost on the working population. As the population ages, this cost per worker will rise.

There is no generally accepted definition of what is an adequate pension. This is a very subjective question which many have argued should be ultimately decided by the individual. Increasingly, however, discussion of this question has centered around what proportion of preretirement income is needed and desired during retirement to prevent a sharp drop in living standards. A significant number of social security systems in developed countries now use mechanisms which not only relate pension benefits to prior earnings but seek to guarantee through these benefits a relatively high level of earnings replacement at retirement. Public pension reforms, for example, in Austria, Belgium, France, Italy, Sweden, and West Germany have resulted in systems embodying the principle of high earnings replacement to provide living standard maintenance. *The trend seems to be toward developing public and private pension systems which will permit the retired population to at least maintain a level of living which approximates that which they enjoyed during their working years.* If this trend continues, it means that income transfers to the aged will rise very sharply in the future.

The Age of Retirement

When a nation establishes by law that a person may receive a full retirement pension at a certain age, the government, in effect, is promulgating a national age of expected or normal retirement. Existing statistics clearly indicate the strong influence of this legislated pension age on the actual age of retirement by persons in the population. In a 1964 survey (David, 1965), for example:

> . . . more than one third of the responding nations stated that the average exact age of initial receipt of pension was either the same as or within one year of normal pensionable age . . . When there was differences between pensionable and actual retirement age the latter was higher, but for schemes having 65 as the pensionable age the variation was generally small (Kreps, 1968).

Thus, for example, in the U.S.A. the participation rate for males over age sixty-four has dropped from 57 percent in 1920 to 26 percent in 1970.

Economic growth resulting from technological innovation, rising levels of education, the growth of capital, etc. has permitted living standards in the industrialized countries to increase while, at the same time, workers generally have had to work less to help produce the rising output of goods and services. Thus, as workers' lifetime earnings have increased, hours worked per week or the number of days worked have fallen; the length of vacations has increased; and the period of retirement has generally lengthened.

It is usually assumed that continued economic growth in the future will presumably make it possible to reduce work effort still further while continuing to raise living standards (Kreps, 1971). This means that hours worked per week could continue to fall, and vacations could be lengthened. The question arises, however, as to whether the normal age of retirement should also be reduced and workers allowed to retire earlier. All workers, whether young or old, should seriously consider when and how they want to take the leisure available to them throughout their lifetime. A fundamental problem, however, is how to operationalize this question so that workers can make meaningful choices.

While there is general recognition and research evidence that people would like to stop working at different ages (Barfield and Morgan, 1969), little has been accomplished toward achieving the goal of flexible retirement (OECD, 1970; Schulz, 1971). Instead, there seem to be mounting pressures for early and mandatory retirement and, most importantly, for social security and private pension full pension eligibility at earlier ages. The motivations for these pressures are not entirely clear and no doubt vary from one country to another, but two factors stand out; the political popularity among middle-aged persons of reducing the social security eligibility age and the economic popularity among businesses, unions, and younger workers of early retirement in order to deal with declining job opportunities due to stagnating industries or high rates of aggregate unemployment.

Recent events in a few countries illustrate the situation. In Sweden a 1969 private pension agreement was reached between the Swedish Employers' Confederation and the salaried employees' union to provide private pensions at age sixty-five equal to public old-age pensions to be paid at sixty-seven (to be reduced when the public pensions came into effect). This agreement was quickly followed by a similar agreement last year between employers and blue-collar workers. In the Federal Republic of Germany one of the major pension debates is currently over whether to increase pension levels or increase the level of pensions paid before the normal retirement age of sixty-five; current sentiment, according to observers, appears to favor earlier payment. In 1971 French trade unions called for two major pension changes—an increase of 40 to 55 percent in old-age pensions under the regime general and a lowering of the retirement age from sixty-five to sixty for all workers (Weise, 1972); the government, guided by the recommendations of the Commission on Social Benefits for the Sixth Plan, proposed legislation (subsequently passed) to significantly raise benefits but rejected the proposal to lower the normal retirement age. In the United States, a number of universities laboring under the general education cost squeeze which pervades all higher education have announced early retire-

ment policies as a means of keeping an age-balanced teaching staff.

To reduce the normal retirement age results in a very large increase in the magnitude of the funds required to provide for each person's retirement. This arises not only as a result of the increased transfers required from the working population but also because of the smaller total national output resulting from the reduced size of the labor force, assuming a full employment economy and that the people retiring are employable.

Current practice in most nations is to allow retirement three to five years before the normal retirement age with reduced pension benefits. While the advantage of this procedure is that it provides some flexibility and a measure of individual choice, such early retirement provisions also tend to encourage institutionalization of the *early* retirement eligibility age as the *normal* age for retirement. At least this seems to have been the experience in the United States where more than one-half the workers now retire early. Within four years of the 1961 amendment to the US Social Security Act, which made men eligible for reduced old age benefits at age sixty-two, one third of the private pension plans studied by the US Bureau of Labor Statistics reduced the normal retirement age, in most cases from age sixty-five to sixty-two. In addition, many US corporations now offer early retirement financial incentives, mainly in the form of supplemental benefits over and above the regular pension; this supplemental benefit continues until social security benefits begin or until the worker is eligible for his full social security benefit at the normal retirement age of sixty-five.

As aging in a population occurs, one way to reduce the cost problems arising from a sharply rising retirement population is by discouraging movement out of the work force. This can be done, for example, by instituting one or more of the following policy measures:

1. Liberalizing (but not necessarily eliminating) "retirement test" provisions associated with social security;

2. Exempting workers over the normal retirement age from social security taxes;

3. Removing tax exemption privileges for employer private pension contributions to finance "early retirement" pension incentives;

4. Outlawing or liberalizing mandatory retirement age rules;

5. Making the work experience and work environment more enjoyable to the worker;

6. Developing "flexible retirement" job opportunities.

This list is certainly not exhaustive but, hopefully, shows the range of policy avenues available. Of course, the experience in almost all countries indicates that change in this policy area to help reduce retirement costs is not very likely.

France, the Federal Republic of Germany, Israel, the United Kingdom and Japan, when facing imbalances between the increase in pension outgo and income [due to the demographic situation], were compelled to seek ways of increasing the income. Only in rare cases expenditures could be reduced by such means as increasing the retirement age (e.g. Argentina).

Concluding Observations

What are the implications of the above discussion and the trends as they seem to be developing? A number of implications seem to be indicated:

1. In trying to predict how soon and how great will be the economic burden of aging populations in various nations, we are faced with the difficulty that the key variables, fertility, pension levels, and the age of retirement, are in a state of flux and essentially unpredictable. This means that long-range planning becomes very difficult. However, at the same time, all these variables are subject to influence by national policy, and, therefore, the magnitude of future problems are subject to control.

2. The increasing transfer costs of an aging population together with rising social costs associated with urbanization and the economic production of a technologically-oriented society will make it increasingly difficult in the future to raise living standards during the working years in the highly developed nations of the world.

3. The trend of a lengthening retirement period resulting from medical advances and, more importantly, from retiring at an earlier age needs to be watched closely. Serious thought should be given to reevaluating or, in many cases, establishing a national policy in this area.

4. As the aging of a population develops, there will be a need for a greater awareness of the intra- and intergenerational equity considerations arising out of developing pension systems. As the national cost of aged income maintenance rises, greater attention to equity issues will be necessary in order (a) to maintain public confidence in and support for the systems and (b) to use with maximum effectiveness the retirement funds available.

REFERENCES

Atkinson, A. B. National superannuation: Redistribution and value for money. *Bulletin of the Oxford University of Economics & Statistics,* 1970, *32,* 171-85.

Barfield, R., and Morgan, J. *Early retirement: The decision and the experience.* Ann Arbor: Braun-Brumfield, 1969.

Brittain, J. A. The real rate of interest on lifetime contributions toward retirement under Social Security. In US Joint Economic

Committee, *Old Age Income Assurance,* Part III. 90th Congress, 1st session. Washington: GPO, Dec., 1967.

Campbell, C. D. Social insurance in the United States: A program in search of an explanation. *Journal of Law & Economics,* 1969, *12,* 249-65.

Chen, Y.P. Inflation and productivity in tax-benefit analysis for Social Security. In US Joint Economic Committee, *Old Age Income Assurance,* Part III. 90th Congress, 1st session. Washington: GPO, Dec., 1967.

David, A. M. Problems of retirement age and related conditions for the receipt of old-age benefits, Report IX of the 15th General Assembly. *Bulletin of the International Social Security Association.* Feb.-April, 1965, *18,* 97-109.

Friedman, M. *Social Security: Universal or selective?* In Rational Debate Seminar. Washington: American Enterprise Institute, 1971.

Goldin, K. D. Social insurance finance. *Rivista di Diritto Finanziario e Scienza delle Finanze,* 1971, *30,* 355-79.

Kreps, J. *Lifetime allocation of work and income.* Durham, NC: Duke University Press, 1971.

Kreps, J. *Lifetime allocation of work and leisure.* Research Report No. 22, Office of Research and Statistics, Social Security Administration. Washington: GPO, 1968.

OECD. *Flexibility of retirement age.* Paris: OECD, 1970.

Projector, D. S. Should the payroll tax finance higher benefits under OASDI? A review of the issues. *Journal of Human Resources,* 1969, *4,* 61-75.

Rosset, E. *Aging process of population.* New York: Macmillan, 1964.

Samuelson, P. Social Security. *Newsweek,* Feb. 13, 1967, p. 8.

Samuelson, P. An exact consumption-loan model of interest with or without the social contrivance of money. *Journal of Political Economy,* 1958, *66,* 467-482.

Sauvy, A. The "old world" grows older. *Interplay,* 1970, *3,* 26-28.

Schulz, J. *Retirement—background and issues.* Prepared for the 1971 White House Conference on Aging. Washington: GPO, 1971.

Schulz, J. Statement in US Senate Special Committee on Aging. *Economics of aging: Toward a full share in abundance.* Part 10A —Pension Aspects. Washington: GPO, 1970.

United Nations. *Demographic yearbook 1970.* New York: UN, 1971.

US Senate Special Committee on Aging. *The stake of today's workers in retirement security.* 91st Congress, 2nd session. Washington: GPO, April, 1970.

Weise, R. W. Higher old-age pensions in France. *Social Security Bulletin,* May, 1972, *35,* 30-32.

Chapter 11

FINANCIAL ADEQUACY IN RETIREMENT: PERCEPTIONS OF OLDER AMERICANS

David A. Peterson

THE ECONOMIC CIRCUMSTANCES of older Americans are of national concern today, both among the older people themselves and among professionals concerned with their welfare. The fact that persons over sixty-five have annual incomes less than 50 percent of their younger counterparts, that over 25 percent of all older people live in poverty, and that the fixed incomes of older people subject them more acutely to the ravages of inflation have lead policy makers and researchers to label economics as the number one problem of older people (US Congress, 1969).

Awareness of this situation has led to numerous attempts to raise the economic position of older people to a level that could be considered adequate. One hindrance, however, has been the lack of a measure of financial adequacy that could satisfactorily determine when adequacy was reached. Several approaches have been developed, the best known being a budget which attempts to "translate a generalized concept of some specific standard of living into a list of commodities and services that can be priced" (US Dept. of Labor, 1966). The Bureau of Labor Statistics' "Retired

Reprinted by permission from the *Gerontologist*, 1973, *12*, 379-383.

Couple's Budget" and "Three Budgets for a Retired Couple" are the most widely used attempts of this type. The original budget prices a moderate standard of living in various parts of the country while the three budgets indicate lower, intermediate, and higher level of living (US Dept. of Labor, 1970).

As comprehensive and meticulous as these BLS budgets are, they have certain weaknesses common to all budget approaches, the most critical being the tremendous amount of time and energy required to bring the budget up-to-date. The latest BLS budget was priced in the spring of 1967. Thus, the prices as well as the quantity and quality of goods and services involved are several years behind actual rates of consumption and income.

A more basic shortcoming of the budget approach, however, is that it must be limited by certain assumptions in order to keep it within reasonable bounds. Since the budget is prepared for couples, neither of whom work, it actually excludes a majority of older people. It also excludes the person with an unusual situation, expense, or past level of living.

Thus the budget can only apply to typical individuals and provides no way to incorporate the unusual circumstances which make many older people unique.

Older People's Perception of Income Adequacy

If one wishes to judge the financial adequacy of any individual's position, a different approach is required. The perceptual approach is one alternative that has been used. This method rests on the assumption that an individual can determine the adequacy of his own finances; in fact, he is probably the only person who is in a position to do so since only he can incorporate consideration of his past level of living, his changing needs, his housing situation, the number of persons he must provide for, his assets, medical expenses, debts, etc. The perceptual method is employed by asking older people how adequate they think their financial situation is and accepting their judgment as the measure of financial adequacy. Use of this approach has been reported in the literature, but it has typically been restricted to small surveys in which the researcher was primarily interested in other data (Barfield and Morgan, 1969; Hansen, 1962, 1965; Hunter and Maurice, 1952; McCann, 1967, Shanas, 1962; Youmans, 1967).

Several questions about the validity and reliability of the perceptual approach may be expressed by those unfamiliar with the procedure. In the survey reported here, face validity was checked for each of the scales used in addition to tests of construct validity. These latter tests were accomplished by making predictions about the relationship between the variable being measured and other variables. For example, it was predicted that persons who were identified by the study as perceiving their finances to be inadequate would have lower monthly incomes, a smaller proportion of perceived needed monthly income, a lower adjusted monthly income, and less likelihood of owning their own home. These predicted relationships occurred for each perceptual variable.

Reliability of one scale was measured through the use of the split-half technique. Other scales included only three questions and consequently did not lend themselves readily to this measure. The split-half method consists of dividing the scale into two halves, assigning odd-numbered questions to one-half and even-numbered ones to the other, then considering the two halves as alternative forms of the same scale and correlating them to estimate the extent to which they are equivalent. The correlation of equivalence was computed to be .94, which indicates that the two halves were adequately equivalent. This survey and others have revealed that older persons are willing to indicate honestly and accurately the amount of money they need to reach an adequate level of living; they do not ask for unreasonably large amounts of money; and they do seem to agree on a general level of adequacy.

In fact the greater danger is in the understatement of need. Older persons tend to make very minimal requests for money. In one study the average annual income was $1130, yet only 40 percent of the respondents indicated that they went without things because they lacked money (Youmans, 1963). Thus, the main drawback to the use of the perceptual approach to the determination of financial adequacy is that older people will tend to understate what might be viewed as reasonable income needed. This factor was minimized in the study reported here by asking a series of questions, each of which probed for an evaluation of adequacy in a different area.

The Study Problem

The study problem was to determine the perceptions of older Americans on their financial adequacy in retirement. The study undertaken was a descriptive survey of retired persons in southeastern Michigan. A fixed-alternative questionnaire was prepared by the investigator and administered to fifteen groups of retirees participating in multi-service senior centers or senior citizen clubs in the Detroit metropolitan area. The individual participant was defined as the sampling unit, and 462 such persons responded to the questionnaire. This was an overall response rate of 83 percent.

A purposeful sample of older persons was selected which included high, middle, and low income groups; urban, suburban, and rural groups; whites and blacks. The sample was compared with existing demographic data on persons over sixty-five years in the United States and in southeastern Michigan (Detroit Regional Transportation and Land Use Study, 1969). It was found to vary only slightly from either of these measures in income, age distribution, marital status, home ownership, employment, race, and sex. Only in the amount of education was the purposeful sample significantly different from the other two populations. The respondents in this study had significantly longer exposure to formal education programs than did persons in the other populations.

Eight different scales were developed by the investigator for this study. These were measures of perceived income adequacy in the present, savings adequacy in the present, financial adequacy in the present, financial adequacy in the past, financial adequacy in the future, and three financial trend scales, past-present trend, present-future trend, and a combination of these, financial trend scale. Hypotheses were not tested; rather fourteen study questions were posed and answered.

The data were collected in May of 1969 by the investigator who personally administered the questionnaire to groups of senior citizens. Pretests of the administration procedure provided information on the best method to use, and this method was standardized and closely adhered to in dealing with each group of older persons.

Perception of Needs

The findings indicate that 57 percent of the retirees surveyed perceived their present finances to be inadequate, while 5 percent saw theirs as adequate, and 8 percent viewed theirs as partially adequate. This determination was made through a series of six questions on income and savings adequacy. If respondents perceived their present income and savings to be adequate, they were judged to have adequate finances; if neither was perceived to be adequate, their finances were considered inadequate; if one was adequate and the other not, the respondent's finances were considered to be partially adequate.

As was expected, the nonmarried, females, blacks, those renting or buying a home, persons with low income, those living alone, and those with less education were all significantly more likely than others to perceive their finances to be inadequate.

Respondents were also asked to indicate the amount of money that would be required in order to meet all of their family's needs. The median amount reported was $400 monthly. The range was fairly large, but it was found that respondents were relatively consistent in the additional amount that they perceived as needed. When a comparison of the respondents' present income was made with the income needed to meet the family needs, the average respondent indicated a desire for 33 percent more than he had. This percentage held very firm for all families with incomes under $6,000 annually. Thus, significantly smaller amounts of income were perceived as needed by some groups, specifically by blacks, persons with low monthly incomes, persons living alone, persons retired for a greater number of years, and persons over age eighty.

On another set of questions respondents indicated the adequacy of their finances in the past and predicted their financial adequacy five years in the future. A comparison of these data provided a trend scale which showed the direction of perceived financial adequacy from the past to the present to the future.

Fifty-one percent of retirees viewed their finances of five years in the past as adequate. In the present, 35 percent saw their finances as adequate, and the percentage dropped to 25 percent when retirees looked five years into the future.

A comparison of the trend of perceived financial adequacy from past to present and present to future confirmed that individual retirees tend not to perceive improvement in their financial position over time. Forty-five percent saw their position as declining from past to future while an additional 45 percent viewed their situation as remaining the same. A significant number fell into this second category because the scale used did not allow for persons who saw their position as inadequate in the past to indicate that it would deteriorate any further in the future. Thus many of this 45 percent may have perceived decline but were not able to note this because of the system used.

Comparisons of Financial Adequacy

The findings of this study clearly indicate that many older people do not perceive their finances to be adequate to meet their present needs. It is obvious that those persons who fell into the demographic categories normally considered most likely to be poor (females, blacks, uneducated, etc.) are the respondents who perceived their financial situation to be inadequate. This provides a crude check on the perceptual method.

A second check was also done. Individual respondents were compared with the standards provided in the BLS budgets to determine their financial adequacy in another way. The moderate level of living (1966 budget) and the intermediate level (1970 budget) are quite comparable ($3869

and $3857 yearly) and may be considered to provide a measure of financial adequacy. After adjustments were made for cost-of-living increases from 1966 to 1969 in Detroit, and each respondent's income was translated into dollars-per-couple (to be equivalent to the budgets) the comparison was made.

Since both the budget method and the perceived adequacy method showed a 5 percent inadequacy rate, it seems reasonable to predict that persons who were determined to have inadequate finances by one method would be the same as those who were determined to have inadequate finances by the other. It was found that the relationship between the two measures was highly significant although far from perfect. Only 22 percent of those below the adequacy level set by the budget ($35 monthly) perceived their income to be anything more than inadequate, but 45 percent of those with adjusted incomes over $350 saw their incomes as less than adequate. Thus, the budget method and the perceptual method do arrive at somewhat different conclusions about the financial adequacy of individual older people.

A third comparison was made by relating the measure of perceived income adequacy to the Social Security poverty index, a minimum income based primarily on the US Dept. of Agriculture economy food plan (Orshansky, 1968). When adjustments were made for increases in the cost of living, the poverty threshold was found to be approximately $2160 annually or $180 monthly. Eighty-four percent of the persons who had incomes below this level viewed their incomes as inadequate while 48 percent of those with more than $1 monthly income also saw their incomes inadequate. Thus the poverty threshold was not as good a predictor of perception of adequacy as were the BLS budgets

Poverty and adequacy appear to denote two separate levels of living.

It was also found that persons with lower incomes typically had much lower financial aspirations than did others. They perceived that a small increase in their income would raise them to a level which they considered to be adequate. They were not demanding great increases but were willing to live on only slightly more than they had, even though this totaled a very modest amount.

One might conclude, then, that financial adequacy is best viewed in relative terms rather than in specific dollar amounts. This may be caused by variations in preretirement income or by the adequacy of adjustment to retirement income. Whatever the reason, the older people in this study who had annual incomes below $6,000 annually indicated a need for 33 percent more income to bring them to a level they perceived as adequate.

For policy purposes then, it is possible to view an attempt to raise the income of most older people as preferable to attempting to bring all older persons up to an arbitrary level. This is the direction that the Social Security program has been taking, and it would appear to be the one that older people in this sample would support.

Future Financial Adequacy

The rising cost of living has caused older people who live on fixed incomes to be increasingly squeezed in recent years as their answers to the questions on past, present, and future financial adequacy indicate. Before retirement, or five years ago, they tended to see their financial situation as adequate, but the present has brought a significant decline in this position, and they do not look to the future with optimism.

Thus, older people now feeling the in-flation pinch, see the future as holding nothing better. They continue to see younger persons improve their position while they actually slide backward. The resulting frustration and anger may well be a force which will lead older persons to collectively demand a greater share of the wealth of this nation in the future.

Summary

A survey of 462 older persons in southeastern Michigan was conducted to determine how they perceived their financial situation. Over one-half perceived the current finances to be inadequate and indicated that they were declining. The average older person regardless of present level of income stated that to reach adequacy, his family income would need to be increased by 33 percent. Definite policy considerations are apparent if the finances of older people are to be raised to a level that they will consider to be adequate.

REFERENCES

Barfield, R., and Morgan, J. *Early retirement: The decision and the experience.* Ann Arbor: Institute for Social Research, University of Michigan, 1969.

Detroit Regional Transportation and Land Use Study, I. J. Rubin, Dir. Unpublished data, Detroit, 1969.

Hansen, G. D. *Chronic illness, disability and aging in Morrison County, Minnesota.* Minneapolis,: University of Minnesota, 1962.

Hansen, G. D. Older people in the Midwest: Conditions and attitudes. In A. M. Rose W. A. Peterson (Eds.), *Older people and their social world.* Philadelphia: F. A. Davis, 1965.

Hunter, W. W., and Maurice, H. *Older people tell their story.* Ann Arbor, Div. of Gerontology, University of Michigan, 1952.

McCann, C. W. *Senior Americans speak out.* Denver, Metropolitan Council of Community Service, 1967.

Orshansky, M. The shape of poverty in 1966. *Social Security Bulletin,* 1968, *31,* 3-32.

Peterson, D. A. *Financial adequacy, retirement, and public policy: A study of the perceptions of older Americans.* Unpublished doctoral disseration, 1969.

Shanas, E. *The health of older people: A social survey.* Cambridge, Mass: Harvard University Press, 1962.

US Congress. Senate Special Committee on Aging. *Economics of aging: Toward a full share in abundance.* Part I—Survey Hearings. Special Committee Print. Washington,: Government Printing Office, 1969.

US Dept. of Labor, Bureau of Labor Statistics.

Retired couple's budget for a moderat standard of living. Bull. No. 1570-4. Wasl ington,: Government Printing Office, 196(

US Dept. of Labor, Bureau of Labor Statistic: *Three budgets for a retired couple in urba areas of the United States,* 1967-68. Bul No. 1570-6. Washington,: Governmen Printing Office, 1970.

Youmans, E. G. *Aging patterns in a rural an an urban area of Kentucky.* Lexington: Un versity of Kentucky Agriculture Experimen Station, 1963.

Youmans, E. G. Disengagement among olde rural and urban men. In E. G. Youman (Ed.), *Older rural Americans.* Lexingtor University of Kentucky Press, 1967.

Chapter 12

THE GENERALITY OF HOUSING IMPACT ON THE WELL-BEING OF OLDER PEOPLE

M. POWELL LAWTON AND JACOB COHEN

IN THIS AGE OF burgeoning housing for the elderly, it is necessary to keep asking the question, "Does it help?" The present project began several years after Carp's (1966) study of a successful project lit by the fire of an extremely gifted team that included architect, housing authority director, administrative and social service personnel, and a research staff intimately associated with the housing. Was the success story of Victoria Plaza the one-occasion result of an unduplicatable team, or is there reason to feel that the basic idea lends itself to replication by other teams?

While there has been considerable study of various aspects of housing for the elderly, only one is known that attempted to assess impact by means of a before-and-after design. Carp's study utilized applicants to a single public housing project for the elderly, assessing them in a variety of areas presumed to be related to their well-being. Her study compared successful applicants who became tenants with unsuccessful applicants; both groups were assessed at the same time prior to occupancy of the building and again about a year after the tenants had moved into the new

Reprinted by permission from the *Journal of Gerontology*, 1974, *29*, 194-204.

building. Her study showed very few differences among successful and unsuccessful applicants at the time of the premove assessment, contrasted with a large number of favorable changes after a year in the rehoused compared to those who stayed in the community. Her tenants were more satisfied with their housing, with their amenities and services, were higher in morale, in perceived health, and more socially active than the unsuccessful group.

Other research approaches to the same issue have been reported by Bultena and Wood (1969), Lipman (1968), and Sherman (1973). These studies found an association between indices of well-being and moving to a new housing environment, but their comparisons with nonmoving groups were cross-sectional, rather than longitudinal, which limits one's capacity to speak about change.

The research reported here is essentially a test of the generality of the favorable impact reported by Carp. One purpose of the current study, not reported here, was to determine possible selective factors that might influence whether an older person wishes to live in planned housing for the elderly. Therefore, it utilized several comparison groups of community-resident elderly who had never applied to housing for the elderly, in contrast to the comparison between successful and unsuccessful applicants as made in Carp's study.

Method

Five new housing sites were assessed in terms of the change experienced by tenants during their first year of occupancy, compared to change in groups of community residents who did not move into new housing.

The *housing sites* consisted of two low-rent public housing sites and three lower-middle income federally-assisted projects (the former HUD Section 202 housing program), all high-rise buildings limited to occupancy by people sixty-two or over, or a few physically handicapped younger people.

Blueberry Acres is low-income housing in a poor but "respectable" location in Jersey City. It opened in July, 1966 and, while predominantly Irish Catholic, has a heterogeneous group of occupants including a small number of blacks. The two buildings of Blueberry Acres are within two blocks of each other and share a very committed manager and a senior-citizen club with a relatively active program.

Ebenezer Towers is a 202 project in a somewhat substandard black neighborhood, sponsored by what is perhaps the most progressive black home for the aged in the country. The 140-unit building opened in the summer of 1968, but had considerable difficulty renting despite the allocation of 10 percent of the units to a rent supplementation program and 25 percent to Philadelphia Housing Authority clients.

Golden Years opened in June, 1966, built under the 202 direct loan program. It is sponsored by two synagogues and a Jewish Community Center, but the population is not entirely Jewish. It is in a very desirable location one block from the boardwalk at Atlantic City, though it was at the time an urban renewal area surrounded by a mixture of condemned structures and already-demolished blocks. No services are offered but some assistance is given to an activity program.

President House is a public housing site opened in a low-income area of Reading, Pa. in July, 1966. Many occupants are "Pennsylvania Dutch" but others are of various ethnic strains. No services are offered, but a community senior citizens

club operates there once a week. The manager serves several buildings but maintains a close relationship with most tenants.

Sholom Aleichem House opened in June, 1968, sponsored by a fraternal organization. Its population is predominantly Jewish. It is a 202 project but includes a noonday dinner in its basic fee. It is in a highly desirable upper-middle class Philadelphia location, though tenancy is limited to lower-middle income people.

The tenants were sampled from lists made available by management about six weeks prior to each building's opening; the sampling interval was adjusted so as to yield somewhere in the neighborhood of 100 to 120 interviews. It proved to be quite impossible to maintain the sample in its original form. Inevitably, applicants would withdraw and be replaced by new prospective tenants. In the case of the three 202 sites, some applicants lived in other cities and could not be interviewed, while others could not be located or scheduled for appointments. Thus, some deviations from the 100 tenants sought occurred, as indicated by the sample size range from 89 to 143 (Table 12-I).

All tenants interviewed prior to occupancy were sought for the twelve-month follow-up interview. Table 12-I shows the follow-up status of the 574 housing subjects. Follow-up interviewing in the housing sites was eminently successful, with an overall reinterview rate of 83 percent.

The Comparison Groups: The community-residents were constituted in different ways. One of our housing sites was located in Jersey City, and it was possible to draw a probability sample of community-resident elderly from the census tracts that furnished the largest number of tenants to this particular project. A sample of 100 white community residents was sought, and, because of our interest in the housing

TABLE 12-I
SUBJECT GROUPS ASSESSED FOR IMPACT STUDY

	Total number of units	First Occasion Names Drawn	First Occasion Inter-viewed	Second Occasion Did not move in	Second Occasion Inter-viewed	Moved	Died	Refused	Other
A. Housing sites									
Blueberry Acres	156	139	119	3	97	4	2	3	10
Ebenezer Towers	140	105	100	1	78	9	6	2	4
Golden Years	208	182	143	11	113	2	1	4	12
President House	143	130	123	9	91	6	1	2	14
Sholom Aleichem House	310	110	89	0	64	9	3	10	3
Totals	957	666	574	24	443	30	13	21	43
B. Community residents									
Jersey City (white)		128	100	—	51	6	3	27	13
Jersey City (black)		112	101	—	69	12	4	8	8
Philadelphia A		84	66	—	28	9	4	8	17
Totals		324	267		148	18	11	43	59

problems of black elderly, a similar sample of aged black community residents was also sought. Residential segregational patterns made it impossible to find 100 black elderly in the originally specified census tracts. Therefore, new adjacent tracts were added to increase the total pool of black subjects.

The Philadelphia group was planned to match the tenants of a 202 project sponsored by a black organization (though not all tenants were black). Since many of these tenants had incomes that were above average for black elderly, locating a predominantly black comparison group through any kind of household sampling method would have been prohibitively expensive. Therefore, each interviewed applicant was told of our wish to compare movers with nonmovers, and asked to suggest three friends of his own sex and approximate age who did not want to move, for possible interview. Opportunities for biased selection are major in such a method, of course, though some other factors may have been equalized through the tendency of people to name friends of similar status, background, and interests.

At follow-up time, the project was operating under major budgetary restrictions. While contact was attempted with all originally interviewed subjects, call-backs and other time-extended means of scheduling appointments were severely curtailed.

Thus, whatever original comparability each comparison group had to its analogous rehoused group no longer existed due to the uncontrolled attrition of the community-resident groups. However, the data-analytic technique utilized, multiple regression analysis, was chosen partly because it is suited for the comparison of groups that are not equated on background variables by virtue of its ability to "partial out" such variables (Cohen, 1968).

Table 12-II shows the background characteristics of the interviewed subject groups. It is clear that race and religion were confounded with subject group. The Ebenezer and Philadelphia comparison groups were black, the Golden Years and Sholom Aleichem groups Jewish, President House tenants predominantly Protestant, and Blueberry Acres had a majority who were Catholic. One Jersey City comparison group and the Philadelphia comparison group were black, and the other Jersey City group completely white.

Procedure

The housing management furnished applicant lists. All subjects were first contacted by a letter which explained briefly the purpose of the study and suggested a time for the interview. They were interviewed in their homes prior to entering the new housing by project staff members, graduate students employed temporarily, or in the case of the Jersey City community dwellers, by trained interviewers from a private national research organization.

The interview schedule was designed to obtain a wide variety of information about the subjects' background characteristics, attitudes toward moving, expectations about the new housing, family relationships, social interaction, activity patterns, self-rated health, morale, and housing attitudes. The interviews lasted from sixty to ninety minutes. The twelve-month follow-up interview repeated much of the earlier interview and inquired, in addition, into many facets of life in the new housing.

The Measurement of Well-Being: The dependent-variable pool began as 334 items that were (a) particularly important to the well-being of older people, or (b) of intrinsic interest on their own account, and (c) relatively nonredundant with one another. In order to develop multi-item indices to be utilized as criteria, a factor-

TABLE 12-II

BACKGROUND CHARACTERISTICS OF INTERVIEWED SUBJECT GROUPS

Group	Age	Mean Monthly Income	Median Occ. Level	Educ.	% Who Are						
					Female	US Born	White	Married	Jewish	Prot.	Cath.
Blueberry Acres	71.4	$192	3.1	8.2	70	76	97	44	7	23	70
Ebenezer	72.0	130	1.7	8.5	78	95	1	12	1	91	8
Golden Years	73.4	198	4.2	9.8	80	33	100	35	96	0	4
President House	72.9	89	2.6	8.1	82	91	99	12	1	72	27
Sholom Aleichem	74.5	232	4.2	—	74	18	100	18	99	1	0
J.C. — White	71.5	250	3.0	8.4	57	67	100	45	9	25	66
J.C. — Black	72.2	164	1.7	6.8	61	100	0	42	0	93	7
Phila. A.	69.0	—	2.6	10.5	81	98	2	31	0	100	0

TABLE 12-III

INDICES OF WELL-BEING DERIVED FROM COMPONENT ANALYSIS

Name of Factor	Representative Item	No. of Items		Direction of High Score	Cronbach Alpha, FU
		Pre	Fu		
1. Functional Health	Still healthy enough to walk half a mile	13	24	Poor health	.83
2. Morale	I get mad more than I used to	12	16	Poor morale	.90
3. Change for the better	Now is the happiest time of my life	8	20	Negative change	.83
4. Loner status	Number of living children	9	6	Low level of contact	.67
5. Orientation to children	How often sees most frequently seen relative	5	10	Many activities	.68
6. Housing satisfaction	Where would you like to live? (Here + response)	8	8	Satisfied	.71
7. External involvement	Spends much time outdoors	4	8	High involvement	.39
8. Continued breadth of activity	Employed now	4	6	High activity	.47
9. Satisfied with status quo	It is better to live for today	3	5	Satisfied	.31
		66	101		

analytic procedure was used on the responses of the first available pool of subjects large enough to yield relatively stable factors. The responses of the first 313 subjects to be interviewed on two occasions were subjected to a principle-components analysis, utilizing forty-one items that appeared only in the preoccupancy interview, 140 that appeared in both interviews, and 124 that appeared only in the follow-up interview. Twenty-two factors with eigenvalues greater than 2.0 were rotated to the varimax criterion. From the resulting factors, nine were selected that (a) contained items whose content reflected well-being, (b) were relevant to both interview occasions and (c) applied both to rehoused and comparison groups. Items retained for the final factors included fifteen from the preoccupancy schedule, fifty-one from both schedules, and fifty from the postoccupancy schedule. Table 12-III lists the factors by name, plus other identifying information. Having defined the factors on the basis of the first 313 subjects, the items were then utilized in constructing scores for each of the 831 housing and community subjects on every factor. The highest-loading items were used to represent each factor, and any given item was used only in the factor where it had the highest loading. Factor scores were computed by weighting each standardized item score by its factor loading and summing all items in each factor. The factors thus defined were considered to represent our best effort at measuring the abstract quality indicated by the item content. This abstraction may be indexed by using any number of the items with high loadings on the factor; one simply increases the reliability of the index as more items are used. The twelve-month follow-up interview was longer and contained more relevant items than the preoccupancy

schedule. In order to take advantage of the greater number of items in the follow-up schedule, separate indices were constructed to measure the same factor on the two occasions, with more items always being used in the follow-up index. The factors were as follows:

(1) *Functional health* is composed of the largest number of items and clearly refers to the frequency and vigor with which the person performs various tasks. All six of the Rosow and Breslau (1966) health scale items load highly on this scale, as do several self-perceived health items.

(2) *Morale* consists of twelve items from the PGC Morale Scale (Lawton, 1972). The items in this factor include most PGC items that refer to neurotic and depressive symptoms.

(3) *Change for the better* consists of twenty-one items, eighteen of which contain a time comparison allowing people to say whether their current state of well-being is better or worse than at some earlier period of life. Five PGC Morale Scale items are also in the factor, most of them with the time comparison, and all expressing satisfaction or dissatisfaction with some facet of the tenant's daily life. These are clearly ideological, in contrast to the symptom items of the morale factor.

(4) *Loner status* in its negative direction describes people with few familial and peer relationships, and with few occasions on which they interact. It seems less than ideally useful because it mixes three separate aspects of the social networks of older people: presence of family, interaction level with family, and interaction level with peers.

(5) *Orientation to children* contains items related explicitly to children, contrasted with the broader social focus of loner status. The items tend to describe

actual behavior either implicitly or explicitly involving children, such as cooking for visitors, visiting the previous Sunday, going to church, and taking trips.

(6) *Housing satisfaction* has a diverse set of items with the very clear common thread of both a positive evaluation of the residential setting and the possession of the basic amenities necessary to a well-equipped household.

(7) *External involvement* is defined by a relatively few items whose common thread is the investment of time in activities that maintain a link to the world outside of themselves, whether that be watching TV, keeping up with the news, going outdoors, or becoming involved in organizational activities.

(8) *Continued breadth of activity* is defined by a small number of loosely related items indicating good functional health, especially emphasizing current employment, though reasons for its independence from the *functional health* factor are obscure.

(9) *Satisfaction with the status quo* contains five items totally different in content, all expressing the tendency to like whatever one has today.

Method of analysis: The longitudinal control-group design has the problems that are inherent in any attempt to measure change (Harris, 1964). In the present state of the art, one useful approach to measuring change is to treat the original criterion measurement as a covariate, or an independent variable in a multiple regression analysis, and remove its effect before examining group differences in the outcome, the follow-up criterion measure. In the present study, the effect of initial state on the dependent variable was removed by using the preoccupancy factor score as the covariate; the dependent variable was the same char-acteristic measured twelve months after occupancy, but indexed by a larger number of items. So treated, the dependent variable becomes a measure of regressed change, i.e. outcome from which original score has been partialled out.

The same principle in multiple regression allows one also to remove from the dependent variable the variation attributable to any other trait or characteristic of the subject. Many of our factor-score indices may well be related to various demographic status characteristics. Since the eight subject groups differ systematically in some of these background characteristics, some method is required to separate the effect of these differences from the critical tests of the experimental effect. The multiple regression model, used hierarchically, allows one to utilize controls in the form of independent variables introduced in a predetermined order designed to partial out the effects of these background differences prior to consideration of the experimental variable. Thus, background characteristics and initial level of the dependent variable are treated identically, in effect as covariates. The criterion score of each subject at the follow-up time is adjusted so as to statistically equate all subjects on these characteristics. The experimental variable (rehousing vs. continued community residence) is reserved as the final independent variable to be entered into the regression equation. When the analysis is so designed, any variance in the dependent variable accounted for by the experimental variable is in addition to and independent of any of the prior-entering variables.

Since the method of calculating factor scores creates indices that are no longer orthogonal, the nine criteria are by no means independent. While they are treated as separate criteria, there is undoubtedly

TABLE 12-IV
DESCRIPTIVE STATISTICS ON INDEPENDENT AND DEPENDENT VARIABLES

		Mean	*S.D.*	*N*
Functional health	–Pre	3.77	1.68	473
	–FU	—.71	5.72	591
Morale	–Pre	.01	4.13	591
	–FU	—.61	4.09	591
Change for better	–Pre	.05	1.55	591
	–FU	—.43	3.74	591
Loner status	–Pre	.73	1.06	591
	–FU	.97	.78	591
Orientation to children	–Pre	.03	1.03	591
	–FU	—.54	1.50	591
Housing satisfaction	–Pre	.08	1.30	591
	–FU	.23	1.19	591
External involvement	–Pre	—.70	.70	591
	–FU	—.58	.89	591
Activity breadth	–Pre	.07	.97	591
	–FU	—.25	1.00	591
Satisfaction — *status quo*	–Pre	.01	.61	591
	–FU	.01	.89	591
Age		72.8	6.32	568
Sex (1 = male, 2 = female)		1.75	.43	584
Marital status (1 = not married,				
2 = married)		1.29	.45	588
Race (1 = black, 2 = white)		1.70	.46	585
Income		180.1	130.36	471
Income II (0 = not reported, 1 = reported)		.77	.42	591
Jewish				184
Catholic				139
Protestant				235
Longstat (1 = rehoused, 2 = community)		1.25	.43	591

some redundancy in prediction among criteria.

Results

Table 12-IV shows the means, standard deviations, and numbers of subjects with information available on each of the independent and dependent variables.

The variable sets, in the order they were introduced into the regression equation, were as follows:

(1) *The prelongitudinal score* (Prelong) on the dependent variable. Factor scores were calculated as the sum of weighted (by the factor loading) standardized item scores. Not all subjects had scores on all items. Means were assigned in these instances, so that Table 12-IV shows no missing factor scores, except for the Prelong health index, where the Rosow and Breslau (1966) health index was not obtained for the Golden Years group.

(2) *Background demographic variables*
   a. Age
   b. Sex (1 = male, 2 = female)
   c. Marital status (1 = not married, 2 = married)
   d. Race (1 = black, 2 = white)
   e. Income, in dollars per month
   f. Income II, dummy-coded vari-

able indicating whether or not the subject gave information on income (Cohen, 1968). Income was the only variable where a significant number of subjects had missing data.

g. Religious background.

(3) The final critical independent variable, *rehoused vs. community-resident* ("Longstat"—1 = rehoused, 2 = community comparison).

The *dependent variables* (FU-Long) are the factor scores for the second occasion, approximately twelve to thirteen months following the occasion on which the Prelong information was gained.

Table 12-V shows the results of the multiple regression analysis in condensed form, for each of the nine dependent variables. All independent variables entered into each regression, but only the combined variance increment of the demographic variables as a set is presented, along with that associated with the critical variable Longstat. The variance increments ($\triangle R^2$) attributable to the Prelong, the set of demographic variables, and the Longstat variables, respectively, are shown for each dependent variable. This figure represents the proportion of variance in the dependent variable that is accounted for by the named variable set with the influence of all other prior-entering independent variables removed. In the case of the final variable, Longstat, the $\triangle R^2$ is the variance uniquely associated with rehousing status. The F values are the statistics associated with the variance increments, for the number of degrees of freedom listed in the last line of Table 12-V. Finally, the last two columns show the total amount of variance accounted for by all three variable sets, and its associated F value.

Table 12-V shows that after removing the variation attributable to the original (Prelong) score on the criterion and the background characteristics, after a year in the new housing, the rehoused were as follows:

(a) Significantly poorer in functional health than the community comparison subjects.

(b) Significantly higher in morale, perceived more change for the better, were more satisfied with their housing, were more involved in external activities, and more satisfied with the *status quo* than the community comparison subjects.

(c) Not significantly different from the community comparison subjects in loner status, orientation to children or continued breadth of activity.

Since physical health is typically so strongly related to all types of well-being, an analysis was also done utilizing score on the Rosow and Breslau health scale (1966) prior to occupancy as a covariate, in effect statistically equating subjects on health prior to testing the effect of rehousing on well-being. Table 12-VI shows the results of the relevant regression analyses, introducing, in order: (a) the Prelong criterion measure, (b) the demographic background variables, (c) the Rosow and Breslau health scale, and (d) Longstat, the rehoused vs. comparison group (experimental-effect) variable. Thus controlling for initial degree of health, the effect of rehousing on morale dropped below the level of statistical significance. The magnitude of the favorable effect of housing on all other factors increased after the control for health.

Discussion

With such a relatively large number of subjects, the size of the effect required to be statistically significant at the .05 level is quite small. In fact, both morale and housing satisfaction are significantly higher

TABLE 12-V

PERCENTAGE OF VARIANCE IN WELL-BEING ACCOUNTED FOR BY PREOCCUPANCY MEASURE, DEMOGRAPHIC VARIABLE SET, AND HOUSING STATUS

Dependent variable	Prelong[a]		Demographic		Longstat		Cumulated variance (3 sets)[a]	
	ΔR^2	F	ΔR^2	F	ΔR^2	F	R^2	F
Functional health	.233	116.75	.076	5.02**	.019	10.08**	.308	16.75
Morale	.168	89.97	.019	1.07	.008	4.25*	.192	10.34
Change for better	.085	41.13	.124	7.92**	.069	37.92**	.209	11.49
Loner status	.056	26.39	.103	6.66**	.022	.91	.160	9.15
Orientation to children	.178	96.25	.079	5.86**	.000	.49	.258	15.13
Housing satisfaction	.092	45.32	.029	1.77	.009	4.33*	.092	6.49
External involvement	.076	36.59	.044	2.71**	.014	7.09**	.135	6.83
Activity breadth	.205	114.72	.056	4.16**	.001	.76	.262	15.52
Satisfaction — *Status quo*	.026	11.80	.040	2.38*	.053	26.43**	.120	5.92
df	1,445		8,427		1,436		10,436	

[a]All F values in these columns significant at .01 level.   *p<.05   **p<.01.

TABLE 12-VI

PERCENTAGE OF VARIANCE IN WELL-BEING ACCOUNTED FOR BY PREOCCUPANCY MEASURE, DEMOGRAPHIC VARIABLES, HEALTH, AND HOUSING STATUS

Dependent variable	Prelong[a]		Demographic		Health		Longstat		Cumulated variance (4 sets)[a]	
	R^2	F	R^2	F	R^2	F	R^2	F	R^2	F
Morale	.140	71.16	.008	.56	.018	9.02**	.006	3.06	.171	8.85
Change for better	.076	36.00	.063	4.66**	.017	8.71**	.081	45.46**	.237	13.33
Loner status	.058	27.03	.015	1.14	.001	.24	.001	.50	.175	9.08
Orientation to children	.167	87.31	.078	6.34**	.003	1.93	.002	.94	.249	14.22
Housing satisfaction	.316	48.54	.037	2.62*	.001	.39	.012	6.07*	.150	7.53
External involvement	.066	30.86	.064	4.54**	.009	4.52*	.016	8.04**	.155	7.85
Activity breadth	.226	127.28	.027	2.14*	.014	8.14**	.004	3.30	.270	15.84
Satisfaction — *status quo*	.195	17.23	.035	2.15*	.000	.05	.067	33.59**	.141	7.00
df	1,437		7,430		1,429		1,428		10,428	

[a]All F values in these columns significant at .01 level.   *p<.05.   **p<.01.

among the rehoused with a partial r of only .10 and hence less than 1 percent variance increment is independently contributed by them. Even the strongest contribution to perceived change for the better accounted for only 7 percent of the variance.

The point to be made is that we need to be very humble in our expectations about the extent of the potential effect a change in housing may have. The person's given biological, psychological, and social characteristics endure, for the most part. The point of entry that the environment has into this ongoing system lies in its potential for changing the role functions and degree of satisfaction the individual takes in these role performances. As stated in greater detail elsewhere (Lawton, 1970; Lawton and Nahemow, 1973), older people, and particularly the older people with housing problems and other problems, are likely to be more vulnerable to environmental influences than people in general might. Therefore, we do have some hope that a favorable effect on the criterion measures might occur. The favorable effect has been confirmed, in the face of the large number of other and more powerful factors that might influence well-being.

Some implications of the findings are as follows:

(1) Positive advantage can be expected from rehousing the elderly especially when the judgment is made by the older person evaluating his current condition as it may have changed over the past year. This kind of evaluation is very likely to be positive partly because of the adjustive value to the respondent that is involved in simply *saying* that he is better off this year than last. That the rehoused say this more frequently than the comparisons is not difficult to accept, since they no doubt experience a need to make their evaluations consonant with the fact of having a new residence. There

is no doubt some tendency also to be afraid to respond other than in a positive way, a not uncommon feeling that one may be asked to move if anything negative is said against the authorities.

(2) Self-perceived change for the better is the most marked indicator of a positive housing effect, but not the only one. The items in the morale factor inquired about subjective feelings of well-being at two points in time, but did not offer the time span as a frame of reference for making the judgment. There was no relationship to rehousing on a zero-order level, but the successive controls for demographic status allowed the small partial correlation between morale and rehousing to emerge. The satisfaction with *status quo* factor is of similar meaning, as is housing dissatisfaction, each a different aspect of expressed life satisfaction, and all in the direction of increased satisfaction among the rehoused.

(3) Involvement in the activities of the external world was greater among the rehoused, though not in all of the ways this behavior could have been measured. That is, the external involvement factor scores were significantly higher, but other kinds of involvement as shown in loner status, activity breadth, or orientation to children did not reflect this change.

(4) The relative decline in functional health among the rehoused is substantial and in need of explanation, inasmuch as this finding runs counter to the general improvement in well-being found in other measures.

Several interpretations may be proposed. One might assert that in spite of the statistically-achieved equivalence of the Prelong functional health scores of the rehoused and comparison groups, those recruited by the new housing were physically more vulnerable. The critical test of this hypothesis would require measurement at a time period prior to our preoccupancy measure, so that differences in the slopes of the health vs. time curves of the rehoused and comparison groups could be tested, as in Figure 12-1. It has been suggested elsewhere (Lawton, 1969) that people tend to assess potential environmental situations in terms of whether they are likely to be consonant with their assets and liabilities.

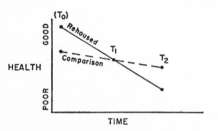

Figure 12-1. Hypothetical slopes of changes in rehoused and comparison groups.

It is entirely possible that housing applicants may have perceived a physical vulnerability in themselves that led them to apply to the more protected living situation found in the planned housing. However, at this point, this is purely a hypothesis for later testing.

It is equally possible that the new environment may have actually curtailed the tenants' functional capacity. Some items in the health factor that do decline significantly more in the rehoused than in the comparison subjects may be essential aspects of the new living situation: frequency of leaving the housing site and frequency of leaving the neighborhood. If such items reflected environmental barriers to mobility, the apparent decline would not be an indicator of personal decline. Also, an item like frequency of climbing steps would inherently decrease with a move into an elevator building. However, other items represent subjective estimates of the difficulty or ease with which physical energy is expended; the criterion thus seems to be a self-estimated functional health index.

The mechanism associated with a direct negative effect of rehousing is obscure. It is possible that following successful occupancy, the tenant may be better able to admit physical limitations than he was as an applicant, when such an admission might have jeopardized his acceptance. Conceivably the "protected environment" might discourage striving. Rosow (1967) has hypothesized that the more facilities that are provided within a housing site, the greater the tendency for withdrawal of tenants from the community. A reduction of energy expenditure would be implied here. If further research, including a study of the form illustrated in Figure 12-1, supported the idea of an erosion of functional health as the result of a move into new housing, it would seem to be particularly important to attempt to predict which people might be more vulnerable to this erosion. Is it the dependent, the psychiatrically disturbed, or the deprived? Particular vigilance would be required to develop counteractive measures to stimulate continued performance of instrumental tasks, geographic movement, and even prescribed exercise.

Regardless of the reason for the decline in health, if health declines, all previous research in aging should lead us to expect that there would be a concomitant decrease in other forms of well-being. Nothing is more regular than the correlation between health and morale, health and social behavior, or health and leisure-time activity (reviewed by Adams, 1971). Yet, in this case, in spite of the greater decline of health among the rehoused than among the controls, the net change in several other indices of well-being was in favor of the rehoused. If the decline in measured health is accepted as representing a true physical decline, one might speculate that the total impact of the new housing was to buffer the individual against a decline in health, so that his attitudes, affect, and even some forms of social involvement could remain at relatively favorable levels.

With the exception of the health variable, the findings of this study over five housing environments are very consistent with Carp's findings at Victoria Plaza. While it is difficult to compare the relative magnitude of the positive effect over two studies that differed in measuring instruments, in type of control group, and in statistical analysis, it nonetheless seems evident that the effect was less marked in the present research. Possible explanations are several. One may speculate that the large amount of national focus on the housing and the research at Victoria Plaza led to an enhanced willingness of tenants to reinterpret their life situations in a favorable light following their move. It is also possible that the major contrast of the new environment with their previous housing situation greatly amplified the tenants' normal positive response. Or, it may be that the currently reported environments are about average in quality and Victoria Plaza superior. Each of these possible reasons may contribute to the difference in magnitude of major effect.

Summary

The longitudinal control-group method was utilized to test the impact of new housing on the well-being of elderly tenants during their first year as tenants. Utilizing factor scores as criteria and controlling for original level on the criteria and for several background factors, positive housing impact was measured in indices of morale, perceived change for the better, housing satisfaction, external involvement, and satisfaction with the *status quo*, compared with change over one year in a group of older people remaining in their homes in the community. A relative decline in functional health was associated with the new housing, and no effect on indices measuring loner status, orientation to children, or activity breadth. Reasons for the decline in health are obscure, but the possibility must be faced that the new housing undermines the tenants' energy expenditure. The relative improvement (or lesser decline) in other criteria despite the decline in health, however, points to a buffering effect of the housing environments in keeping tenants' psychological state buoyed up. The size of the favorable effect is relatively small, however, and caution is advised in the extent to which even the best housing environment can be expected to solve lifelong or current problems of the tenants.

REFERENCES

Adams, D. L. Correlates of satisfaction among the elderly. *Gerontologist*, 1971, *11*, 64-68.

Bultena, G. L., and Wood, V. The American retirement community: Bane or blessing? *Journal of Gerontology*, 1969, *24*, 209-217.

Carp, F. M. *A future for the aged.* Univ. of Texas Press, Austin, 1966.

Cohen, J. Multiple regression as a general data-analytic system. *Psychological Bulletin*, 1968, *70*, 426-443.

Harris, C. W. (Ed.) *Problems in measuring change.* Univ. of Wisconsin Press, Madison, 1964.

Lawton, M. P. Supportive services in the context of the housing environment. *Gerontologist*, 1969, *9*, 15-19.

Lawton, M. P. Ecology and aging. In L. A. Pastalan, and D. H. Carson (Eds.), *The spatial behavior of older people.* Univ. of Michigan Institute of Gerontology, Ann Arbor, 1970.

Lawton, M. P. The dimensions of morale. In D. Kent, R. Kastenbaum, and S. Sherwood (Eds.), *Research, planning, and action for the elderly.* Behavioral Publications, New York, 1972.

Lawton, M. P., and Nahemow, L. Ecology & the aging process. In C. Eisdorfer and M. P. Lawton (Eds.), *Psychology of adult development and aging*. American Psychological Assn., Washington, 1973.

Lipman, A. Public housing and attitudinal adjustment in old age: A comparative study. *Journal of Geriatric Psychiatry*, 1968, 2, 88-101.

Rosow, I. *Social integration of the aged*. Free Press, New York, 1967.

Rosow, I., and Breslau, N. A. Guttman health scale for the aged. *Journal of Gerontology*, 1966, 21, 556-559.

Sherman, S. R. Housing environments for the well elderly: Scope and impact. New York State Dept. of Mental Health, Albany, 1973. (mimeo).

Chapter 13

THE AMERICAN RE-TIREMENT COMMUNI-TY: BANE OR BLESSING?

Gordon L. Bultena and Vivian Wood

Widely divergent views prevail as to the desirability of older persons segregating themselves in planned retirement communities. These places have been criticized as unnatural and stultifying environments as well as heralded as offering an exciting new concept in meeting the needs of the aged. Residents of retirement communities have been pictured as bored and disillusioned persons who lead shallow lives dominated by a hedonistic pursuit of happiness (Davis, 1966; Paulson, 1967; Peck, 1963; Trillin, 1964). It has been argued that many would return to their home communities were it not for their financial investments and the stigma of having earlier rejected retirement among friends and relatives. An opposing view is that retirement communities offer the aged a unique opportunity to remain physically and socially active and to avoid the isolation and loneliness that plague many of their peers in more conventional settings.

Little study has been made of the situation and attitudes of older persons residing in planned retirement communities compared to those retiring in places with younger families (recent studies of retirement communities include Hamovitch,

Reprinted by permission from the *Journal of Gerontology*, 1969, *24*, 209-217.

1966; Herbert, 1966; Peterson and Larson, 1965; Sherman, Mangum, Dodds, Walkley, and Wilner, 1968). Findings are reported here from a study of older persons who migrated after retirement from the Midwest to two types of communities in Arizona: one which encompasses all age groups (age-integrated or regular communities) and the other designed exclusively for the aged (age-segregated or planned retirement communities). Comparative data are also reported on persons who retired in their home towns in Wisconsin. Our purpose is to assess the role of planned retirement communities in American life, as revealed in the adaptation of their residents to the retirement role.

Background

Although the concept of special communities for the aged is an ancient one, it has been only in recent years that these places have appeared in the United States. Today, they evidence considerable growth, both in number and in size. In 1966 it was estimated that in the previous ten years the number of retirement communities in California had grown from none to thirty-five, in which were housed over 54,000 elderly persons (Barker, 1966). Sun City, Arizona, one of the first and more successful developments, has mushroomed in size since its founding in 1960 to over 12,000 aged residents by 1969.

The recent popularity of retirement-community living has posed a challenge to some long-standing beliefs as to what constitutes a desirable community setting for the aged. A pervasive view both in the public mind and among many professionals working with the aged is that older persons are happiest when they remain in their home towns after retirement (Kleemeier, 1963; Mumford, 1956; Vivrett, 1960). The segregation of older persons in special communities has been widely condemned as invidious and undemocratic and as an extension of undesirable trends in American society in which older persons increasingly have been removed from participation in instrumental activities and isolated within the social structure.

Of course, much of the criticism of retirement communities is not addressed to the concept of age-grading *per se,* but rather to the unscrupulous selling practices and poorly planned facilities which have been evident in the rapid expansion of this housing market (Barker, 1966; Cooley, 1965). Much criticism also is predicated on a simplified and often faulty perception of the situation of the aged in more conventional settings. Recent studies have revealed that the mere physical propinquity of older and younger persons is no assurance of meaningful intergenerational interaction and that the social interests of older persons may be best served in residential settings in which there is a high concentration of their age-peers (Rosow, 1967). However, little scientific attention has been paid to structural alternatives to the age-integrated environment. Studies of the factors associated with morale among the aged, for example, have dealt primarily with personal attributes (i.e. age, sex, income, occupation, health status) and largely have ignored the way in which the relationship of these variables to morale may be mediated by different social structures. Important exceptions are Blau (1961) and Neugarten (1967).

This study was designed (*a*) to investigate differences in the personal adjustment of older persons who have moved to age-integrated and to age-segregated communities in a retirement state, and (*b*) to examine some of the factors which may account for differential adjustment.

Sample and Procedures

The data on migrants are from interviews in 1967 and 1968 with 521 retired males residing in three age-integrated communities (Tucson, Tempe, Mesa) and in four planned retirement communities (Green Valley, Sun City, Dreamland Villa, Youngtown) in Arizona. The respondents have moved permanently to Arizona following their retirement in the Midwest.

The sample of migrants (N = 199) to age-integrated communities was drawn randomly from city directories listing all permanent residents in these places. The sample of those in planned retirement communities (N = 322) was drawn randomly from lists of residents. A screening interview was employed to determine eligibility for inclusion in the study of those whose names initially were drawn in the sampling process (i.e. they had to be migrants from a midwestern state).

The average length of residence of the respondents in the two types of communities was similar, 4.0 years in the regular communities and 4.1 years in the retirement communities. The median age of the respondents in the two types of communities was sixty-eight and seventy, respectively.

Some comparative data are presented from a sample of males (N = 284) who have retired in their home towns in Wisconsin. These respondents were selected through two procedures: (*a*) a random sample drawn from lists of all retired persons compiled as part of a larger study of the aged in two small communities (3,000 and 10,000 population), and (*b*) an area-probability sample coupled with a screening interview for obtaining retirees in a metropolitan community (170,000 population).

A modified form of the Life Satisfaction

Scale was used as one measure of morale in our study. The form we employed contained thirteen agree-disagree items designed to tap the respondent's assessment of his life-situation. The scores obtained by our respondents on this scale ranged from zero to twenty-six, with a median score of twenty. The scores were utilized in their raw form in the correlational analysis, but were combined in the contingency tables, following previously established standards, into three categories: low morale (0-12), medium morale (13-21), and high morale (22-26).

χ^2, correlation, and partial correlation were employed in the analysis of the data. Differences are reported as significant if at the .05 level.

Observations

Morale, as measured by the Life Satisfaction Scale, was significantly higher for respondents in the planned retirement communities than for those in the age-integrated communities (Table 13-I). Over twice as many of the retirement-community residents obtained a high score (57% and 27%), and a smaller proportion had a low score. The median scores for the two types of communities were twenty-two and eighteen, respectively.

That residents in the planned retirement communities were not disenchanted with their situation is further pointed up in their responses to several other questions which were posed in the study. When all of the migrants were queried with regard to their satisfaction with retirement living in Arizona, two-thirds, (68%) indicated that they were very satisfied. However, the proportion expressing this satisfaction was significantly higher for persons in retirement communities than for those in regular communities (75% and 57%, respectively). Similarly, a significantly higher proportion of those in the retirement communities noted that their wives were very satisfied with their retirement in Arizona (64% and 51%). A high level of satisfaction with retirement community living also is found by Hamovitch (1966), Herbert (1966), Peterson and Larson (1965), and Sherman *et al.* (1968).

Only 3 percent of those in the planned retirement communities expressed any misgivings over having retired in their present location rather than in their home towns in the Midwest. While reluctance to speak disparagingly of their present community or situation may reflect a certain amount of self-justification of their earlier decision, our analysis indicates that there is not the disaffection with retirement community living which often is attributed to this popu-

TABLE 13-I

PERCENTAGE DISTRIBUTION ON LIFE SATISFACTION SCORES OF AGED MIGRANTS IN RETIREMENT COMMUNITIES AND REGULAR COMMUNITIES IN ARIZONA

Life Satisfaction	Retirement Communities	Regular Communities
	(N = 322)	*(N = 199)*
Low morale (0 — 12)	3	10
Medium morale (13 — 21)	40	63
High morale (22 — 26)	57	27
Total	100	100

$\chi^2 = 51.44$; $df = 2$; $p < 0.001$.

lation. A small proportion (13%) did indicate that they had given some thought to moving in the near future, but the motivations underlying this decision typically reflected a desire to find a cooler climate or to lower living costs rather than a rejection of age-segregated living. Only five respondents in the retirement communities indicated a desire to return permanently to the Midwest.

The higher levels of morale found for those in the retirement communities than in the regular communities may be attributed to two factors: (*a*) the differential personal attributes of migrants locating in these two types of communities, and (*b*) structural features associated with retirement that migrants make to the retirement role and to their residential move.

Personal Attributes

SOCIOECONOMIC STATUS: Retired migrants to both regular and planned communities in Arizona, although drawn from all class levels, disproportionately came from the higher occupational and educational levels of the aged population. Migrants to planned retirement communities, in particular, represent an elite group, with 52 percent previously having been employed in professional or managerial positions and 43 percent having completed one or more years of college. Almost one half (47%) of the respondents in planned communities had an annual retirement income in excess of $5,000 compared to 36 percent of those in the regular communities; less than one-half as many had incomes of under $3,000 a year (Table 13-II).

Although migrants to the retirement communities were drawn from all socioeconomic levels, each community was found to be characterized by the predominance of a particular social class. Over four fifths of the home owners in Green Valley were

from professional or managerial backgrounds, as were two thirds of those interviewed in Sun City. Youngtown and Dreamland Villa, on the other hand, drew more heavily from the blue-collar rank (59% of those in Youngtown were retired from blue-collar occupations). Status selectivity also was found for persons moving into Leisure World at Laguna Hills, California (Peterson and Larson, 1965). The striking differences between retirement communities in the class origins of their residents suggest that important differences may be masked when these communities are treated collectively for analytical purposes. Further, there is considerable danger in generalizing about the role of retirement communities in American society without recognizing the differences in the characteristics of their residents which set them apart.

HEALTH: A larger proportion of migrants to retirement communities perceived their health as being very good or good than did those in the regular communities (75% and 59%). Conversely, only 2 percent of the retirement community residents but 16 percent in the regular communities defined their health as being poor or very poor (Table 13-II).

FAMILY TIES: Physical isolation from children, relatives, and friends often is viewed as a major factor bringing demoralization for those who retire outside their home communities. Our findings, however, suggest that migration seldom precipitates isolation and that the extent of separation from children is exaggerated.

Not having children in the home community or region may have been an important factor in the decision of some of the respondents to migrate. Only one fourth of the migrants with children had a child located in their home community at the time of the interview; 65 percent of the

TABLE 13-II

PERSONAL CHARACTERISTICS OF RESPONDENTS IN RETIREMENT COMMUNITIES
AND REGULAR COMMUNITIES IN ARIZONA

Personal Characteristic	Retirement Communities % (N=322)	Retirement Communities % (N=199)	Distribution for National Aged Population %
Preretirement occupation			
Professional or technical	20	19	8
Managerial or proprietory	32	20	15
Clerical or sales	13	14	14
Blue collar	28	41	54
Farmer	6	6	9
Not ascertained	1	0	—
Total	100	100	100
$\chi^2 = 12.53$; $df = 4$; $p<0.02$			
Educational attainment			
8 years or less	23	35	62
9 — 12	33	28	27
13 or more	43	36	11
Not ascertained	1	1	—
Total	100	100	100
$\chi^2 = 8.65$; $df = 2$; $p<0.02$			
Current income			
Under $3,000	12	26	
$3,000 — 4,999	30	27	
$5,000 — 7,999	28	19	
$8,000 and over	19	17	
Not ascertained	11	11	
Total	100	100	
$\chi^2 = 16.94$; $df = 3$; $p<0.001$			
Perceived health status			
Very good	33	25	
Good	42	34	
Fair	23	25	
Poor or very poor	2	16	
Total	100	100	
$\chi^2 = 36.93$; $df = 3$; $p<0.001$			

Note: National data on occupational status are for white males aged fifty-five to sixty-four employed in this occupation in 1960 (U. S. Bureau of the Census, 1960). Occupations were classified according to the U. S. Bureau of the Census (1963). Educational data are from Brotman (1967).

Wisconsin respondents, on the other hand, had one or more children in their home town. Nearly all (96%) of the Wisconsin retirees with children had at least one child living in the Midwest. This compares with 71 percent of the migrants to planned retirement communities and 56 percent of those in the regular communities. If the migrants with children had retired in their home communities, almost three-fourths would not have had children located nearby; one-half would have had no children living in their home state.

Migrants tended to have smaller families than the Wisconsin retirees. Also, a larger proportion were childless. In fact, one third of those entering retirement communities had no living children (compared to 21% of those in the regular communities and 18% in Wisconsin).

While persons retiring in their home communities in Wisconsin were more likely than migrants to have had at least one child located nearby, nearly one fifth (17 %) of those in retirement communities and one-half (52%) in regular communities reported at least one child presently living within twenty miles. In fact, over one half (54%) of the migrants had one or more of their children living closer now than before their move, and two-fifths (43%) reported having one-half or more of their children nearer now than if they had retired in their home towns. It is significant in this regard that the majority of the migrants' children who had left the Midwest were located in the Mountain or Pacific regions.

Retirees remaining in their home communities were more likely than migrants to maintain frequent contact with at least one child. However, it cannot be inferred that the Arizona migrants would have had a comparable level of interaction had they retired instead in their home towns for, as we have pointed out, they had smaller families and there was a greater likelihood of their children having settled elsewhere. Frequent contact with children was found to be more pronounced in the regular communities than in the retirement communities. One half of those in the regular communities, but only 16 percent in the retirement communities, reported at least weekly contact with a particular child (Over two thirds of the Wisconsin respondents had at least weekly contact with a particular child). The presence of a child in the retirement area appears to be a salient factor influencing the decision of some migrants to settle in regular communities rather than in an age-segregated setting.

Structural Effects

In addition to the fact that the community differences in morale may reflect the differential personal attributes of migrants locating in these two types of places, the effects of the differing social structure of these communities also should be considered. The higher morale of those in retirement communities may be a function not only of the fact that they are drawn, to a greater extent than migrants to regular communities, from those segments of the aged population which generally evidence high morale, but also that the features of retirement communities are such as to contribute positively to the adaptation by their residents to the retirement role. Two structural features of these communities, in particular, seem important to our findings: (a) a physical concentration of age-peers of similar social backgrounds which serves to expedite the formation of new friendship ties, and (b) the promulgation of a leisure orientation in these places which is more compatible with the life situation of residents than is an extension of the work ethic into the role definitions of the retiree.

FRIENDSHIP TIES: A study in Cleveland (Rosow, 1967) revealed that older persons in age-segregated environments had more friendship interaction than those in neighborhoods with younger families. Our results are consistent with this finding. A significantly smaller proportion of the migrants to retirement communities than of those in age-integrated communities reported: (*a*) a decline in close friends as a result of their move (34% and 58%, respectively), and (*b*) dissatisfaction with the number of friends that they had made in their new community (11% and 25%).

This is not to say that migrants to the regular communities were isolated socially, for nearly one-half reported as many close friends now as when they were living in their home communities, and three-fourths expressed satisfaction with their current level of friendship interaction. Also important is the fact that almost three-fourths (72%) had one or more children, relatives, or close friends from their home towns living within a short drive.

Advancing age has been found in previous research to bring a shrinkage in the friendship ties of the aged (Blau, 1961; Bultena, 1968). However, social disengagement with advancing age may not occur as early in the planned retirement communities as elsewhere. Our oldest respondents in the retirement communities reported having as many close friends as did those retirees who were younger. The older respondents generally had been situated longer in their present community, with the result that they had cultivated a wider range of associates than their more recently arrived, and younger, neighbors. Also these age-concentrated environments provided a sizable cohort of potential replacements for friends lost late in life through migration, ill-health, or death, thus staving off a constriction in life-space occasioned by factors other than one's own increased physical incapacities.

LEISURE ACTIVITY: Probably no aspect of retirement-community living has drawn greater public condemnation than the hedonistic perspective or fun-morality often attributed to residents of these places. The profusion of leisure-oriented groups in many retirement communities and the emphasis on recreational activity stand in sharp contrast to the normative prescriptions based on the work ethic which commonly hold in age-integrated settings.

Our analysis revealed that migrants to Arizona, particularly those in the planned retirement communities, held more liberal or permissive attitudes toward the behavior of their age-peers than did those of comparable status retiring in their home towns in Wisconsin (Bultena and Wood, 1967). Migrants were found to place greater importance than nonmigrants in their retirement decision on the desirability of having more leisure time and they took a more positive view generally of the retirement role.

The retirement communities, with their relatively permissive atmospheres, served to insulate their residents from a set of normative expectations commonly operative in regular communities in which instrumental or productive functions are emphasized. The retirement community residents, in effect, comprised a reference group which legitimized behavior which was compatible with their own orientations with regard to appropriate and desirable conduct in old age. As such, these communities likely mitigated some of the psychological conflicts that their residents might otherwise have experienced had they retired instead in their home towns.

This view is commensurate with the argument of Eisenstadt (1956) and Messer (1965) that the individual's adaptation to a new set of role behaviors may be eased by his participation in social systems in which many others are undergoing similar role transitions. The identity crisis precipitated at retirement in American society is particularly severe given the extension of norms governing middle-age into the retirement period, coupled with the structural impediments which preclude older persons from performing productive functions. A persistence of instrumental values among the aged, as often occurs in regular communities, has been found (Clark, 1967) to engender a hostile competitiveness with the young and to serve for some as a source of demoralization in old age.

That there is a widespread acceptance among retirement-community residents of a leisure-oriented role is suggested in the response to the question: "Do you personally think that retired persons should take part in some type of community or public-service activity, or do you think they deserve the right to relax and should feel free now to avoid activities of this type?" One fourth (28%) of the respondents felt that it was best if older persons remained active in some form of service-oriented or community activity. Most, however, felt that avoidance of these types of activities should not reflect adversely on the retiree and that older persons have earned the right to a life of leisure and should feel under no obligation to become involved in activities other than those of a purely social or recreational nature. An analysis of the respondents' participation in formal groups revealed that most had reduced their involvement in instrumentally-oriented groups after their move (i.e. business, political, charitable, or community-service groups), but had increased their participation in consummatory or leisure-oriented groups (social clubs, hobby groups, and sport groups).

Those in retirement communities over whelmingly rejected the idea that resident spend too much time on leisure activitie or that there is undue social pressure fo persons to become involved in the socia life of the community. However, many i these communities came from background characterized by relatively high levels o social participation and they undoubtedl were attracted to a retirement communit by a predilection to lead an active socia life in their retirement. Thus, any pressur to be active which they experienced ap pears to be compatible with their ow orientations with regard to the desirabilit of involvement in social activities.

Testing Structural Effects

In order to examine the influence o structural factors, correlations were com puted between type of community and lif satisfaction, controlling on several persona attributes which have been identified i previous research as associated with moral and which distinguish the populations i these two types of communities. If struc tural effects obtain, the relationship be tween community type and morale shoul persist when controlling on these factors.

The association between type of com munity and life satisfaction (.36) remained relatively stable when controlling, in turn on age, occupational status, income, educa tional attainment, and perceived healt status, and when controlling on all five o these factors simultaneously (Table 13-III) Controlling on perceived health status had the most marked effect on this relationshi (dropping it from .36 to .30), but the rela tionship of community type to life satisfac tion, nevertheless, remained statisticall significant.

While the analysis reported in Tabl 13-III does not permit a definitive state ment as to the contribution of structura

TABLE 13-III

ASSOCIATION BETWEEN COMMUNITY TYPE AND LIFE SATISFACTION, CONTROL-
LING ON AGE, OCCUPATIONAL STATUS, INCOME, EDUCATIONAL ATTAINMENT,
AND PERCEIVED HEALTH STATUS

Control	Association Between Community Type and Life Satisfaction
Zero-order correlation	.36
Control (partial correlation)	
Age	.34
Occupational status	.36
Educational attainment	.36
Income	.36
Perceived health status	.30
Simultaneous control	
on all 5 personal characteristics	.29

Note: The zero-order and partial correlations reported in this table are significantly different from zero at the .001 level.

factors to morale, the findings are consistent with the argument that retirement communities provide a social milieu that is more conducive than that in regular communities to the achievement by migrants of a happy retirement. It is impossible with these data to assess the relative morale levels of migrants prior to their entering these two types of communities. A longitudinal analysis providing such data is essential to isolate adequately structural from individual effects.

Discussion

Our analysis indicates a higher level of morale and satisfaction with retirement among older males from the Midwest who settle in planned retirement communities than for those selecting regular communities in Arizona. This finding may reflect both the differential social composition of these communities and the effect on morale of their structural features.

Just as an earlier analysis (Bultena and Wood, 1967) revealed substantial differences in the characteristics of aged migrants and persons who had retired in their home

communities, these data indicate that migrants to planned retirement communities and to regular communities in Arizona differ in several respects. A larger proportion of those in retirement communities come from the higher occupational and educational levels, have higher incomes, and fewer are in poor health. Similarly, they are more likely to be childless, and of those with families, they are less likely to have children living in the vicinity.

The greater homogeneity in age, socioeconomic status, and value orientations toward the retirement role in the planned retirement communities than in the regular communities can be seen as facilitating social interaction and the formation of new friendship ties. Most of the migrants would not have been able to maintain a high level of personal contact with their children had they retired in their home towns, and many were no more isolated physically from their children now than before their move. Finding new friends to replace those lost through death, illness, or as a result of the move to Arizona appears to be expedited in an environment in which neighbors evidence common characteristics and values.

Planned retirement communities not only provide an opportunity for older persons to continue an active social life but also serve as a supportive reference group for those committed to a leisure-oriented life style in retirement. Persons holding a strong leisure orientation find a positive endorsement of activities in these settings which in other places might be subject to strong criticism or condemnation.

An important consideration in our findings is the self-selection that operates in migration. Persons entering the retirement communities largely were those who could be expected to benefit most from the social and recreational opportunities available in these places. On the other hand, persons selecting regular communities might be unhappy in an age-segregated setting. About three fourths of our respondents in the regular communities in Arizona held negative attitudes toward retirement communities, with the most frequent criticism being the absence of younger persons in these places and the "abnormality" in living patterns which this was taken to imply. Those who take the position that they would "rather be dead than live in a retirement community" may become demoralized in these places, and in any case would be unlikely residents because of their values.

Research has indicated that older persons, just as those of other ages, have a diversity of social-interaction styles and that these require differential social structures to maintain morale (Rosow, 1965). Although only a small proportion of the national aged population is now living in retirement communities, we have found no evidence in our study that these places have a detrimental effect on morale, satisfaction with retirement, or level of social interaction; quite the contrary. Obviously, retirement communities are not a universal solution for older persons, but neither do we find them to be ghettos of ill-adjusted, frustrated, and alienated old people.

REFERENCES

Barker, M. B. *California retirement communities*. Special report No. 2, Center for Real Estate and Urban Economics, Institute of Urban & Regional Development. Berkeley: University of California, 1966.

Blau, Z. S. Structural constraints on friendship in old age. *American Sociological Review*, 1961, *26*, 429-439.

Brotman, H. *Educational attainment of the older population*, Useful facts No. 28. Washington: Administration on Aging, 1967.

Bultena, G. L. Age-grading in the social interaction of an elderly male population. *Journal of Gerontology*, 1968, *23*, 539-543.

Bultena, G. L. Rural-urban differences in the familial interaction of the aged. *Rural Sociology*, 1969, *34*, 5-15.

Bultena, G. L., and Wood, V. Tolerance of unconventional behavior among migrant and nonmigrant retirees. Paper presented at the 20th Annual Meeting of Gerontological Society, St. Petersburg, Fla., Nov. 8-11, 1967.

Clark, M. *Culture and aging*. Springfield, Ill.: Charles C Thomas, 1967.

Cooley, L. F. *The retirement trap*. Garden City, N.Y.: Doubleday, 1965.

Davis, C. Death in Sun City. *Esquire*, Oct., 1966, *133*, 135-137.

Eisenstadt, S. N. *From generation to generation*. Glencoe, Ill.: Free Press, 1956.

Hamovitch, M. Social and psychological factors in adjustment in a retirement village. In F. M. Carp (Ed.), *The retirement process*. PHS Publ. No. 1778. Washington: PHS, HEW, 1966.

Herbert, M. *The older adult: Life in a retirement community compared to life in a city*. Berkeley, Calif.: Bureau of Community Research, 1966.

Kleemeier, R. W. Attitudes toward special settings for the aged. In R. H. Williams, C. Tibbitts, and W. Donahue (Eds.), *Processes of aging.* Vol. II. New York: Atherton Press, 1963.

Messer, M. The third generation: An extension of Eisenstadt's age-homogeneity hypothesis. Paper presented at the meeting of Society for Social Science Research, Chicago, 1965.

Mumford, L. For older people—not segregation but integration. *Architectural Record,* 1956, *119,* 191-194.

Neugarten, B. L. Disengagement reconsidered in a cross-national context. Paper presented at the 20th Annual Meeting of Gerontological Society, St. Petersburg, Fla., Nov. 8-11, 1967.

Paulson, M. C. Are all the days balmy in retirement cities? *National Observer,* Oct. 2, 1967, 24.

Peck, J. H. *Let's rejoin the human race.* Englewood Cliffs, N.J.: Prentice-Hall, 1963.

Peterson, J. A., and Larson, A. Social-psychological factors in selecting retirement housing. In F. M. Carp and W. M. Burnett (Eds.), *Patterns of living and housing of middle-aged and older people.* PHS Publ. No. 1496. Washington: PHS, HEW, 1965.

Rosow, I. Housing and local ties of the aged. In F. M. Carp and W. M. Burnett (Eds.), *Patterns of living and housing of middle-aged and older people.* PHS Publ. No. 1496. Washington, PHS, HEW, 1965.

Rosow, I. *Social integration of the aged.* New York: Free Press, 1967.

Sherman, S. R., Mangum, W. P., Dodds, S., Walkley, R. P., and Wilner, D. M. Psychological effects of retirement housing. *Gerontologist,* 1968, *8,* No. 3, Pt. I, 170-175.

Trillin, C. Wake up and live. *New Yorker,* April 4, 1964, *40,* 120-177.

Vivrett, W. Housing and community settings for older people. In C. Tibbitts (Ed.), *Handbook of social gerontology.* Chicago: University of Chicago Press, 1960.

U.S. Bureau of the Census. *U.S. Census index of occupations and industries.* Washington: U.S. Government Printing Office, 1960.

U.S. Bureau of the Census. *U.S. Census of population: 1960. Detailed characteristics. U.S. summary.* Final report PD (I)—ID. Washington: U.S. Government Printing Office, 1963.

Chapter 14

COMPREHENSIVE HEALTH CARE FOR THE ELDERLY: AN ANALYSIS

The Continuum of Medical, Health, and Social Services for the Aged

STANLEY J. BRODY

COMPREHENSIVE HEALTH services is the slogan for the seventies. "True to our pluralistic nature, we have a veritable plethora of uncomprehensive, comprehensive, and sometimes incomprehensible plans" (Brody, 1970). Currently Congress is considering at least sixteen different programs all labeled comprehensive health services. Evaluating these proposals without any benefits criteria, particularly for the elderly, adds to the confusion (Wylie, 1970).

Criteria are measuring devices against which program evaluations are made. One widely circulated criterion is "efficient and effective services." Without an acceptable standard of performance couched in terms of health status, such a criterion is meaningless. Establishment of health program goals gives meaning to such measurements. They reflect the indices of need against which indices of benefits become relevant. Such goals can be deduced from the definition and understanding of health itself. Accordingly, a conceptual framework con-

Reprinted by permission from the *Gerontologist*, 1973, *13*, 412-418.

structed on the basis of understanding of the definition of health is a basic requirement for evaluating any program which asserts that it is a comprehensive health plan.

Goals of a Health System

The most widely accepted definition of health is that of the World Health Organization. "Health is a state of complete physical, mental, and social well-being and not merely the absence of disease or infirmity" (WHO, 1946). Dubos (1968), in attempting to limit this vague definition traces the word health to its Anglo-Saxon root which means "hale," "sound," "whole." Thus health describes the ability "to function well physically and mentally, and to express the full range of one's potentialities."

Historically, medicine has been concerned with the understanding and management of disease (Richmond, 1969). Preventive efforts have been primarily based on disease prevention rather than health maintenance and optimum functioning. The medical system has been concerned with quantity rather than the quality of life. If the new understandings of health are to be implemented, the traditional emphasis of medicine on disease and the institutions developed for its treatment must be augmented by new institutional forms and emphases. Movement from a focus on pathology to a focus on pathogenesis and the preservation of social and biological effectiveness requires a shift from the acute illness setting to a new operational base. The hospital, with its dramatic emphasis on acute episodic care, has consumed the major share of fiscal, manpower, and facility resources. Like the automobile gasoline engine, it has been refined to the point where it no longer is responsive to he ecological needs of the community.

The nature of the new institutional and structural arrangements for health delivery will be shaped by the totality of community programs.

The relationship of the individual to a comprehensive health system is that of an open subsystem to a complex of interlocking systems. This includes not only the general environment, but the many protective subsystems such as the family, and more broadly, the public-private organizations of income maintenance, housing, and health care delivery. The individual's index of health and his ability to rally from insults depend not only on his own capacities but also on the supports necessary and available to achieve optimum functioning. Accordingly, the effectiveness of comprehensive health programs must be measured in terms both of the elderly person's response to the insults to which he is exposed and of the extent to which the health system enables him, or proposes to enable him, "to rally," respond, or function. An acceptable index will be found in the considerable research which has gone into the development of a scale for evaluating the activities of daily living.

Health Problems of the Elderly

Morbidity statistics are useful to a health index based on functioning only to the extent they help describe disability.

What is significant is that while 81 percent of the over sixty-five suffer some chronic illness, 33 percent have no physical limitation on their activities; 7 percent have some limitations, but not on their major activity; 26 percent have limitations on major activity; and about 16 percent are unable to carry out their major activity. Thus, approximately one half of the elderly are somewhat disabled because of a chronic illness (National Center for Health Statistics, 1969).

Of particular importance is the specific level of mobility; 80 percent of the non-institutionalized elderly are bed-fast or house-bound. In addition, 6 percent have limited physical ability to move in the community. But overall, more than 30 percent report difficulty in walking stairs (Shanas, Townsend, Wedderburn, Friis, Milhoj, and Stehouwer, 1968). In an environment where those with limited income live in a world of steps (steps within residences, to board buses or streetcars, to descend into subways) the ability to negotiate stairs becomes critical to mobility. Thus, physical disability as a correlate of aging has been extensively documented.

Mental impairment also imposes limitations of function. Estimates of the incidence of mental impairment among the elderly vary from 10 to 25 percent (S. Brody, 1971). Rates of psychosis, symptoms experienced as physical illness and organic mental disorders, as with physical disabilities, rise with advancing age.

A system of comprehensive health care delivery should not only provide medical and health resources but should also include those support services that would enable the elderly who are physically disabled and/or mentally impaired to utilize those resources.

A recent senate committee report (Special Committee on Aging, 1970) points out the environmental problems of concentrations of the elderly poor isolated in neighborhoods which have experienced radical changes; locked in by what has been euphemistically described as substandard, low-cost housing; frequently among alien ethnic groups; subject to malnutrition; lacking appropriate transportation to the sources of medical care and other services; and often imprisoned in their own homes by an intense fear, based on fact, of being subject to robbery and attack (E. Brody, 1971a; Clark, 1971; Lawton, Kleban, and Singer, 1971).

Lack of information can also be characterized as an environmental hazard. Even when services are available, they are either complexly organized, physically dispersed, inadequately advertised, or encrusted with eligibility requirements all of which deter and discourage their utilization by the elderly and the families for whom they were hopefully designed (Brody and Brody, 1970; Brody, Finkle, and Hirsch, 1972; Leyhe and Procter, 1971).

By any of these measures of physical, mental, and environmental disability, older people in our society are as a group at high risk (Ivarson, 1971). The nature and number of their problems are beyond individual and family resources, thus requiring public coordination and support through services and programs. Shanas (1971) estimates that the target population of elderly needing services to maintain them at home is one in seven. It is suggested that is a conservative estimate. When considerations of mental impairment and environmental hazards are added to those of physical disability, the need for services is possibly one in three (29.9% of over sixty-five had a limitation on one or more activities of daily living) (Comm. on Chronic Illness, 1957).

Population Explosion of the Elderly

Of prime consequence is Brotman's (1971) report based on the 1970 census that the rate of increase of those seventy-five and over has escalated to three times as great as that of the sixty-five to seventy-four group.

The seventy-five and over group is substantially more vulnerable to all three classes of insults (i.e. mental, physical, and environmental). While 35 percent of those sixty-five to seventy-four with chronic illness were subject to significant impairment of function, 53 percent of those over seventy-five were similarly limited (National Center for Health Statistics, 1966). Riley and Foner's (1968) summary of research findings indicate that rates of all types of psychosis rise steadily by age. This reinforces the conclusion that given a functional approach to needs for comprehensive health services, more than one third of the elderly may require health support service (Goldberg, 1970).

Health-Social Services

While the aged have need for acute medical care, their major requirement is in the continuum of services for the chronically disabled that will enable them to function optimally. Any health system which continues to be limited to a disease orientation will not meet the increasing needs of the aging community. Medical service must take their place as a part, and only part, of the continuum of health care. Health-social services are at least equal and certainly not ancillary to any other service. The etiology of ancillary from the Greek meaning "slave-hand maiden" indicate why the term should be eliminated from the health lexicon particularly when referring to health-social services. This does not imply a denigration of medical care but rather an elevation of the health-social service care professions to equality, visibility and recognition.

Health-social services in the community closely conform to parallel functions in the inpatient acute hospital. The five components of health-social services, personal services, supportive medical services, personal care, maintenance, counseling and linkages are common to both in-patient and community care. Between the extremes of the hospital and independent living are a variety of settings where some of these services may be delivered on a semi-institutional basis:

1. *Personal services* are keyed to personal hygiene including grooming, dressing, and bathing. Hospital personnel performing these services are licensed practical nurses, nurses' aides or orderlies. Home-health aides perform these services in the home.

2. *Supportive or extended medical services* are the role of the registered nurse, physicians' assistant and physical, recreational, or occupational therapist in or out of the hospital (Cosin, 1967). In addition to carrying out physicians' orders, observation and feedback to monitoring physician is a key function.

3. *Maintenance services* including housekeeping, environmental hygiene, and food preparation are also closely parallel. While a number of housekeeping and dietary hospital personnel are engaged in these tasks, they are usually the work of the homemaker in the community.

4. The *counseling* function may be performed in both settings by a variety of staff, but training and concentration places these services most appropriately in the social work orbit. It involves listening skillfully, extending help, mobilizing existing resources, and enabling the utilization of these resources.

5. Increasingly *linkages* are being recognized as a vital set of services without which available health care is not utilized. Linkages are any services that help connect the elderly to the needed services. Outreach, information, referral, and education are bound together by communication and transportation in assuring utilization and executiveness of health services. In this respect Titmuss (1959; 1968) points out that removing payment barriers to access to health care was not enough: under the National Health Service in Britain, the higher income groups made better use of services than lower income groups who need them more. For a like Swedish view see Ivanson (1971).

These five categories of health-social services are vital to the continuum of care for the aged. For a similar list see Titmus, 1968. (Report of the Comm. on Local Authority and Allied Personal Soc. Serv., 1969). Any measure of current or proposed programs of comprehensive care must evaluate the extent to which the benefit structure enables the elderly to be informed about, gain access to, and utilize a full range of health-social services.

Medicare

With these criteria in mind, to what degree do Medicare and the proposed health programs before Congress quality as comprehensive health care programs for the elderly?

Medicare provides for home health service benefits both under Part A, Hospital Insurance (HI), and Part B, Supplementary Medical Insurance (SMI). The act limits the patient to 100 incidents of service under either part, with a co-pay provision under Part B.

Three major limitations are imposed by legislation and regulation. The home health agency must be primarily engaged in providing skilled nursing care; services must be provided on a part-time intermittent basis; and it must be demonstrated that "personal care" is needed and that the patient is severely limited in function (Meyers, 1970).

The average benefit claim reimbursed for all home health service in 1969 was $77.00 against an in-patient day claim cost of $667.00. Of the 20 million subscribers, less than 3 percent were reimbursed for home health care (Soc. Sec. Bull., 1969). An undifferentiated number of claims was .032 percent. The utilization rates clearly demonstrate the underutilization of the home health service program under Medicare.

Catch-22 Syndrome of Medicare

The administration of the program appears to have been governed by a reluctance to fund those services related to patient maintenance because they seemed too closely related to funding a housekeeper and inappropriate to a health program (Trager, 1971). Similar services rendered in an acute setting or an ECF are freely reimbursed. Paradoxically many patients in hospitals and ECF's are able to provide their own personal care. The setting rather than the service controls the reimbursement pattern. The disease orientation of the program virtually forces patients into institutional facilities as the only alternative to hazardous living in the community. The elderly disabled person, like Catch-22's Yosarian, is put into the bind that unless he is sick enough to require institutional care he cannot receive the identical services in his own home.

The agencies too are trapped in the Catch-22 syndrome.

> It is all too risky, to find that charges are disallowed if the major portion of the time is not related to bathing, shampooing, and personal hygiene. A clean body in a dirty house may not be good health care, but that is what they pay for. If you have standards, it is just as well not to provide service at all (Trager, 1971).

Legislative Proposals and the Elderly

The significance of the Medicare experience with health-social services is not only in its failure to assure a continuum of health-social services but in its effect on new comprehensive care proposals.

The Javits proposal extends Medicare to the entire population, reaffirming the entire Title 18 experience. Only to the extent that it proposes authorizing contracts with "comprehensive health service systems," specifying the linkage services of transportation and health education, does it advance the delivery of health-social services. For the addition of benefits above those authorized by Title 18, approval of the Secretary of HEW is required, again reinforcing the Medicare experience (S. 836, 1971).

The Nixon proposal simply repeats the benefit structure of the Medicare act. The provisions which encourage Health Maintenance Organizations, likewise limit "other health services (to) . . . the same as when used in Title XVIII (S. 1623, 1971)."

The Health Insurance Association of America's, representing the commercial insurance companies, proposal is embodied in the Burlesan Bill. Again, home health services are identified as in Section 1861 of the Medicare act (H.R. 4349, 1971).

Similarly Senator Long's proposal for catastrophic health insurance restrict "home health services (as defined in 186 (m))," that is the current Medicare provision (S. 1376, 1971). The earlier catastrophic bill introduced by Senator Boggs defined insurable medical costs as those deductible under Section 213 of the Internal Revenue Code (S. 191, 1971). The Code includes "Transportation primarily for . . . medical care" as a deductible (Int. Rev. Code, 1968).

Even more extreme is the American Medical Association's proposal which equates health coverage with medical and inpatient care. The proposal takes the same position for insurance against catastrophic illness (S. 987, 1971).

At the other end of a very short spectrum is the Kennedy-Griffith Bill. Included in covered benefits are "such nonemergency transportation services as the Board finds essential to overcome special difficulty of access to covered services." Other supporting services specifically included are physical therapy, nutrition, social work, or health education and those others performed b agencies approved by the proposed administrative Health Security Board. On the other hand, home health agencies may be qualified only if they are primarily engaged in furnishing, on an intermittent basis, skilled nursing and other therapeutic services, language which again takes its words and tone from Title XVIII (S. 3, 1971).

Perhaps the most promising of proposals as they effect the extension of health-social services is that of Ameriplan by the American Hospital Association which has not as yet been formally legislatively introduced. A Health Care Corporation is proposed which would assure for each of its registrants:

> continuity of care . . . providing . . . home-health care, counseling for the individual and his family with resepct to his health and health-related problems.

Conclusions

Money is not the issue. This country spends many times what comparable western societies expend for health. The issue is the restructuring of our health delivery system. It is suggested that the first step is establishing the goals of our health system. The health field is projecting, through comprehensive health legislative proposals, a continuation of its concentration on the quantity of life to the exclusion of the quality of life. The goal of efficient and effective services is being pursued through these proposals without confronting the ultimate purpose.

If the current disease-oriented approach to health is continued as the single approach, then the needs of the elderly will be unmet. On the other hand, if a functional as well as a disease orientation is to be the basis of a comprehensive health care program, then legislative proposals must reflect a balanced health system which integrates augmented health social services with reorganized medical institutions.

REFERENCES

Brody, E. M. High risk groups among the elderly and their communities. *Proceedings*. Madison: Univ. of Wisconsin, 1971.

Brody, E. M., and Brody, S. J. A ninety-minute inquiry: The expressed needs of the elderly. *Gerontologist*, 1970, *10*, 99-106.

Brody, S. J. Maximum participation of the poor. *Social Work*, 1970, *15*, 68-74.

Brody, S. J. Prepayment of medical services for the aged: An analysis. *Gerontologist*, 1971, *11*, 152-156.

Brody, S. J., Finkle, H., and Hirsch, C. Benefit alert. *Social Work*, 1972, *17*, 14-22.

Brotman, H. Facts and figures on older Americans. SRS-Administration on Aging Publication 182. Washington: HEW, 1971.

Clark, M. Patterns of aging among the elderly poor of the inner city. *Gerontologist*, 1971, *11*, 58-66.

Commission on Chronic Illness. *Chronic illness in a large city, the Baltimore Study, Chronic Illness in the U.S.* Cambridge: Harvard Press, 1957.

Cosin, L. Z. Rehabilitation of the elderly. Paper presented at the Third Dinner Meeting of the Hunterian Society. London, 1967.

Dubos, R. *Man, medicine and environment.* New York: Frederick A. Praeger, 1968.

Goldberg, E. M. Helping the aged. In *National Institute for Social Work Training Services.* No. 19. London: Allen & Unwin, 1970.

H. R. 4349, 92nd Congress, 1st Session, *National Health Care Act of 1971.* Washington: USGPO, 1971, Title V, Sec. 501. (a)

Internal Revenue Code. Chicago: Commerce Clearing House, 1968.

Ivarson, K. Social issues in the field of health. (Report to the 6th European Symposium of the International Conference on Social Welfare, Commission 8) Stockholm: Social Welfare Planning Dept. National Board of Health & Welfare, 1971, *1*, 23.

Lawton, M. P., Kleban, M. H., and Singer, M. The aged Jewish person and the slum environment. *Journal of Gerontology*, 1971, *26*, 231-239.

Leyhe, D. L., and Procter, R. M. Medical patient satisfaction under a pre-paid group practice. In Sch. of Public Health, Univ. of California, Los Angeles, Medi-Cal Project Report No. 3, 1971.

Meyers, R. M. *Medicare. Bryn Mawr:* McCahan Foundation, 1970.

National Center for Health Statistics. *Age patterns in medical care, illness and disability, U.S. July, 1963-June, 1965.* (Series 10) Washington: HEW, 1966.

National Center for Health Statistics. *Chronic conditions causing activity limitations, U.S., July, 1963-June, 1965.* (Series 10) Washington: HEW, 1969, No. 51.

Report of the Committee on Local Authority and Allied Personal Social Services, July, 1968. London: Her Majesty's Printing Office, 1969.

Richmond, J. B. *Currents in American medicine: A developmental view of medical care and education.* Cambridge: Harvard Univ. Press, 1969.

Riley, M. W., and Foner, A. *Aging and society,* Vol. 1. New York: Russell Sage Foundation, 1968.

S. 3, 92nd Congress, 1st Session, *Health Security Act.* Washington: USGPO, 1971, Title 1, Part A, Sec. 27 (a), 5, (b), Sec. 46 (a).

S. *191,* 92nd Congress, 1st Session. *National Catastropic Illness Prevention Act of 1971.* Washington: USGPO, 1971, adding to the Social Security Act, Title XX, Part A, Sec. 2003, (1), (2).

S. *836,* 92nd Congress, 1st Session, *National Health Insurance and Health Services Improvement Act of 1971.* Washington: USGPO, 1971, Title I, Part A, Sections 102 & 103; Part G, adding to Title 18 of the Social Security Act, Part D, Sec. 1883 (b) (2) (5), (d).

S. *987,* 92nd Congress, 1st Session, *Health Care Insurance Act of 1971.* Washington: USGPO, 1971, Sec. 3, adding to the Social Security Act, Title XX, Sec. 2009 (a), (b) Sec. 2010.

S. *1376,* 92nd Congress, 1st Session, *Catastrophic Illness Insurance Act.* Washington: USGPO, 1971, adding to the Social Security Act, Title XX, Sec. 2203, (1) (C).

S. *1623,* 92nd Congress, 1st Session, *National Health Insurance Partnership Act of 1971.* Washington: USGPO, 1971, Title I amending Title VI of the Social Security Act, Sec. 603 (a) (6); Sec. 604 (b) 2; Sec. 608, (6).

Shanas, E. Measuring the home health needs of the aged in five countries. *Journal of Gerontology,* 1971, *26,* 37-40.

Shanas, E., Townsend, P., Wedderburn, D., Friis, H., Milhoj, P., and Stehouwer, J. *Old people in three industrial societies.* New York: Atherton Press, 1968.

Social Security Bulletin, Annual Statistical Supplement, 1969. Washington: USGPO SSA, HEW, 1970, Tables 113 and 114.

Special Committee on Aging, United State Senate. *Older Americans and transportation: A crisis in mobility.* Washington: USGPO 1970, *Report 91-1520.*

Titmuss, R. M. *Commitment to welfare.* New York: Pantheon Books, 1968.

Titmus, R. M. *Essays on the welfare state.* New Haven: Yale Univ. Press, 1959.

Trager, B. Home health services and health insurance. *Medical Care,* Jan.-Feb., 1971, 89 98.

World Health Organization. *Constitution o WHO,* Preamble. Geneva, 1946.

Wylie, C. M. The definition and measuremen of health and disease. *Public Health Report,* 1970, *85,* 100.

Chapter 15

MOBILE MEDICAL CARE TO THE ELDERLY: AN EVALUATION

BILL D. BELL

T HE HEALTH CARE NEEDS of older Americans has been a topic of interest to social gerontologists since well before the advent of Medicare. By and large, the work of individuals, such as Confrey and Caldstein (1960), Lowenthal (1964), Rothenberg (1964), Gray (1965), Busse (1965), Shanas (1965), and Travis (1966), has been sufficient to sketch the extent of the physical and mental difficulties facing the elderly. For the most part, these writers report frequent instances of chronic and debilitating conditions among older persons regardless of sexual or racial characteristics. On the other hand, however, few writers or public agencies venture beyond the realm of enumerating or describing those health care services available to older persons (Reynolds and Barsam, 1967; Shanas, 1971; Van Zonneveld, 1962; HEW, 1971). In general, few medical delivery systems are presently available for older individuals in the population.

The purpose of the present paper is two-fold. First of all, it is the intention of the writer to present a new and potentially unique innovation in health care delivery to the aged. The task in this regard will consist in a detailed discussion of this new

Reprinted by permission from the *Gerontologist*, 1975, *15*, 100-103.

concept along with the theoretical and practical justification for such a system. Secondly, it will prove most helpful to potential employers of this method to carefully evaluate this program in terms of its effectiveness and cost-efficiency.

The Geographical Setting

The setting for the present system of health care delivery is the State of Arkansas. Recent estimates (HEW, 1973) place Arkansas second in the nation with respect to the proportion of persons in the population over sixty-five years of age (12.7%). Of this population of older persons, 45.3 percent currently fall below the most recently established poverty levels. In addition, given the rural nature of the state, 50 percent of Arkansas' 2 million inhabitants live in predominantly rural areas, the majority of these individuals are found in the rural areas of the northwestern, northcentral, and southeastern portions of the state. Racially, the aged population in the two northern areas is generally white; in the southeastern region, blacks tend to predominate (IREC, 1973).

Although the aged tend to be distributed throughout the state and chiefly in the rural areas, medical facilities, on the other hand, are centralized. Over 45 percent of the state's physicians, for example, are located within the two urban counties of Pulaski and Sebastian (IREC, 1973). In addition, within the seventy-five counties comprising the state, fifty-eight have no internist, sixty-two have no pediatrician or obstetrician, and forty-five have no surgeon (SRC, 1974). Further, while 85 percent of the aged population have one or more chronic conditions to contend with (AHSC, 1974), the state has developed no county-based system of health clinics.

The questions to be confronted, then,

145

involve the problems of suitable medical facilities, adequate financial resources, and transportation availability. For the most part, surveys of the Arkansas scene have revealed finances to represent the greatest barrier to health care (IREC, 1973). On the other hand, transportation has ranked a close second. By and large, older rural residents must travel considerable distances to obtain medical services easily available in urban areas. With these facts in mind, there appears a definite need for an innovative approach to health care delivery.

The MERCI Project

The MERCI (Multiphasic Examinations to Reduce Chronic Illnesses) project developed from an experimental program entitled Community Activities for Senior Arkansans (CASA), began in 1968. One phase of CASA's work was a single mobile medical clinic staffed by a physician, a registered nurse, two licensed practical nurses, and a driver/maintenance man. This mobile clinic functioned to screen elderly persons for a number of chronic conditions. In its two-year existence (1968-69), the CASA clinic examined nearly 10,000 persons sixty years of age and older. For the purpose of gathering comparative data on health conditions in the state, individuals in both urban and rural settings were screened.

The present MERCI project was begun under the auspices of the Arkansas Office on Aging with a federal grant of approximately $125,000. The Arkansas Health Systems Foundation was made the grantee agency in July of 1973. Within a period of two months, the CASA mobile unit was rebuilt, the necessary staff hired (e.g. a director, a project coordinator, a secretary, a registered nurse, a licensed practical nurse, a medical technician, and a driver/maintenance man), and the project was under-

way. The MERCI program, consistent with the medical conditions described above, differs chiefly from the CASA project in directing primary attention to the rural aged.

In general, this mobile unit travels extensively to those rural areas of the state which are at least twenty miles from the nearest physician. The unit is designed especially to screen those persons over sixty years of age for specific chronic illnesses. The services in this instance are free and there is no income for the unit other than state and federal funding.

The Screening and Referral Process

After a brief registration process and the taking of a urine sample, the patient enters the medical unit. A short medical history is taken and visual acuity and blood pressure are checked. At the second station in this converted sixty-six-passenger school bus, the clinical laboratory work is done. Here, the urine sample is tested, and blood is collected for analysis. Finally, the patient's temperature is taken and his vital capacity determined prior to his leaving station two. At the third station, the registered nurse requests the patient to place himself on an examining table and an electrocardiogram tracing is made. While the patient is relaxing, the nurse utilizes the opportunity to double check the information that has already been gathered. The entire process of examination takes approximately fifteen minutes. On the average day, the unit examines between thirty and forty-five patients.

At the end of a week's work in the field unit personnel return to the main office in Little Rock. The physician and registered nurse on the team go over each patient file to determine whether that person should be referred to a local physician. Efforts are made to avoid needless referral s such are regarded as jeopardizing the finances of the patient as well as overburdening the schedules of local physicians. Upon the termination of the initial field contact, the patient is told that if he does not hear from the project within a specified period of time (generally two weeks), all tests performed were negative. Where there is doubt regarding specific tests, a letter is sent advising the person to consult medical help as soon as possible. In addition to the letter advising further medical consultation, a copy of all medical data gathered by the unit is forwarded to the physician of the patient's choice.

Project Utilization—The First Six Months

Within the first six months of operation, the MERCI unit processed and screened 2,738 persons. Of this number, 95.3 percent were sixty years of age and older. The men comprised 42.7 percent of those examined; 57.3 percent were women. The mean age of these persons was 69.5 years. White patients comprised 66.8 percent; 33.2 percent were black. By and large, the majority of project utilizers had total family incomes of less than $3,000 per year (76.4%). The backgrounds of these persons were rural in nature and reflected little in the way of geographic mobility.

For the most part, MERCI data indicate significant incidences of high blood pressure (31.0%), heart trouble (21.9%), and eye problems (17.3%). Secondarily related problems include diabetes (7.4%), arthritis, bursitis, etc. (6.6%), and a variety of "nervous conditions" (3.7%). These findings are not unlike those observed in previous health inventories (MLIC, 1968; White and Gordon, 1969; USPHS, 1960).

Of the persons seen, 98.1 percent were presently utilizing Medicare. Nevertheless, the mean length of time since the last visit to a physician was 11.4 months. Whites tended to see their physicians more often than did blacks. Blacks, however, exhibited more serious medical conditions than found among whites. By and large, a much higher proportion of blacks were subsequently selected in the referral process for such conditions as high blood pressure (25.3%) and diabetes (8.7%). In general, those persons who consulted their physicians regularly were less likely to need subsequent referral.

Project Effectiveness—The Evaluation Phase

The effectiveness of the MERCI project can be examined on a number of levels. First and foremost are those questions relating to the concerns which first initiated the project. Specifically, has the project reached the kind of older person envisioned in the planning phases of the program?

An examination of the first six months of project activitiy indicates that the mobile unit has processed and screened a significant number of older persons (2,738). For the most part, these persons have been over sixty years of age (95.3%) and subsisting on incomes well below the $3,000 level (76.4%). As initially hypothesized, three major factors have been disclosed to influence the health picture of rural Arkansans, lack of transportation, medical facilities, and personal finances. On the other hand, the project has met with considerably more success among older whites (66.8%) than among blacks (33.2%). These findings are noteworthy in light of the data which indicate blacks to have significantly more serious medical problems. This picture is made even clearer when it is observed that even in predominately black counties, the majority of project utilizers are white.

The results of follow-up interviews with these older persons suggest part of the inequities in utilization to rest in the mode of media dispersal relative to the project as well as certain normative features inherent to rural Arkansas. In the first instance, much of the information dispersal is under the control of a retired business executive. It is the task of this individual to travel in advance of the unit and discuss the unit's function with local newspapermen, members of the medical community, radio announcers, and civic leaders. It is this person who selects the proper placement of the unit and displays posters and signs in key points throughout the community. From relevant data, however, it is clear that certain modes of media dispersal are more appropriate than others. In addition, an approach with respect to one community has been found ineffective relative to another. In the case of whites, the most effective source of information about the MERCI unit and its function is gleaned from newspapers, close friends, posters, and the radio, in that order. For blacks, on the other hand, the most effective forms of media dispersal have been the radio, close friends, school notes sent home with small children, and the newspaper, in that order. For the most part, then, the failure of alternating media modes is partially responsible for the differential participation of blacks and whites.

In addition to the mode of media dispersal, there are certain normative aspects of rural Arkansas to be considered. Specifically, those interviewed indicated what can best be described as a concern for "medical racism," a legacy of the past. This "atmosphere" manifests itself in terms of a white medical establishment; secondly, in the provision of limited services to racial and minority groups in general; and, finally, in a reluctance to treat a racially-mixed clientele. Evidence from MERCI records suggests this perspective more typical in the

southeastern delta area; a place where blacks have traditionally located. Although most persons interviewed suggest the image of medical services to be changing toward a more positive perspective, the white medical staff of the MERCI unit, its broad base of middle class support, and the past history of medical racism in the state, all operate to reduce the overall effectiveness of the unit. By and large, an integrated unit (from the standpoint of staff) along with broader community support (both socially and racially) are seen as necessary components in a viable health program of this nature.

Perhaps the weakest aspect of the MERCI program is the referral process. As indicated previously, the staff physician and registered nurse determine together those cases requiring further medical attention. Following this determination, a letter is sent to the patient advising him to consult his local physician and necessary data from MERCI records is forwarded to that physician. Only one attempt, however, is made to gauge the effectiveness of the referral process. Specifically, individuals are sent a letter containing a postage-paid card upon which the person simply checks whether or not he or she has taken the unit's advice and actually seen a physician. No effort is made, on the other hand, to contact any of the physicians in question. Consequently, there is no means presently available to corroborate the indications of consultation received at the MERCI office. It seems essential that a random sampling be made of those physicians potentially involved in subsequent referrals to determine the effectiveness of this segment of project work.

Related to both the screening process and the matter of referral effectiveness is the ultimate question of cost. Early estimates on behalf of MERCI personnel suggested the possibility of screening 7,500 per sons in a twelve-month period. Such a number would bring the overall per person cost of the project to $16.00. Although present figures indicate this goal a possibility, rising material and manpower expenses suggest the cost will be somewhat higher, perhaps $18 to $19. In addition, this figure can be expected to rise further should the above-mentioned revisions be incorporated within the program.

Finally, evidence from interview data suggests the acronym "MERCI" may be a negative factor relative to project utilization. By and large, this acronym connotes a patronizing attitude toward the clientele in question. In addition, the suggestion of dependence is implicit in the term. It would seem more appropriate to rename the project in line with the aged's understanding of their needs in an effort to assure the widest possible participation in the project.

The Future of Mobile Medical Delivery

From the data gathered thus far, it is evident that mobile medical delivery works in practice as well as in theory. A significant segment of the aged in rural Arkansas has been advised of the availability of free medical evaluations and have greeted this innovation favorably. The cost of this project has remained relatively low and early indications suggest these costs will stabilize at somewhat less than $20 per person. This is less than cost estimates for a system of country-based medical clinics. It seems clear, then, that an adjunct medical system, such as this contributes significantly to the maintenance of the health and well-being of an elderly population.

REFERENCES

Arkansas Health Statistics Center. *An overview of the 1973 Arkansas health interview survey.* Little Rock, AHSC Publication No. 3, 1974.

Busse, E. W. The aging process and the health of the aged. In F. C. Jeffers (Ed.), *University council on gerontology: proceedings of seminars, 1961-1965.* Durham, North Carolina: Duke University Regional Center for the Study of Aging, 1965.

Confrey, E. A., and Caldstein, M. S. The health status of aging people. In C. Tibbitts (Ed.), *Handbook of social gerontology.* Chicago: University of Chicago Press, 1960.

Gray, R. M. Stress and health in later maturity. *Journal of Gerontology,* 1965, *20,* 65-68.

Industrial Research and Extension Center. *A changing Arkansas: population and related data.* Little Rock, College of Business Administration Publication No. L-7, 1973.

Lowenthal, M. F. Social isolation and mental illness in old age. *American Sociological Review,* 1964, *29,* 54-70.

Metropolitan Life Insurance Company. Health characteristics of the elderly, *Statistical Bulletin of the Metropolitan Life Insurance Company,* 1968, *49,* 2-4.

Reynolds, F. W., and Barsam, P. C. *Adult health: services for the chronically ill and aging.* New York: Macmillan Co., 1967.

Rothenberg, R. E. *Health in the later years.* New York: New American Library, 1964.

Shanas, E. Health care and health services for the aged. *Gerontologist,* 1965, *5,* 240; 276.

Shanas, E. Measuring the home health needs of the aged in five counties. *Journal of Gerontology, 1971,* 26, 37-40.

Southern Regional Council. *Health care in the south: a statistical profile.* Atlanta, SRC Publication No. 2, 1974.

Travis, G. *Chronic disease and disability.* Berkeley, California: University of California Press, 1966.

U.S. Department of Health, Education, and Welfare, Social and Rehabilitation Service, Administration on Aging. *Health services working with older people.* Washington, AoA Publication, Vol. 1, 1971.

U.S. Department of Health, Education, and Welfare, Office of Human Development, Administration on Aging. *New facts about older Americans.* Washington, DHEW Publication No. 73-20006, 1973.

U.S. Public Health Service. Older persons, selected health characteristics, United States, July, 1957 to June, 1959. *Health Statistics,* Series C, No. 4, 1960.

Van Zonneveld, R. J. *The health of the aged.* Baltimore, Md.: Williams and Wilkins, 1962.

White, E. L., and Gordon, T. Related aspects of health and aging in the United States. In M. F. Lowenthal and A. Zilli (Eds.), *Colloquium on health and aging of the population.* New York: S. Karger, 1969.

Section IV

WORK, RETIREMENT, AND LEISURE

T HE ISSUES OF WORK, retirement, and leisure were scarcely new to the gerontologists of the 1930s and early 1950s. On the other hand, the impetus to
fully explore the many ramifications of these phenomena can properly be ascribed to the Social Security Act of 1935. With the promulgation of this legislation, both government and privately sponsored research began to focus on such
questions as the meaning of work, the matter of retirement planning, and the
problems attendant upon a newly acquired leisure status. Accordingly, a number of surveys were conducted to: (1) assess the extent of the problems associated
with retirement, and (2) evaluate the effectiveness of current ameliorative programs aimed at this segment of the older population. One outcome of these efforts
was the shedding of considerable light on the relationship of income, health, and
attitudinal predisposition to retirement adjustment.

Perhaps the most earnest efforts of the period were manifested in attempts
to explicate the nature of work and its part in the social and psychological makeup of the older person (Caplow, 1954; Morse and Weiss, 1955). For the most
part, work was regarded as the central integrative factor in the self-conception
and emotional stability of the mature adult, especially the older male. Subsequent research, however, was to question the intrinsic meaningfulness of this
role area. Friedmann and Havighurst (1954), for example, found the importance
attached to work to vary among class and occupational groupings. For these
authors, work took on an intrinsic character with rising social status and white
collar employment. Among lower status, blue collar individuals, work assumed
a more instrumental quality. In still other instances where work loss was found
to be accompanied by negative psychological reactions, researchers often located
the explanation for such effects in the termination of significant relationships
associated with the work experience rather than in the loss of the work role
per se (Burgess, 1954; Barnes and Ruedi, 1942).

While the importance of work might vary given social class and occupational
differences, the matter of leisure became a more critical issue. Leisure, in contrast
to a productive ethic, was to impose a new and negatively valued burden upon
the elderly. No longer able to achieve in an achievement-oriented society, un-
trained and unprepared for a life of leisure, and unable financially and psycho-

151

logically to cope with the experience, older individuals began to associate leisure with uselessness and disrespect. Leisure more often assumed the dimensions of a curse than a blessing to the aged, a fact which served to make the transition to retirement a traumatic event for many older persons.

Retirement itself was viewed principally as an *event,* rather than a process. As such, the major interest of researchers came to center on the preparation for and subsequent adjustment to retirement (Havighurst, 1954; 1955). As preparation programs were largely to await a later time frame, the major thrust during this phase of gerontological development was on adjustment to the immediate life circumstances confronting the aged (i.e. lowered income, poor health, and reduced mobility). The "successfully adjusted" were those who had supposedly made the best of a bad situation.

It goes without saying that the research of this era was essentially descriptive in nature. Data were generally amassed through extensive surveys. For the most part, these were atheoretical efforts aimed toward building the foundations for future programs of aid and assistance. On the other hand, the information gleaned from such research forced attention not only upon retirement as an *event in time,* but also delineated the nature of the retirement role and emphasized the importance of the reactions of others in the shaping of this role. In addition, these early works generated a base of empirical information for the development of a host of social theories regarding retirement.

The late 1950s and early 1960s saw renewed interest in each of these areas. Technological developments during this period not only brought about numerous changes in the types of work available, but also called for a reevaluation of the character and meaning of the work experience (Bloomberg, 1957; Riesman, 1958). By the same token, efforts were made to assess the relationship between the older worker's attitudes toward work and his eventual adjustment to work loss (Burgess *et al.,* 1958; Heron, 1963; Johnson, 1958). In addition, the psychological effects of work loss were explored relative to several behavioral contexts, the family, voluntary associations, and the community (Anderson, 1958; Streib and Thompson, 1957).

Following on the heels of the previous research was a new concept of retirement. No longer an isolated event in the life course, retirement was now seen as *a social process* (Donahue *et al.,* 1960; 1958; Hart, 1957; Roe, 1956). As a process rather than an event, retirement assumed the character of a social role. As is true of all role relationships, however, this one, too, required socialization and/or prior preparation. As a consequence, a number of efforts were made to acquaint older workers both with the expectations of the retirement role and the limitations implied in this experience. During this era, for example, several handbooks on retirement made their appearance. Many of these dealt with the social and psychological implications of retirement (Buckley, 1956; Kleemeier, 1961). Others, however, focused on problems attendant upon a newly acquired life of leisure (Dumazedier and Ripert, 1963; Hoar, 1961; Martin, 1963). At still another level, business and industry began to institute training programs to accomplish the goal of a smooth transition from work-related tasks.

Another change to be observed during this period was a decline in the negative associations of leisure. Although influenced by a work ethic, the social and technological changes brought about in the late 1950s and early 1960s necessitated a new definition of leisure. With more and more individuals entering the ranks of the retired and large amounts of free time becoming available, it was no longer possible to ignore the difficulties wrought on previous generations by leisure time (Miller, 1965; Kaplan, 1958). As a consequence, leisure came to be viewed not as a unique experience in the life of the retired, but rather as an extension or continuation of a previously-developed pattern of behavior (Kaplan, 1960; Cowgill, 1962; Neumeyer and Neumeyer, 1958; Smigel, 1963). That is, the most creative and meaningful forms of leisure were observed to be reflections of the previous life experience of the individual. As such, leisure was seen to involve both an element of "work" and a dimension of "freedom-from-work." Given such a view, leisure not only lost most of its negative cast, but could be planned and prepared for in a fashion similar to retirement.

The methodological approaches employed in the above studies reflect developments in many areas of gerontology. The psychological interest in attitudes, for example, is seen not only in attempts to develop more sophisticated measuring devices, but also in efforts to relate these measurements to role adaptation and social stability in late life. In addition to these developments, longitudinal designs became recognized as the most effective means whereby to judge the overall implications of the changes brought about by retirement. In a similar fashion, the formulation of viable theoretical orientations made possible the meaningful investigation of numerous variables within an explanatory context. As a consequence, the research of this era began to assume a more analytic character.

The evaluation of work, retirement, and leisure has continued apace through the late 1960s and early 1970s. While work remains an important facet of personal identity for many older persons (Ellison 1968), it is beginning to share the spotlight with numerous leisure endeavors. This fact is attested by the increase in voluntary as opposed to compulsory retirement (Barfield and Morgan, 1969; Bortz, 1968; Epstein, 1966), participation in work-related leisure programs (Maddox, 1968), and the creativity evidenced by numerous older persons (Cunningham, 1968; Campbell, 1969). Cross-national and comparative studies have revealed similar findings (Kreps, 1968). Leisure, then, no longer appears tinged with the stigma of earlier times. Instead, it now assumes a meaning and value it its own right (Pfeiffer, 1971; Rosow, 1969).

Retirement, on the other hand, continues to be studied as a social process (Carp, 1968). Attention is given not only to the delineation of the retirement role, but also to one's attitudes toward retirement, especially as these relate to the individual's "success" in later life. In addition, the effectiveness of preretirement programs has now been evaluated (Charles, 1971) as have the effects of early retirement upon subsequent adjustment (Atchley, 1971; Barfield and Morgan, 1969). In essence, the transition to retirement has not reflected the trauma postulated in previous research. The institutionalization of this experience through governmental and private programs has led to a fairly clear understanding of role expectations by older workers. As a consequence, the social and psychological deficits hypothesized to follow this event have largely not materialized (Streib and Schneider, 1971). The utilization of longitudinal designs and parametric statistical techniques (e.g. multiple regression) have added considerably to the validity of these findings.

From still another standpoint, the contemporary approach to work, retirement, and leisure has been of an integrative nature. Not only have efforts been made to relate isolated variables to retirement phenomena, but cross-national efforts have also provided valuable data useful in the formulation of social theories. Such formulations have given the student of aging greater insight into the role changes of later life as well as made possible a greater appreciation of individual differences. These theoretical and methodological contributions have also provided a realistic foundation for policy planning and program implementation.

In the papers which follow, most of these themes are in evidence. There is a clear attempt in each, for example, to understand both retirement and leisure as developmental processes. In addition, there is also a concern for the phenomenological aspects of aging and retirement. In this regard, full weight is given to the psychological as well as the sociological dimensions of the problem at hand. Finally, the new definitions of work and leisure are spelled out in such a way that the reader can fully grasp the implications of both with respect to their impact on the older person.

The paper by Fillenbaum examines the relationship of one's attitude toward work to his subsequent attitude toward retirement. The author argues that attitudinal consistency would suggest that the opportunity to give up a burdensome task would be welcomed, whereas giving up a meaningful activity should be regarded with some degree of dismay. As much of the previous research on this issue is contradictory in character, Fillenbaum proposes that a more comprehensive test of this relationship calls for responses from a wide variety of occupational levels.

Employing a mailed questionnaire, the author reports data from 243 randomly selected nonacademic employees from a total population of nearly 6,000 at an eastern university and medical center. The findings indicate that of the job attitudes examined, only one variable, possibility of achievement, appears to be related to retirement. In addition, this relationship holds true only for white males. Apart from this, little relationship is evidenced between job attitude and retirement attitude. Those individuals with a positive attitude toward retirement express essentially the same job attitudes as those having a negative view of retirement.

For the most part, studies of early retirement have shown poor health to be the major element in the early retirement decision. The paper by Pollman, however, questions the predominance of this factor in light of both medical developments and improvements in retirement benefit programs. The author observes that previous studies have shown the relationship between poor health and retirement to vary according to job class. In addition, policies regarding retirement are frequently related to occupational differences. As a consequence, Pollman's study seeks to determine which factor or factors figure most strongly in the matter of early retirement.

Data were obtained from a group of 442 retired factory employees (age range 60-65) who were members of the UAW. The findings suggest an adequate retirement income to be the major consideration in early retirement. Poor health proved a second factor in prevalence, closely followed by the desire for more free time. Job and work group dissatisfaction do not appear significant influences in the decision. Poor health as a retirement influence was found to be related to job class.

The paper by Palmore considers one of the most controversial issues in contemporary gerontology, compulsory retirement at a fixed age versus flexible retirement based on ability. Acknowledging compulsory retirement policies to affect almost one half of the wage and salary workers in this country, the author examines the theories and facts supporting both flexible and compulsory forms of retirement.

In his argument, Palmore notes age to be a poor criteria for retirement given the wide variation in abilities observed among aged persons. Accordingly, "flexible retirement would better utilize the skills, experience, and productive potentials of older persons and thus increase our national output." Further, flexible retirement would increase the financial well-being of the aged and thus reduce the transfer of payments necessary for income maintenance. In addition, flexible retirement would not only improve life satisfaction and longevity by providing more employment, but might also reduce the hostility and resentment engendered by compulsory retirement. The author suggests a number of proposals for encouraging flexible retirement policies.

The paper by Fillenbaum focuses attention on the 30 percent of American males over the age of sixty-five who are still employed, i.e. the working retired. The author notes that insufficient data are available to characterize this group of men. As such, her paper represents an exploratory study to determine from a wide range of variables those most closely associated with work after retirement.

Data for the study were obtained from 469 persons interviewed initially by Simpson, Back, and McKinney in 1966. Additional data were collected five years later from 107 individuals in the sample who had been previously classified as preretired. The findings indicate that the working retired differ chiefly from the nonworking retired in terms of having received a greater amount of schooling, intending to work when retired, and being less likely to report a decline in health. In addition, the working retired also had less financial need to work and held memberships in a larger number of voluntary associations. The author suggests a greater involvement in work along with success and recognition on the job to be major factors in inducing certain persons to continue working after officially retiring.

In examining the social-psychological impact of retirement on American men, Thompson explores the utility of two current theoretical positions in social gerontology. The first suggests that separation from work at retirement leads or

can lead to demoralization, "because it represents the loss of a culturally dominant social role and the acquisition of a culturally devalued one." The second
position argues that, "positive role realignment is possible upon retirement and
that leisure and/or citizenship-service roles can replace work roles and provide
a sense of usefulness, personal satisfaction, and positive social support."

The data were obtained from interviews with a multistage probability sample
of 1589 noninstitutionalized men sixty-five years of age and older living in the
continental United States. The findings indicate that variations in the morale
of the retired can be explained in terms of a combination of four variables, perception of health, age, income, and functional disability. The author proposes
that while work no doubt remains a major factor in the integration of one's
personality and social stability, leisure roles function as an adequate substitute
for many older persons.

REFERENCES

Anderson, J. E. Psychological aspects of aging. In W. Donahue, W. W. Hunter, D. H.
    Coons, and H. K. Haurise (Eds.), *Free time: challenge to later maturity*. Ann Arbor:
    University of Michigan Press, 1958.

Atchley, R. C. Retirement and leisure participation: continuity or crisis. *Gerontologist*,
    1971, *11*, 13-17.

Barfield, R., and Morgan, J. *Early retirement: the decision and the experience*. Ann
    Arbor: Institute for Social Research, 1969.

Barnes, H. E., and Ruedi, O. M. *The American way of life: our institutionalized pat-
    terns and social problems*. New York: Prentice-Hall, 1942.

Bloomberg, W., Jr. Automation predicts change: for the older worker. In W. Donahue
    and C. Tibbitts (Eds.), *The new frontiers of aging*. Ann Arbor: University of Mich-
    igan Press, 1957.

Bortz, E. L. Retirement and the individual. *Journal of the American Geriatrics Society*,
    1968, *16*, 1-15.

Buckley, J. C. *The retirement handbook: a complete planning guide to your future*.
    New York: Harper & Bros., 1956.

Burgess, E. W. Social relations, activities, and personal adjustment. *American Journal of
    Sociology*, 1954, *54*, 352-360.

Burgess, E. W., Corey, L. G., Pineo, P. C., and Thornbury, R. T. Occupational differences
    in attitudes toward aging and retirement. *Journal of Gerontology*, 1958, *13*, 203-260.

Campbell, D. E. Analysis of leisure time profiles of four age groups of adult males.
    Research Quarterly, 1969, *40*: 266-273.

Caplow, T. *Sociology of work*. Minneapolis: University of Minnesota Press, 1954.

Carp, F. M. (Ed.) *The retirement process*. Washington, D. C.: United States Department
    of Health, Education & Welfare, 1968.

Charles, D. C. Effect of participation in a preretirement program. *Gerontologist*, 1971,
    11, 24-28.

Cowgill, D. O., and Baulch, N. The use of leisure time by older people. *Gerontologist*,
    1962, *2*, 47-50.

Cunningham, D. A. Active leisure time activities as related to age among males in a total
    population. *Journal of Gerontology*, 1968, *23*, 551-556.

Donahue, W., Hunter, W.W., Coons, D. H., and Maurice, H.K. *Free time: challenge to
    later maturity*. Ann Arbor: University of Michigan Press, 1958.

Donahue, W., Orbach, H. L., and Pollak, O. Retirement: the emerging social pattern. In C. Tibbitts (Ed.), *Handbook of social gerontology*. Chicago: University of Chicago Press, 1960.

Dumazedier, J., and Ripert, A. Retirement and leisure. *International Social Science Journal*, 1963, *15*, 438-447.

Ellison, D. L. Work, retirement, and the sick role. *Gerontologist*, 1968, *8*, 189-192.

Epstein, L. A. Early retirement and work life experience. *Social Security Bulletin*, 1966, *29*, 3-10.

Friedmann, E. A., and Havighurst, R. J. *The meaning of work and retirement*. Chicago: University of Chicago Press, 1954.

Hart, G. R. *Retirement: a new outlook for the individual*. New York: Harcourt, Brace, and Co., 1957.

Havighurst, R. J. Flexibility and the social roles of the retired. *American Journal of Sociology*, 1954, *59*, 309-311.

Havighurst, R. J. Employment, retirement, and education in the mature years. In J. Webber (Ed.), *Aging and retirement*. Gainesville: University of Florida Press, 1955.

Heron, A. Retirement attitudes among industrial workers in the sixth decade of life. *Vita Humana*, 1963, *6*, 152-159.

Hoar, J. Study of free time activities of 200 aged persons. *Sociology and Social Research*, 1961, *45*, 157-163.

Johnson, D. E. A depressive retirement syndrome. *Geriatrics*, 1958, *13*, 314-319.

Kaplan, M. Pressures of leisure on the older individual. *Journal of Gerontology*, 1958, *13*, 36-41.

Kaplan, M. *Leisure in America: a social inquiry*. New York: John Wiley & Sons, 1960.

Kleemeer, R. W. (Ed.) *Aging and leisure*. New York: Columbia University Press, 1961.

Kreps, J. M. Comparative studies of work and retirement. In E. Shanas and J. Madge (Eds.), *Methodology problems in cross-national studies of aging*. New York: S Karger, 1968.

Maddox, G. L. Retirement as a social event in the United States. In B. L. Neugarten (Ed.), *Middle age and aging: a reader in social psychology*. Chicago: University of Chicago Press, 1968.

Martin, A. R. *Leisure time: a creative force*. New York: National Council of Aging, 1963.

Miller, S. J. The social dilemma of the aging leisure participant. In A. M. Rose and W. A. Peterson (Eds.), *Older people and their social world*. Philadelphia: F. A. Davis, 1965.

Morse, N. C., and Weiss, R. S. The function and meaning of work and the job. *American Sociological Review*, 1955, *20*, 693-700.

Neumeyer, M. H., and Neumeyer, E. S. *Leisure and recreation*. New York: Ronald Press Co., 1958.

Pfeiffer, E., and Davis, G. C. The use of leisure time in middle life. *Gerontologist*, 1971, *11*, 187-195.

Reisman, D. Leisure and work in post industrial society. In E. Larrabee and R. Meyersohn (Eds.), *Mass Leisure*. Glencoe, Illinois: Free Press, 1958.

Roe, A. *The psychology of occupations*. New York: John Wiley & Sons, 1956.

Rosow, I. Retirement, leisure, and social status. In FF. C. Jeffers (Ed.), *Duke University council on aging and human development: proceedings of seminars, 1965-1969*. Durham, North Carolina: Duke University Center for the Study of Aging and Human Development, 1969.

Smigel, E. O. (Ed.) *Work and leisure*. New Haven, Conn.: College and University Press, 1963.

Streib, G. F., and Thompson, W. E. Personal and social adjustment in retirement. In W. Donahue and C. Tibbitts (Eds.) *The new frontiers of aging*. Ann Arbor: University of Michigan Press, 1957.

Streib, G. F., and Schneider, C. J. *Retirement in American society: impact and process*. Ithaca, New York: Cornell University Press, 1971.

Chapter 16

ON THE RELATION BE-TWEEN ATTITUDE TO WORK AND ATTITUDE TO RETIREMENT

GERDA G. FILLENBAUM

JOHNSON AND STROTHER (1962) boldly state that, "The kind and degree of orientation the individual has toward his job affects his orientation to retirement." Little has been published directly testing this assumption. Studies which are available suggest that it is only partly true. Friedmann and Havighurst (1954) indicate that there are exceptions to their general finding that those who are less involved in work have a greater willingness to retire. Saleh and Otis (1963) found that for older managerial level employees the mean level of anticipated satisfaction with forthcoming retirement was higher for those for whom work held extrinsic interest than for those for whom work held intrinsic interest, although the latter still had a positive orientation to retirement. The work of Simpson, Back, and McKinney (1966) indicates that this finding is not general. They found that only among upper occupational status persons was there the expected relationship between attitude to retirement and such job factors as work commitment and intrinsic interest in work. Upper occupational status persons who are high on these measures did not look forward to re-

Reprinted by permission from the *Journal of Gerontology*, 1971, *26*, 244-248.

tirement, while for middle and lower occupational level persons no relationship was found between job involvement and preretirement attitude.

Throughout these studies there is the expectation that since retirement means the end of the job, attitude to the job will be related in some meaningful, consistent way to attitude to retirement. Insofar as we expect consistency among attitudes we would expect that the opportunity to give up an activity which has become burdensome might be welcomed, while giving up an activity which is enjoyed might be treated with dismay. It therefore seems reasonable to suggest the simple hypothesis that those who are satisfied with their jobs will have a negative attitude to retirement, while those who are dissatisfied with their jobs will have a positive attitude to retirement. We shall examine this hypothesis.

Since previous work indicates that the relationship between job attitude and retirement attitude may differ with occupational level, the responses of persons from a wide range of occupational levels need to be examined, and since factors extrinsic to the job may affect attitude to the job and to retirement (e.g. adequacy of expected retirement income (Thompson and Strieb, 1958), health and difficulty in getting to work (Tuckman and Lorge, 1953)), these need to be controlled.

Materials and Methods

SUBJECTS: Approximately 100 Ss within each of the age spans twenty-five to thirty-four, thirty-five to forty-four, forty-five to fifty-four, and over fifty-four were selected at random from the entire population of nearly 6,000 nonacademic employees at a university and medical center. Persons of both sexes, both races and all occupational levels were included. Ss were mailed a ninety-five-item questionnaire whose main interest was to determine acceptance of a proposed retirement planning program, but which included items on job satisfaction, attitudes to, plans for, and beliefs about retirement. Anonymity was requested. Of the questionnaires 56 percent were returned, returns varying with the age group (25-34: 47%; 35-44: 54%; 45-54: 69%; over 54: 58%). The responding population is representative of the contacted group on race, occupational status and length of time employed, but does contain a disproportionately larger number of females.

MEASURES USED: *Ss* were asked about their health, ease of getting to work, and adequacy of expected retirement income.

JOB SATISFACTION: Following Herzberg, Mausner, and Snyderman's (1959) concepts of motivator variables and hygiene variables, questions were drawn up which were designed specifically to reflect those matters which these variables represent, i.e. for the motivator variables: achievement, recognition for achievement, work itself, responsibility, advancement; for the hygiene variables: company and administration, supervision, pay, interpersonal relations, working conditions. Motivator variables may also be considered as intrinsic aspects of the job, and the hygiene variables as extrinsic aspects.

ATTITUDE TO RETIREMENT: The first two items of Thompson's three-item Attitude to Retirement Scale (Thompson, 1956) were used. The third item (If it were up to you alone, would you continue working for your present employer?) was not used since analysis of responses to it indicated that movement away from the job reflected ease of getting another job rather than a lack of desire to work.

Results

These people enjoy good health. Only 13 percent (31/240) rate their health as being less than good, 9 percent (21/237) have experienced some change for the worse in the past year, and 17 percent (40/239) report some health problem. Very few days have been lost from work. Only 6 percent (15/243), all females, report difficulty in getting to work. No relationship was found between attitude to retirement and either health or difficulty in getting to work.

Because of the relative youth of most of this group, retirement income is not known, and few could estimate whether it would be adequate. It is, therefore, unlikely that this factor would influence retirement attitude for these *Ss*.

While questions dealing with ten job satisfaction variables were included in the questionnaire, only five variables could be used in analysis since the response range of the others was too limited. The job variables used, and the percentage of *Ss* indicating greatest satisfaction with each variable are achievement, 47 percent; responsibility, 40 percent; advancement, 59 percent; not in dead-end jobs; pay, 43 percent; working conditions, 51 percent. Where attitude to retirement is concerned, 81 percent consider retirement to be a good thing, 68 percent look forward to retirement, 65 percent both think it is good *and* look forward to it, and 16 percent think it is a bad thing *and* do not look forward to it.

The responses to each of the five job variables were compared by means of χ^2 analysis with the responses to each of the three measures of retirement attitude (i.e. (*a*) retirement is a good thing vs. retirement a bad thing; (*b*) looked forward to vs. not looked forward to; (*c*) good thing *and* looked forward to vs. bad thing *and* not looked forward to).

Only one job satisfaction variable, achievement, bore any relationship to retirement attitude. Those who reported that they had less chance of increasing their skills were more likely to view retirement as a good thing ($\chi^2 = 5.07$, 1 df, $p<0.05$), to look forward to retirement ($\chi^2 = 4.91$, 1 df, $p<0.05$), or to hold a consistently positive view of retirement, i.e. to believe retirement is a good thing *and* to look forward to it ($\chi^2 = 9.14$, 1 df, $p<0.01$).

It is possible that the relationship between job attitudes and retirement attitudes is different for persons having different characteristics. It is conceivable, for instance, that there is one relationship between job attitude and retirement attitude for older persons and a different relation in the case of younger persons. If these persons are treated as members of the same group and the data pooled, no relationship between retirement attitude and job attitude would be found, whereas if they were kept separate a relationship might be found within each group.

Because of this possibility the data were reanalyzed, emphasis being placed on examining the possible effects of four S characteristics: age, sex, race, and occupational status. We first tried to determine whether there was any relationship between a particular S characteristic and either retirement attitude or job attitude. For instance, do older persons differ markedly from younger persons in their attitude to retirement or in their attitude to work? We then controlled retirement attitude in order to further ascertain whether there were differences in job attitude, e.g. if we consider only persons with a positive view of retirement, will we find that the job attitudes of older persons differ from those of younger persons? Last, we examined the relationship between job attitude and retirement attitude when S characteristic was controlled, e.g. if we consider only data from older persons, will we find that there is a significant relationship between retirement attitude and job attitude? When the analysis is repeated for younger persons will a similar relationship hold?

Analysis was by means of χ^2. The specific variables used in the analyses were as follows:

A. S characteristics
1. age (25-44, N = 106; 45 and over, N = 137)
2. sex (males, N = 72; females, N = 171)
3. race (white, N = 186; black, N = 53; no information on 4 persons)
4. occupational status (upper, N = 61; middle, N = 109; lower, N = 71; no information on 2 persons)

B. Three pairs of retirement attitudes
1. retirement a good things vs. retirement a bad thing
2. look forward to retirement vs. not look forward to retirement
3. retirement good *and* look forward to it vs. bad *and* not look forward to it it

C. Five job variables
achievement, responsibility, advancement, pay, working conditions.

The specific analyses performed were as follows:
1. Each of the four S characteristics by each of the three pairs of retirement attitudes.
2. Each of the four S characteristics by each of the five job variables.
3. With retirement attitude controlled (i.e. separately for retirement a good thing, retirement a bad thing, etc.) each of the four S characteristics by each of the five job variables.
4. With S characteristics controlled (i.e. separately for older persons, younger persons, males, whites, etc.) each of the three pairs of retirement attitudes by each of the five job variables.

The results of these analyses should enable us to determine whether age, sex, race, or occupational status might have masked the expected relationship between job attitude and retirement attitude, and if so, to indicate where this has occurred. In brief, the results of these more detailed analyses support our earlier findings. Those differing in age, sex, race, or occupational status did not differ in attitude to retirement and showed few differences in job attitude, those differences which were present probably being due to a close association between the job attitude and occupational status. Only minimal differences were found when job attitude was examined with retirement attitude controlled. Those differences which did not reflect the close association between job attitude and occupational status were related to both positive *and* negative retirement attitudes, and consequently gave no support to the hypothesis. The only statistically significant findings in the last set of analyses, where S characteristics were controlled and the relation between job attitude and retirement attitude was examined, indicated that high achievement was significantly associated with a negative view of retirement among older persons. In general, then, these analyses support the findings reported above.

Discussion

Of the job attitudes examined, only one variable, possibility of achievement (referring to possible acquisition of further knowledge and skills), appears to be related to retirement attitude, and then only among the elderly, among whites, and among males. Apart from this there appears to be no relationship between job attitude and retirement attitude. Those having a positive attitude to retirement express the same job attitudes as those having a negative view of retirement. Such a finding could arise if the range of re-sponses were severely restricted. While some restriction in response range is present, this is gross in only one case (retirement as a bad thing), and the size of the group is such that a relation between retirement attitude and job attitude should have been manifested if present.

Various explanations could account for the present findings. We do not know the reasons for the particular retirement attitude held. In the Introduction we suggested that when retirement signals the end of a burdensome situation it will be anticipated with pleasure. But a positive attitude to retirement should also be held if retirement is accepted as an appropriate stage in the life cycle, if it is seen as a reward for work, a time to devote to other interests, a time when one is at last one's own master. When retirement has such strong positive connotations, attitude to work may be quite unimportant in determining attitude to retirement. If among our group some people look forward to retirement as a release from work, whereas others have a positive view of retirement regardless of their attitudes to their jobs, for the group as a whole the effect of job attitude on retirement attitude would be reduced and no consistent, significant relations would be obtained. It is, then, necessary to determine *why* a particular retirement attitude is held.

Matters other than beliefs about retirement, or attitude to the job, may also influence attitude to retirement. One attitude should only affect another if the matters to which they refer have something in common. It is possible that for our Ss work and retirement have little in common; that, in fact, their retirement attitudes are influenced by nonwork factors rather than work-related factors.

Only when the job is of prime importance as the central organizing factor of a person's life should it affect his retirement attitude. It reaches such a level of importance for only a few people, typically for self-employed and upper-echelon businessmen, for self-employed professionals, and for academics. This may explain why Simpson *et al.* (1966) found a relationship between job attitude and retirement attitude for their upper occupational status *Ss,* whereas we did not. Their *Ss* were persons for whom the integration of work into the total life is quite complete, whereas this is not the case for our *Ss.* Our upper occupational status *Ss* are not self-employed, and little that they do outside their working hours will affect their jobs.

Most people have interests in addition to their work. These interests tend to be of three types: (*a*) strictly work connected, where membership implies that one has a particular type of job or a particular work interest, e.g. membership in a professional society or Trade Union, (*b*) connected with work, insofar as one is encouraged to join a particular group because of the type of work or work career which one has, e.g. where work acts as a means of social integration (Ross, 1962; Wilensky, 1961), and (*c*) interests unrelated in any way with work.

While the "strictly work connected" interests may be sharply reduced or eliminated when the job ends, the other interests need not be discarded. Simpson *et al.* (1966) point out that relationships which originally developed because of work and which have helped to integrate the person into society need not necessarily be discarded on retirement. Even before retirement such interests may be pursued for their own ends, and the member be welcomed in his own right.

The ability and desire to continue these interests, and especially the ability and desire to continue those interests which are totaly unrelated to work, may influence attitude to retirement.

Summary

The relationship between the job attitudes and retirement attitudes of 243 randomly selected nonacademic employees from a total population of nearly 6,000 at a university and medical center was examined. Ss ranged in age from twenty-five to sixty-seven, were of both sexes and races, and all occupational levels. A very limited relationship was found between job attitude and retirement attitude. The general lack of relationship could not be attributed to differences in age, sex, race, or occupational status.

It is suggested that only where work holds the central organizing position in a person's life should job attitudes influence retirement attitudes.

REFERENCES

Friedmann, E. A., and Havighurst, R. J. *The meaning of work and retirement.* Chicago: University of Chicago Press, 1954.

Herzberg, F., Mausner, B., and Snyderman, B. B. *The motivation to work.* New York: John Wiley & Sons, 1959.

Johnson, J., and Strother, G. B. Job expectations and retirement planning. *Journal of Gerontology,* 1962, *17,* 418-423.

Ross, A. D. Philanthropic activity and the business career. Reprinted in S. Nosow and W. H. Form (Eds.), *Man, work, and society.* New York: Basic Books, 1962.

Saleh, S. D., and Otis, J. L. Sources of job satisfaction and their effects on attitudes towards retirement. *Journal of Industrial Psychology,* 1963, *1,* 101-106.

Simpson, I. H., Back, K. W., and McKinney, J. C. Orientation toward work and retirement, and self-evaluation in retirement. In

I. H. Simpson and J. C. McKinney (Eds.), *Social aspects of aging*. Durham, NC: Duke University Press, 1966.

Thompson, W. E. The impact of retirement. Unpublished Ph.D. dissertation, Cornell University, 1956.

Thompson, W.E., and Streib, G. F. Situational determinants: health and economic deprivation in retirement. *Journal of Social Issues,* 1958, *14,* 25-34.

Tuckman, J., and Lorge, I. *Retirement and the industrial worker.* Columbia University, Teachers College, Bureau of Publications, New York, 1953.

Wilensky, H. L. Orderly careers and social participation. *American Sociological Review,* 1961, *26,* 521- 539.

Chapter 17

EARLY RETIREMENT: A COMPARISON OF POOR HEALTH TO OTHER RETIREMENT FACTORS

A. William Pollman

D URING THE 1960s the option to retire before the commonly accepted age of sixty-five was presented to more and more industrial workers. Moreover, these options often included retirement benefits which made early retirement financially possible, although some reduction in the standard of living was required on the part of most such retirees.

Prior to the 1960s retirement, and especially early retirement, involved a rather painful financial sacrifice for most people. It is not really surprising then that poor health predominated as the major reason given for retirement at any age. An early study of the economic status of the aged (Steiner and Dorfman, 1957) found poor health and declining physical capacity to be the principal retirement factors. Of the voluntary retirees, 79 percent cited health problems as leading to their retirement decision.

Poor health was also the leading reason that was given for retirement (Minister of Labour and National Service, 1954) by 4,834 men who had retired upon reaching

the minimum pensionable age of sixty-five. Of these men, 25.2 percent had retired because of chronic illness, while 24.8 percent did so as the result of a currently disabling illness. Except for slightly more than 28 percent of the men who had retired involuntarily, all other retirement reasons were less than 10 percent each.

Another British study (Townsend, 1957), although far smaller in size, substantiated the verbal expressions of physical incapacity that were given by the retirees. This study of 203 elderly people living in a London borough found health problems to be the major retirement reason for 58 percent of the sample. Poor health was a contributing cause for another 20 percent of these people.

Health factors again took first place among reasons for retirement cited by 1,700 participants in another survey of the economic position of the elderly (Corson and McConnell, 1956). Poor health, an accident, or company initiated retirement for health reasons were mentioned by 25.6 percent of the sample. The next most prevalent reason for voluntary retirement, "more time to myself," totaled only 8.8 percent of these people.

A study of early retirees who joined the social security rolls while in the age range of sixty-two through sixty-four found these men to be characterized by low income, a low employment rate prior to retirement, and poor health (Palmore, 1964). Only about 40 percent of these people, who had not been in the labor force, were well enough to work. Almost 75 percent of the whole group had retired due to poor health or the inability to obtain another job. Markedly fewer of the men aged sixty-five and more retired for the same reasons, although almost 50 percent cited these same reasons for retirement.

Reprinted by permission from the *Journal of Gerontology*, 1971, *26*, 41-45.

The relationship between poor health and retirement also was found to vary according to job class (Steiner and Dorfman, 1957). As the occupational status diminished, there was a greater chance that retirement was occasioned either by poor health or by some physical limitation. Higher job classes were characterized more by mandatory retirement as the result of a formal retirement system. Sixty-five percent of the occupational group classified as operatives retired for health reasons. This statistic dropped to 53 percent for foremen and craftsmen and to only 21 percent for professional and technical people.

Poor health or declining physical capacity thus stands out as the predominant factor for the industrial or blue-collar class of worker. However, this situation may no longer be entirely true. In the 16-month period from September 1, 1965, through 1966, 7,223 employees retired from the Chrysler Corporation. Over 61 percent of these people were early retirees. The liberalized early retirement options took effect on September 1 of 1965. During 1963 and 1964, only 12 percent of the 2,186 retirees were less than sixty-five years old. It would appear from the significant increase in the number of early retirees after September 1, 1965, that perhaps other factors besides poor health might be a large part of the retirement decision (Wall Street Journal, 1967). This study was initiated to determine whether poor health was in fact still the predominant reason for early retirement by these workers.

Subjects

The 1965 period of negotiation for the United Automobile Workers' Union produced contracts which included improved early retirement options. Supplemental early retirement payments, which were in addition to the regular accrued pension benefit, were a part of these agreements. Workers, who are aged sixty to sixty-five with ten years or more of seniority, may retire at their own option and be eligible for this supplemental benefit. The combination of this supplemental benefit, which is paid only until the recipient is eligible for full social security payments, along with the basic accrued pension benefit can reach a total of $400 per month (Shoemaker, 1965).

The *Ss* selected for this study were all retired factory employees who were members of the UAW. They belonged to four midwestern UAW local unions. Only men were selected for inclusion in the sample, since women could well work and retire for quite disparate reasons, especially if they were married. These men were all in the age range of sixty to sixty-five.

Methods

This survey was accomplished through the use of a mail questionnaire. Questionnaires were sent to all of the early retirees in three of the locals and approximately one half of the men in the fourth local. A postage-paid return envelope was included, along with a cover letter from the cooperating union officials. A second mailing of this package of survey materials was made three weeks later. A total of 725 retirees received the questionnaire. Completed questionnaires were returned by 442 of these people for a response rate of 60.9 percent.

Variables included in the survey instrument related to satisfaction with the job and fellow workers, supervision, retirement benefits, health status, and the desire for additional free time. Respondents were asked to consider each of these variables and then to rank them as to the importance of each in influencing their retirement decision.

Job class was determined from the job

description given by each respondent. Skilled jobs would require periods of study and/or apprenticeship; these jobs would not have the work pace controlled by the machine. Machine operators would require some training but not long periods of apprenticeship. These job holders often had some control over the pace of their work effort. Assembly line people required minimum periods of training, but their work pace was entirely under mechanical control. The utility class of job holders required minimum periods of training also, but in this type of work they had complete control over their work pace.

Results

Data analysis indicates that health problems for this group of early retirees were not the leading retirement factor. As Table 17-I shows, the leading primary retirement factor was simply the feeling that an adequate pension benefit was available. Almost one half of these men cited this factor, while slightly less than one out of four, 24.49 percent, felt that poor health was their most important retirement influence. The desire for more free time for hobbies, 19.49 percent of the retirees, was nearly as large a primary retirement influence as was the incidence of poor health. Dissatisfaction with the job, 5.52 percent, and a dislike of the supervisor or the work peers, 3.16 percent, were of distinctly minor influence.

TABLE 17-I
PRIMARY REASON FOR RETIREMENT

Retirement Reason	% of Retirees
Adequate retirement income	47.34
Poor health	24.49
Wanted more free time	19.49
Dissatisfied with the job	5.52
Didn't like the boss or the people on the job	3.16

Since a decision such as the retirement decision has tremendous impact upon the life of an individual, it may well be based upon a serious consideration of several factors. The respondents were thus asked to consider all the elements which entered their retirement decision and to then rank them. The factors, which were designated as being second in degree of influence upon the retirement decision, are found in Table 17-II. The majority of these men, over 53 percent, felt that only one factor was really involved in their decision. The leading secondary retirement influence cited was the desire for more free time for hobbies and other desired activities. Slightly more than 21 percent selected this factor. The leading primary retirement reason, the feeling that an adequate pension benefit was available, was next in prevalence at 13.35 percent. Poor health was the next factor in order of prevalence among these secondary influences. However, it was only slightly ahead of dissatisfaction with the job and with the people on the job as an element in the retirement decision. Less than one in ten, 7.73 percent, cited health as a secondary part of the decision to retire.

TABLE 17-II
SECONDARY REASON FOR RETIREMENT

Retirement Reason	% of Retirees
No second reason	53.40
Wanted more free time	21.08
Adequate retirement income	13.35
Poor health	7.73
Dissatisfied with the job	3.50
Didn't like the boss or the people on the job	.94

Thus, as a motivation for retirement, the job itself appears to be of minimal importance compared to the existence of an adequate retirement benefit, the desire for more free time, or poor health. The men who were eligible for these early retirement options were by this simple fact of eligibility some of the most experienced men in the plant. Many of them held skilled jobs where a definite labor shortage exists. Replacement of these men will not be easy. However, due to the low degree of job dissatisfaction, there appears to be little such employers can do to retain these men on the job.

factor as a second part of their decision to stop working. Less than 12 percent of these men cited poor health.

The desire for more free time was third in prevalence among the primary retirement influences, but it was very close behind poor health in incidence. The leading secondary factor to be combined with it was the feeling of an adequate pension

TABLE 17-III
SECONDARY RETIREMENT REASONS FOR EACH PRIMARY RETIREMENT FACTOR

Secondary Retirement Reasons	Primary Reason For Retirement				
	Adequate Retirement Income	Poor Health	Wanted More Free Time	Dissatisfied With the Job	Didn't Like the Boss or the People On the Job
No second retirement reason	49.23	63.73	53.09	47.82	7.69
Wanted more free time	36.55	10.78		8.70	38.64
Adequate retirement income		18.63	34.57	30.43	23.08
Poor health	11.68		7.41	8.70	15.38
Dissatisfied with the job	2.03	5.88	3.70		15.39
Didn't like the boss or the people on the job	.51	.98	1.23	4.35	

The specific combinations of primary and secondary retirement elements are delineated in Table 17-III. This table thus indicates the prevalence of each factor as a secondary retirement influence in conjunction with each primary retirement factor. The factor most likely to be found in conjunction with the leading primary retirement factor, adequate retirement income, was the desire for more free time. Over 36 percent of these men, who primarily retired due to the pension benefit, gave this

benefit. Over 34 percent selected this factor. Poor health was again next most prevalent, but only 7.41 percent did find it to be a part of their decision.

When poor health was the principal retirement reason, the level of pension benefits was the most prevalent second retirement reason. Over 18 percent selected this factor, while 10.78 percent designated the desire for more free time.

But, for each of these three leading primary retirement reasons, the lack of a second retirement reason occurred with the greatest frequency. Almost 50 percent of those stressing pension benefits and 53.09 percent of those desiring more free time had no second retirement reason. However, among those who retired primarily because of a health problem, a comparatively larger proportion listed no other perceived retirement influence. For 63.73 percent of these workers, health problems constituted the sole retirement reason. Thus, when health was the principal retirement influence, it was more likely to exist as the single factor in the total retirement decision.

As Table 17-IV indicates, the incidence of poor health as the principal retirement reason varied markedly among the four job classifications. The probability that the skilled workers retired primarily as the result of poor health was much less than that for the other job classes. The data for these workers shows that the incidence of poor health was well behind the leading factor, adequacy of retirement income, and in fact ranked third in importance. Slightly more than one of every two skilled men retired due to the money income available, but less than one in five retired due to poor health.

Poor health was a much greater retirement influence among workers from the other job classifications. Approximately equal proportions of the machine operator, assembly line, and utility job class people selected the pension benefits available as their key retirement influence. But, poor health was a much more prevalent consideration for these men, especially for the former assembly line and machine operators. Health problems as the primary retirement reason were mentioned by 33.34 percent of the assembly line people and 30.59 percent of the machine operators. These percentages are less than the leading retirement reason for both groups, which was again the satisfaction with the pension income, but the disparity between the number of assembly line and machine operators citing each of these retirement reasons was much less than among the skilled group of men. This disparity increased again for the utility class of workers as the result of a decrease in the incidence of poor health.

Discussion

Health problems seem to be much more prominent as a retirement influence upon the assembly line people and machine operators than upon the utility and skilled labor classes. The existence of health problems was especially less prevalent among the skilled personnel. Health problems as a retirement influence increased in importance as job class prestige diminished until the utility class of workers was reached. The prevalence of health problems among these

TABLE 17-IV
PRIMARY RETIREMENT REASONS ACCORDING TO JOB CLASS

| Primary Retirement Reasons | | % of Each Job Class | | |
	Skilled	Machine Operator	Assembly Line	Utility
Adequate retirement income	52.45	43.12	41.20	43.96
Poor health	17.86	30.59	33.34	25.23
Wanted more free time	19.41	15.02	17.62	24.27
Dissatisfied with the job	5.72	7.51	5.88	4.67
Didn't like the boss or the people on the job	4.56	3.76	1.96	1.87

men was less than that found in the machine operator and assembly line classes.

The nature of the job itself may be responsible for this situation. In the job classes where health ranks highest as a retirement influence, all or a substantial part of the work effort is controlled by the machine. The skilled and utility job class individuals are able to control and adjust the rate of the work pace as their physical capacities diminish. Older people often tend to work at a slower but also steadier pace. This adjustment is not possible when the machine controls the work pace. Mechanical control of the work pace is particularly evident in the case of the assembly line people.

Poor health as a singular retirement reason seems quite rational, but the adequacy of retirement income as the sole retirement motivation appears logically to be insufficient reason to stop working as the data in Table 17-III indicate to be the case for some men. These men, evidently in good health, must surely have as a secondary retirement goal more free time. Perhaps if forced to state a secondary reason for early retirement, many of these men probably would cite this factor as an implicit part of their decision. Friedman and Havighurst (1954) determined, though, that a rather surprising proportion of workers, as high as 28 percent of the people in one of the samples, found no other meaning to their work than the money involved. If work has no other meaning beside the monetary reward, the adequacy of the retirement benefit could possibly then exist as the only conscious retirement-inducing factor of any consequence. This might well be the case for some of these men. There would be no further need to continue working. In other words, an adequate retirement benefit may exist not only as a necessary precondition for retirement, but also as the sole motiva-tion to retire. The premier valuation placed upon work by the Protestant ethic, if such a widespread valuation does indeed exist, does not seem to widely exist among these men.

Summary

Retirement at any age for industrial workers in the United States has been primarily due to poor health. Financial considerations usually prevented retirement until health problems dictated work cessation. However, during the 1960s early retirement options and pension benefits were vastly improved. This study was undertaken to determine whether health would continue to be the primary retirement factor for a group of industrial retirees in the age range of sixty to sixty-five. These men received a mail questionnaire which drew a response from 442 of them.

The existence of an adequate retirement income was by far the leading retirement consideration with poor health a distinct second in prevalence. Poor health was closely followed by the desire for more free time. Job and work group dissatisfaction were not important influences.

The majority of retirees perceived only one factor to be of any consequence in their retirement deliberations. For those who did perceive a secondary influence, health problems were third in order behind the desire for more free time and the amount of pension income, respectively.

Poor health as a retirement influence was related to job class. Assembly line and machine operators were much more likely to have selected this factor as their main retirement reason, although satisfaction with the pension benefits was still the leading factor. Health problems as the primary retirement reason were less prevalent among the skilled and utility class of work-

:s. This was especially true for the skilled
:dividuals.

REFERENCES

orson, J. J., and McConnell, J. W. *Economic needs of older people.* New York: Twentieth Century Fund, 1956.

:iedman, E. A., and Havighurst, R. J. *The meaning of work and retirement.* Chicago: University of Chicago Press, 1954.

(inister of Labour and National Service. *National insurance retirement pensions: Reasons given for retiring or continuing at work.* London: H. M. Stationery Office, 1954.

Palmore, E. Retirement patterns among aged men: Findings of the 1963 survey of the aged, *Social Security Bulletin,* 1964, *27,* 3-10.

Shoemaker, R. The quickening trend towards early retirement. *AFL-CIO American Federationist.* 1965, *22,* 13-17.

Steiner, P. O., and Dorfman, R. *The economic status of the aged.* Berkeley: University of California Press, 1957.

Townsend, P. *The family life of old people.* Baltimore: Penguin Books, 1957.

Wall Street Journal. Workers at Chrysler said to retire earlier under labor pact plan. March 15, 1967. p. 13.

Chapter 18

COMPULSORY VERSUS FLEXIBLE RETIRE- MENT: ISSUES AND FACTS

ERDMAN PALMORE

THE LOCAL, STATE, and national confer- ences involved in the 1971 White House Conference on Aging have increased concern with one of the most controversial issues in gerontology: that of compulsory retirement at a fixed age versus flexible re- tirement based on ability. Debate on this perennial issue also seems to increase as compulsory retirement policies affect more and more workers who are still able to work and as the national costs of maintain- ing incomes and health care for the retired steadily escalate. Some argue that compul- sory retirement is a clear case of discrimina- tion against an age category and should be banned along with other forms of age, sex, and race discrimination in employment (Gould, 1968).

Various arguments and theories sup- porting one side or the other have appeared in scattered reports and articles (Busse and Kreps, 1964; Havighurst, 1969; Hyden, 1966, Kreps, 1961; Koyl, 1970; Lambert, 1964; Mathiasen, 1953; Palmore, 1969a). This article attempts to summarize these arguments and present the relevant facts as a basis for future private and public policy.

Reprinted by permission from the *Gerontologist*, 1972, *12*, 343-348.

We will first present the facts on the ex- tent of compulsory retirement, then discuss the theories and facts supporting flexible retirement, and third, discuss those sup- porting compulsory retirement. Finally, we will present three proposals for encourag- ing flexible retirement policies.

Extent of Compulsory Retirement

The practice of compulsory retirement apparently became widespread only in this century and grew along with the swift in- dustrialization and growth of large corpora- tions in the early 1900s (Mathiasen, 1953). A series of national surveys conducted by the Social Security Administration and oth- ers show that compulsory retirement poli- cies affect a large and growing proportion of older workers. A comparison of the rea- sons for retirement given in the 1951 and the 1963 Social Security surveys of the aged indicate that the proportions of male bene- ficiaries who retired because of compulsory retirement provisions doubled during those twelve years (11% in 1951 and 21% in 1963 for wage and salary workers retired within the preceeding 5 years [Palmore 1967]). In their 1969 Survey of Newly En titled Beneficiaries, the Social Security Ad ministration found that 52 percent of th nonworking beneficiaries, who had been wage or salary workers and who became en titled at age sixty-five, had retired because of compulsory retirement (Reno, 1971 (Those who retired before they reached 6! about ²/₃ of the new beneficiaries, usual gave poor health or job discontinued as th main reason, rather than compulsory r tirement). A national survey of retiremer policies found that 73 percent of compani with pension plans (which includes mo large companies) had compulsory retir ment at a fixed age for some or all worke (Slavick and McConnell, 1963). The majo ity of these had compulsory retirement at age sixty-five. The 1966 SSA survey of retirement systems in state and local governments found that 79 percent had compulsory or automatic retirement at a fixed age (Waldman, 1968). This is an increase from the less than one half of the systems in 1944.

The Case for Flexible Retirement

1. Compulsory retirement is by definition discrimination against an age category, contrary to the principle of equal employment opportunity. Federal law now prohibits discrimination in employment based on race, sex, or age for persons under sixty-five. It is ironic that the present law against age discrimination in employment is limited to persons under sixty-five, because persons over sixty-five are the ones who are most likely to be discriminated against by such policies as compulsory retirement. It seems possible that restricting this law to persons under sixty-five could be considered unconstitutional in the sense that it does not provide equal protection of the law to all persons.

Supporters of compulsory retirement might argue that such discrimination is as legal and justifiable as child labor laws and policies which restrict the employment of children. However, there seems to be a valid difference in that child labor restrictions are designed primarily for the protection of children while compulsory retirement policies are usually justified on grounds other than those of protecting older persons.

2. Age, as the sole criteria for compulsory retirement, is not an accurate indicator of ability because of the wide variation in the abilities of aged persons. All the available evidence agrees that despite the declining abilities of some aged, most workers could continue to work effectively beyond age sixty-five (Riley and Foner, 1968).

3. Flexible retirement would better utilize the skills, experience, and productive potentials of older persons and thus increase our national output. If the millions of persons now forced to retire were allowed to be gainfully employed, the national output of goods and services could increase by billions of dollars.

4. Flexible retirement policies would increase the income of the aged and reduce the transfer payments necessary for income maintenance. Since the average income of retired persons is about one-half that of aged persons who continue to work (Bixby, 1970), it follows that flexible retirement policies might double the average incomes of those who were forced to retire but are willing and able to work. Similarly, over twice as large a proportion of retired aged persons have incomes below the poverty level as do aged persons who continue to work. Thus the millions of aged persons with poverty incomes might be substantially reduced by flexible retirement, which would increase their employment opportunities. This in turn would substantially reduce the amount of old age assistance and other welfare payments currently given to the aged with inadequate incomes. Similarly, Social Security payments could be reduced substantially because of the provision which reduces retirement benefits for earnings of over $1,680 per year. Considering the fact that over 20 billion dollars a year are paid by Social Security to retired workers and their dependents, it is easy to see that several billion dollars could be saved from income maintenance programs if only a minority of the aged could avoid forced retirement.

5. Flexible retirement, in providing more employment, would improve life satisfaction and longevity of the aged. Most evidence indicates that retirement does

tend to decrease life satisfaction. Streib (1956) found that even for persons with similar levels of health and socioeconomic status, morale still tends to be comparatively higher among the employed. Thompson (1960) found that decreases in satisfaction over two-year period were somewhat greater among older persons who retired than among those who continued to work; and decreases in satisfaction were substantially greater among reluctant retirees. The Duke Longitudinal Study (Palmore, 1968) found that reductions in economic activities including retirement were closely associated with reduction in life satisfaction.

There is less evidence supporting the idea that retirement has negative effects on health and longevity. Most of the association of poor health and greater mortality with retirement is probably due to the fact that people in poor health and with shortened life expectancies are the ones who tend to retire (Martin, Doran, 1966; Riley, 1968). However, we found that work satisfaction was one of the strongest predictors of longevity in our longitudinal study of normal aged (Palmore, 1969b). It may be that lack of work satisfaction, which can occur among the employed as well as among the retired, is the factor which reduces longevity.

6. Flexible retirement reduces the resentment and animosity caused by compulsory retirement. Apparently, many workers bitterly resent being thrown on the trash dump while they are still capable of working. Flexible retirement policies, by allowing such workers to continue work, eliminates this problem.

The Case for Compulsory Retirement

1. Compulsory retirement is simple and easy to administer. Flexible retirement would require complicated tests which would be difficult to administer fairly and difficult to explain and justify to the worker. This may be the main reason for the popularity of compulsory retirement among administrators. Proponents of flexible retirement agree that it would be somewhat more difficult to administer, but many with experience in the administration of flexible retirement plans assert that the complications have been exaggerated and that adequate tests of retirement based on ability are "not the monsters they were made out to be" (Mathiasen, 1953). Various groups have been working on improving techniques for measuring functional ability as a basis for retirement practices (Koyl, 1970).

2. Compulsory retirement prevents caprice and discrimination against individual workers. Proponents of flexible retirement also grant this point, but point out that prevention of individual discrimination is bought at the price of wholesale discrimination against an entire age category. They argue that the net number of workers willing and able to work who are forced to retire would be much less under policies of flexible retirement.

3. Compulsory retirement provides predictability. Both employer and employee know well in advance that the employee must retire on a fixed date. Thus, both can plan ahead better. On the other hand, some predictability can be built into flexible retirement by requiring workers and management to give a certain amount of advance notice to the other party of any intended retirement.

4. Compulsory retirement forces management to provide retirement benefits at a determined age. Most compulsory retirement plans are accompanied by retirement pension systems (Slavick and McConnell, 1963). On the other hand pension systems are often combined with flexible retirement policies with no great difficult

(Mathiasen, 1953).

5. Compulsory retirement reduces unemployment by reducing the number of workers competing for limited jobs. This is especially important in declining or automating industries or plants with an over supply of workers. On the other hand, it could be pointed out that compulsory retirement tends to increase unemployment among older workers by forcing them to leave one job at which they are experienced and seek another job in a new area in which they may be disadvantaged. Using compulsory retirement to reduce unemployment is analogous to firing all women or all blacks in order to reduce the number of workers competing for jobs. A better solution to the unemployment problem is for the government to stimulate the economy or to create additional jobs by being the "employer of the last resort."

6. Compulsory retirement prevents seniority and tenure provisions from blocking the hiring and promotion of younger workers. This is certainly true when seniority and tenure provisions are used to retain workers who have become less efficient and productive. A solution to this problem under flexible retirement would be to eliminate seniority and tenure provisions at a fixed age and require the older workers to compete periodically for their jobs on the basis of ability rather than seniority.

7. Compulsory retirement forces retirement in only a few cases because most workers sixty-five and over want to retire or are incapable of work. This claim is probably not true as shown by the surveys cited earlier.

8. Compulsory retirement saves face for the older worker no longer capable of performing adequately. The older worker does not have to be told and does not have to admit that he is no longer capable of working but can blame his retirement on the compulsory retirement policy. Such a face-saving device undoubtedly has important value for many workers, but the number of such workers should be balanced against the perhaps equal number of capable workers forced to retire by compulsory retirement and the resulting frustration, loss of status, reduction of income and of national productivity.

9. Most workers sixty-five years old have impaired health or only a few years of health left. The facts do not support this argument. Life expectancy for a sixty-five-year-old person is now about fifteen years, and the majority of aged do not appear to have disabling impairments. Only 37 percent of persons sixty-five and over report any limitation in their major activity (National Center for Health Statistics, 1971).

Seventy percent of the Social Security male beneficiaries retiring at age sixty-five because of compulsory retirement report no work limitation (Reno, 1971). Furthermore, despite compulsory retirement and other discrimination against the aged, about one third of men over sixty-five continue to do some work (Bogan, 1969). Thus, it appears probable that the majority of workers age sixty-five can expect a substantial number of years in which they will be capable of productive employment.

10. Most older workers are inferior and cannot perform most jobs as well as younger workers. This appears to be another of the stereotypes about the aged which has little or no basis in fact.

11. Compulsory retirement does little harm because most workers who are forced to retire could get other jobs if they wanted to. Again the evidence is contrary to this theory. When workers sixty-five and over lose their jobs, they have much more difficulty in getting another one than younger men. The proportions of older workers in the long-term unemployed categories are

about twice as high compared to workers age twenty-to thirty-five (Riley and Foner, 1968). Educational differences do not explain these differences in long-term unemployment (Sheppard, 1969). More than one half of all private employees in states without age-discrimination legislation in 1965 admitted age limits in hiring practices and many more probably informally discriminate against older workers (Wirtz, 1965).

12. Most workers forced to retire have adequate retirement income. Again the facts appear to be to the contrary. We do not know exactly what percentage of those forced to retire are in poverty, but 30 percent of all retired couples and 64 percent of the retired nonmarried persons have incomes below the official poverty level (Bixby, 1970). And it is precisely those forced to retire early who have incomes substantially lower than those who retire early voluntarily (Reno, 1971).

Proposals for Increasing Flexible Retirement

The most extreme proposal would be to outlaw all compulsory retirement by removing the age limitation in the present law against age discrimination in employment. The main objections to such a proposal is that at present it would be politically difficult if not impossible to pass such a law and that even if it could be passed it would be extremely difficult to enforce effectively. A counter-argument would be that the difficulty of enforcement should not prevent passage of a just law. We have many excellent laws which are difficult to enforce, such as laws against murder, robbery, and racial discrimination. Another serious objection is that while compulsory retirement may usually be unjust, in some situations it may be less unjust than a system with no retirement criteria or with

completely arbitrary decisions as to who must retire.

A more moderate proposal would be to provide tax incentive for flexible retirement policies. A reduction in the amount of Social Security tax paid by the employer with flexible retirement policies could be economically justified by the savings in Social Security benefits that would result from continued employment of workers not forced to retire.

The most modest proposal would be to encourage some kind of compromise between complete compulsory retirement and flexible retirement based on ability alone. Brown (1950) of Princeton University proposed such a compromise plan over twenty years ago. Under this plan a definite age would be set at which all employees recognize that the promise of continued employment ends. At this time all seniority right and further accumulation of pension credit ends. Then retired employees can be recalled to work as temporary employees, subject to the needs of management.

REFERENCES

Bixby, L. Income of people aged 65 and older. *Social Security Bulletin*, 1970, *33*, 4, 3-34.

Bogan, R. Work experience of the population. *Monthly Labor Review*, 1969, *92*, 44-50.

Brown, J. The role of industry in relation to the older worker. In *The aged and society.* New York: Industrial Relations Research Assn., 1950.

Busse, E., and Kreps, J. Criteria for retirement a reexamination. *Gerontologist*, 1964, *4*, Pt 1, 117-119.

Gould, D. Let's ban retirement. *New Statesman*, 1968, *75*, 411.

Havighurst, R. J. (Ed.). Research and development goals in social gerontology. *Gerontologist*, 1969, *9*, Part II.

Hyden, S. *Flexible retirement age.* Paris: Organization for Economic Cooperation & Development, 1966.

Koyl, L. A technique for measuring functional criteria in placement and retirement practices. In H. Sheppard (Ed.), *Towards an industrial* gerontology. Cambridge, Mass. Schenkman, 1970.

Kreps, J. Case study of variables in retirement policy. *Monthly Labor Review*, 1961, *84*, 587-91.

Lambert, E. Reflections on a policy for retirement. *International Labor Review*, 1964, *90*, 365-75.

Martin, J., and Doran, A. Evidence concerning the relationship between health and retirement. *Sociological Review*, 1966, *14*, 329-343.

Mathiasen, G. (Ed.). *Criteria for retirement.* New York: G. P. Putnam's Sons, 1953.

National Center for Health Statistics. Current estimates from the Health Interview Survey —1969. *Vital & Health Statistics*, Ser. 10. No. 63, 1971.

Palmore, E. Retirement patterns. In L. Epstein and J. Murray, *The aged population of the United States.* Washington: Government Printing Office, 1967.

Palmore, E. The effects of aging on activities and attitudes. *Gerontologist*, 1968, *8*, 259-263.

Palmore, E. Sociological aspects of aging. In E. Busse and E. Pfeiffer (Eds.), *Behavior and adaptation in late life.* Durham: Duke University Press, 1969. (a)

Palmore, E. Predicting longevity. *Gerontologist*, 1969, *9*, 247-250. (b)

Reno, V. Why men stop working at or before age 65: Findings from the Survey of New Beneficiaries. *Social Security Bulletin*, 1971, *34*, 6, 3-17.

Riley, M. and A. Foner, *Aging and Society*, Vol. II. New York: Russell Sage Foundation, 1968.

Sheppard, H. Aging and manpower development. In M. Riley and A. Foner, *Aging and Society*, Vol. II. New York: Russell Sage Foundation, 1969.

Slavick, F., and McConnell, J. Flexible versus Compulsory retirement policies. *Monthly Labor Review*, 1963, *86*, 279-81.

Streib, G. Morale of the retired. *Social Problems*, 1956, *3*, 270-276.

Thompson, W., Streib, G., and Kosa, J. The effect of retirement on personal adjustment. *Journal of Gerontology*, 1960, *15*, 165-169.

Waldman, S. *Retirement systems for employees of state and local governments*, 1968. Washington: Government Printing Office, 1968.

Wirtz, W. *The older American worker.* Washington: Government Printing Office, 1965.

Chapter 19

THE WORKING RETIRED

Gerda G. Fillenbaum

ACCORDING TO THE 1960 U.S. Census, 30.5 percent of males over the age of sixty-five were gainfully employed. Since sixty-five is the accepted retirement age in the USA the question arises as to who these older working persons are and why they continue to work.

It has been reported that those who work at a later age tend to be upper-occupational status (Palmore, 1965) and to be married males (Steiner and Dorfman, 1957). Reasons given for working have included attempting to maintain social status, needing the time structuring which some work provides, and needing the money (Clark, 1966; Donahue, Orbach, and Pollak, 1960; Wentworth, 1968). This is in apparent contradiction with the finding that it is upper occupational status people who work.

Since our present knowledge of the factors which are important in determining which persons will work after retirement is so limited, it seems to be justifiable to do an exploratory study, looking at a wide range of variables in order to determine which are related to work after retirement. In certain areas hypotheses can be formulated. We will concentrate on three of these areas: occupational status and matters closely connected with occupational status, attitude to retirement, and certain aspects

Reprinted by permission from the *Journal of Gerontology*, 1971, *26*, 82-89.

of personality.

Since others (e.g. Palmore, 1965) have found that upper-occupational level persons tend to work to a later age we would expect to find that those who work after officially retiring come mainly from this occupational status and manifest properties typical of this status, i.e. more education, a higher income (and so after retirement are less likely to work purely because they need the money), stronger intrinsic interest in work (Friedmann and Havighurst, 1954), greater organizational membership (Wright and Hyman, 1958), and better health.

Working past retirement age generally involves a definite decision and effort. Such a decision is probably only partially affected by financial position for, if it is now possible to choose whether or not to work, personal desires concerning work and leisure may be expected to become more relevant. If this is so we would expect those who have a positive attitude toward work or a negative attitude to retirement to plan to continue to work when retired and so to be more likely to work when retired.

Work is an activity expected of all males who have completed their studies and who have not yet reached an acceptable retirement age. In a sense, work belongs to the middle-aged. This being so, we would expect retired persons who work to hold attitudes similar to those held by middle-aged persons, to be more likely to consider themselves as middle-aged (rather than old), and to consider middle-age, or the past, a more desirable time of life. The nonworking retired are probably more likely to identify themselves with other older persons and be less likely to view the past in a desirable light.

Older men who work, unlike similar persons who do not work, have been found to have greater internal control and to be less readily influenced by external events (i.e., are less field-dependent) (Karp, 1967). We would, therefore, expect the working retired to have greater confidence in themselves and their abilities and be more likely to see their own actions as determining what happens to them.

In summary, we expect that (*a*) the working retired will tend to come from the upper occupational status and exhibit characteristics related to that status, (*b*) before retirement the working retired will have had a positive attitude to work or a negative attitude to retirement and will have made plans to continue to work, and (*c*) they will perceive the past in a more favorable way, and show a greater belief in their own abilities.

Method

Subjects

The data analyzed were those obtained from *Ss* interviewed by Simpson, Back, and McKinney (1966). The group, all white male long-term residents of the area, consisted of 308 retired workers and 161 workers who were within five years of retirement, located in the Piedmont area of North Carolina and Virginia in 1960 and 1961. They were obtained from lists provided by a tobacco, a textile, and a chemical factory, an insurance company, three universities, and from local membership lists of the American Bar Association, the American Medical Association, and executive directors of a local Young Men's Christian Association. The percentage of those at each occupational level for the retired and the preretired (in parentheses) was upper occupational status: 26 percent (52%); middle: 40 percent (24%); lower: 34 percent (24%). A man was considered to be retired if he was on one of the retirement lists from which *Ss* were chosen. Five years later as many as possible of the 161

preretired workers were reinterviewed. Of those seen 107 had retired.

By analyzing separately data obtained from those retired in 1961 (1961 group) and those retired between 1961 and 1966 (1966 group), we can see whether the findings obtained from one group are consistent with those obtained from the other. In addition, by looking at the preretirement information available from the 1966 group possibly relevant preretirement factors which are associated with work in retirement can be identified.

Of the 1961 group 31 percent (97/308) and of the 1966 group 41 percent (44/107) had worked for pay after retiring.

Information was available on a very wide range of subjects, of which the following were selected for examination: education; health (self-assessment, comparison with that of others, and change over time); matters related to work (intrinsic, generalizability of job skills, number of different jobs held, orderly or disorderly career pattern, occupational status); matters related to retirement (whether *S* had looked forward to it, whether he had made plans, and whether the plans were for work or recreation); source of the good and bad things which had befallen *S* (whether attributed to the self or other sources); adequacy of retirement income (retirement income was considered adequate if it was 50 percent of the preretirement income *and* more than $2,000 p.a. for the 1961 group, 50 percent *and* more than $3,000 p.a. for the 1966 group); achievement of life goals (whether *S* had achieved most, some, a few, or none); age (on retirement, and when interviewed); length of time retired; and ratings of *myself, middle-aged man, working man, retired man,* and *old man* on seven-point scales.

In addition, for the 1966 group, the following items were included from the follow-up interviews: health (self-assessment, comparison with health of others, and change over time) ; intrinsic interest in work, source of control (internal or external, a precursor of the Rotter (1966) Scale was used); ladder scale (Cantril, 1965; rating of own position at age forty-five and also 5 years previously) ; and a repetition of the ratings of *myself, middle-aged man, working man, retired man,* and *old man* on each of the original seven-point scales.

Data Analysis

As is evident in the Introduction, many of the variables in which we are interested are interrelated. An analysis in which we consider each variable separately and note its relationship to work after retirement tells us little, since the effect obtained may not be due to that variable but to the relation of that variable with another or others. In order to cope with this problem, multidiscriminant analysis was used in examining the data, since this technique takes the covariances among variables into consideration and also determines the relative discriminating power of the variables. In addition, by obtaining the intercorrelations among variables, it is possible to see how variables cluster and consequently to determine why some variables appear to have little or no discriminating power.

Multidiscriminant analysis can only be used when information is complete for all *Ss.* Since all *Ss* did not answer all questions, data could only be analyzed for 66 percent of the 1961 group (60/97 working retired, 143/211 nonworking retired) and 72 percent of the 1966 group (31/44 working retired, 46/63 nonworking retired). For both 1961 and 1966 groups *Ss* who gave complete information were compared with those giving partial information on five variables in order to determine whether there were statistically significant differences between

these groups. The variables selected were schooling, occupational status, self-rating of health, length of time retired, and age at interview. For the 1961 group differences between complete and partial respondents were found in occupational status ($x^2 = 13.11$, 2 *d.f.*, $p < 0.01$) and health ($x^2 = 4.26$, 1 *d.f.*, $p < 0.05$), those giving complete information tending to be middle and lower occupational status, who reported having better health. In the 1966 group similar differences were found for occupational status ($x^2 = 7.64$, 2 *d.f.*, $p < 0.05$), in addition those giving complete information had a significantly lower level of education ($x^2 = 4.41$, 1 *d.f.*, $p < 0.05$). To some extent, our respondents may overrepresent middle and lower occupational level persons in these two samples.

Results

While the proportion of working to nonworking retired is similar in both 1961 and 1966 groups (.31 and .41, respectively), the 1966 group has a higher proportion of upper occupational status persons ($x^2 = 6.89$, 2 *d.f.*, $p < 0.05$) and, consequently, of persons with a higher level of education ($x^2 = 6.08$, 1 *d.f.*, $p < 0.05$). Both the average length of time retired and the range are greater in the 1961 group than in the 1966 group (1961, average 5.46 years, range just retired, 18 years; 1966, 3.14 years, just retired, 7 years). There are also differences in mean age and age range (1961, mean age 70.19 years, range 55-91 years; 1966, on reinterview, mean age 68.39 years, range 65-77 years). It is clear that the 1966 group is somewhat more homogeneous in age than the 1961 group and is of a higher occupational level. Because of this additional analysis of the data using only upper occupational status *Ss* was also performed.

Multidiscriminant Analysis Results

In all, six multidiscriminant analyses were run, two on the 1961 group (entire group, and upper occupational level Ss only) and four on the 1966 group of which two were on preretirement data (1 on entire group, 1 on upper occupational level Ss only) and similarly two on postretirement data. In the latter postretirement information, together with preretirement information which had not been superceded by postretirement information was included among the data for analysis (e.g. educational level and number of jobs held were included in both analyses, but postretirement rather than preretirement ratings of health were considered).

1961 Group

Only two variables seem to be relevant in discriminating between those who have and those who have not worked since retiring. In order of importance, these are the original intention to work when retired (15/60 working retired and 138/143 nonworking retired correctly classified) and the length of time retired (classification, variables 1 and 2 combined, 36/60 working retired and 113/143 nonworking retired correctly classified). The next two variables, while having little further discriminating power, are of interest because they are the important discriminating variables in the 1966 postretirement and preretirement analyses. They are level of education and perceived change in health over time.

Retirement plans seem to be more important than any other variable considered in determining whether or not a person will work when retired. This variable bears no correlation of any significance with any of the other variables examined.

Length of time retired, the next most important variable, indicates that those who have been retired a longer time are a little more likely to have worked after retiring. These persons were also slightly older when interviewed (70.68 years in contrast with 69.29 years for the nonworking retired), and were more likely to have an adequate retirement income although overall those who had been retired longer tended to have an inadequate retirement income.

Adequacy of retirement income was also related to amount of schooling, which was the third variable of importance. The working retired had had more education, associated with which was a more adequate retirement income ($r = 0.62$) and membership in a larger number of organizations both before *and* after retirement.

The working retired were more inclined to believe that their health had improved, or remained the same, and reported having better health than the nonworking retired who reported a decline in health.

1966 Group—Post-retirement Data

The variables of third and fourth importance in the 1961 group are of greatest importance in the 1966 group. Level of education alone yielded a correct classification of 21/31 working retired and 40/45 nonworking retired, which combined with the findings on change in health yielded a correct classification of 24/31 working retired and 38/45 nonworking retired.

The working retired have received more education, related to which is a higher occupational status ($r = 0.75$), they have dropped out of a larger number of organizations, have a greater intrinsic interest in their work and hold unfavorable attitudes toward both *working man,* who is seen as being less free to do things, past-oriented rather than future-oriented, and more dissatisfied with life, and to *old man* who is viewed as not being respected. They view *myself* as being more respected than *working man,* the difference for the working retired being much greater than for the nonworking retired.

1966 Group—Preretirement Data

Again, level of education (with 21/31 working retired and 40/45 nonworking retired correctly classified) and change in health (with a cumulative correct classification rate of 24/31 working retired and 38/45 nonworking retired) have the greatest discriminating ability. Interestingly the next two variables in order of importance (though they produce no further improvement in discrimination) are the type of plans made for retirement and attitude to retirement, those making no plans, and those looking forward to retirement being the least likely to work.

Level of education is, as expected, related to occupational status, and is also related to various attitudes held about *working man,* the more educated seeing him as less effective, dissatisfied, and disregarded.

Unlike those who will not work after retirement, those who will work report no adverse change in their health and give their health a better rating than do those who will not work later.

Upper Occupational Status— 1961 Group

The twenty-two *Ss* in each of the working and nonworking retired groups constituted 49 percent (22/45) and 55 percent (22/40) of the entire group of upper occupational status working and nonworking retired. The findings were very similar to those obtained when the entire 1961 group was considered.

The three most important variables, in order of discriminating ability, together with cumulative correct classifications were intention to work after retiring (11/22 working retired and 21/22 nonworking retired correctly placed; those who do not intend to work do not) ; perception of *working man* as being free to do things (14/22 working retired and 17/22 nonworking retired correctly classified; the working retired being *less* likely to see *working man* as being free to do things) ; and level of education (17/22 working retired and 18/22 nonworking retired correctly assigned; the working retired have had more education).

On examining the correlations of these variables with others we find that those who intended to work had definitely not planned a life of recreation $(r = 0.48)$.

The perception of *working man* as being free to do things is related to a similar perception of *middle-aged man* and to having planned leisure pursuits for retirement, all of which are beliefs more likely to be held by the nonworking retired.

Level of education is related to a rather larger complex of variables. Again, those with more education are more likely to have an adequate retirement income $(r = 0.80)$. They belong to more organizations, perceive their health as being better (it is possibly because of this correlation between health and education that health has not emerged as a separate variable in this analysis), had made plans for retirement, and were more likely to view *retired man* as not being respected.

Upper Occupational Status— 1966 Group—Postretirement Data

Complete information is available from 62 percent (18/28) and 53 percent (10/19) of the upper occupational status 1966 working and nonworking retired.

Only two variables had any discriminating power: perception of one's standing in life at age forty-five (12/18 working retired and 8/10 nonworking retired correctly classified, the working retired reporting a much better life at age 45 than did the nonworking retired) ; and level of education (17/18 working retired and 7/10 nonworking retired correctly assigned, the working retired had more education).

Those with a favorable perception of their standing in life at age forty-five also tended to hold a favorable perception of their standing five years previously, and rated *working man* as being less satisfied.

While the working retired were more likely to report that their health was the same as before retirement, or better, the correlation between schooling and this health measure indicates, surprisingly, that there is a tendency for health to deteriorate as level of schooling increases. Again, work had held a greater intrinsic interest for those having more education. Schooling was also related to attitudes concerning others. As amount of schooling increases *retired man* is seen as being less free to do things, *middle-aged man, working man,* and *old man* are less respected, with the latter also being considered useless and the former ineffective. Apparently those with more education (typically the working retired) have a poorer opinion of the abilities of others.

Upper Occupational Status— 1966 Group—Preretirement Data

Once more level of education is the most important discriminating variable; those who will work after retiring have had more education than those who will not (17/18 working retired and 6/10 nonworking retired correctly classified). Inclusion of the two variables next in importance yields little improvement in discrimination; they are, however, of interest since they are similar to variables found to be important in the 1961 group. These variables are the perceived sources of the good things which have happened to *S*, and the intention to work when retired, the working retired being more likely to state that the good things which have happened to them are due to their own actions and that they intend to work when retired (cumulative correct classification rate: 17/18 working retired and 8/10 nonworking retired). The main results are summarized in Table 19-I.

Discussion

Our hypotheses were formulated around three areas: occupational status and the complex of variables related to occupational status; attitude to work and retirement; and the interaction between work and personality.

The evidence available did not wholly support our first hypothesis, since level of education seemed to be more important than occupational status, appearing as a discriminating variable even when only upper occupational level persons were considered. For the 1966 group education and occupational status were correlated ($r = 0.75$). There was no marked correlation for the 1961 group, probably because of the wide age-range (36 years) of this group. Older persons of the 1961 group needed fewer years of education than did younger persons to obtain similar level jobs.

In agreement with our hypothesis, the working retired did not seem to work because of dire financial distress. The working retired of the 1961 group were more likely to have adequate retirement income than were the 1961 nonworking retired, while adequacy of retirement income did not enter as either an important discriminating variable in the 1966 group or as being correlated to a discriminating variable. In these groups those who work do not do so because of extreme need.

TABLE 19-I

RANK ORDER OF IMPORTANCE AND DISCRIMINATING POWER OF DISCRIMINATING VARIABLES

Discriminating Variables	Entire Sample						Upper Occupational Status Only					
	1961		1966 Postretirement		1966 Preretirement		1961		1966 Postretirement		1966 Preretirement	
	W[a]	NW[b]	W	NW	W	NW	W	NW	W	NW	W	NW
Plan to work	1		(5)		(3)		1	1				3
Length of time retired	2											
Level of education	(3)[c]		1		1			3		2		1
Perceived health change	(4)		2		2							
Attitude to retirement					(4)			2				
Working man: free to do things												
Self-perception at age 45										1		
Perceived source of good things												2
No. in group	60	143	31	45	31	45	22	22	18	10	18	10
No. correctly classified	36	113	24	38	24	38	17	18	17	7	17	8

[a] W = work after retiring.
[b] NW = no work after retiring.
[c] ( ) = next in importance, but does not improve discrimination.

In looking at this problem with a more representative sample, that of the 1960 Census 1 in a 1,000 population, those who worked after age sixty-five were found to fall mainly into two income groups, those with the greatest income ($5,000 p.a. and over) and those with the least ($0) (Fillenbaum, unpublished analysis), a finding similar to that reported by Belbin and Clark (1970) using British Census data.

Consistently, both before and after retirement, those who form the working retired group are less likely to report a deterioration in health. The other variables forming the complex generally associated with occupational status did not always emerge as important and when occurring had low correlations with amount of schooling.

Considerable support is available for the second hypothesis. The plans made for retirement do indeed influence retirement activities. The intention to work when retired is the main variable discriminating the working from the nonworking retired in the 1961 group. It is important in a slightly different form in the 1966 preretired group (where the discrimination is on the basis of those who make no plans) and is again relevant after retirement (fifth in order of relevance for the 1966 retired group). Intention to work when retired is, then, extremely important in determining whether an individual will work.

Surprisingly, attitude to retirement appears to be of little consequence, and where it does enter (1966 preretirement data) does not improve the discriminating ability of more important variables. Attitude to retirement is undoubtedly a complex matter; the same attitude may be held by different persons for a variety of different and conflicting reasons.

No data were available to permit all parts of the third hypothesis, which is concerned with some relationships between work and personality, to be examined.

There is little consistent evidence to support the concept that those who work believe they have greater control over what happens to them.

Realizing that the Ss of the 1961 and 1966 groups differed in age range and occupational status, analyses were repeated using only upper occupational level Ss, so controlling for one of the variables on which the groups differed. This should, and in fact does, result in a greater correspondence of findings. It also has the additional effect of removing from consideration an important discriminating variable, so permitting other variables which usually have less discriminating power to become more evident. Those variables which were previously found to be important, level of education and intention to work, are again important. In addition, some confirmatory evidence for the third hypothesis is obtained, the working retired of the 1966 group are, before retirement, more likely to see themselves as being the source of the good things which have happened to them and after retirement hold a more favorable attitude to the past.

The two groups which we have been considering differ markedly in the age range and occupational status of their Ss; nevertheless there is good agreement in the main findings which lead us to believe that these data are generalizable.

The data indicate that those who work after retirement may not only have the mental ability to work at a later age (as evidenced by more schooling), the inclination, and possibly the interest (for they work for some reason other than that of money), but they may also have the physical capacity.

Summary

Multidiscriminant analysis, applied to two groups of *Ss,* indicated that the important ways in which the working retired differed from the non-working retired lay in their having received a larger amount of schooling, intending to work when retired, and being less likely to report a deterioration in health. The working retired also had less financial need to work and held memberships in a larger number of associations, which we interpret to imply a greater involvement in work. The latter, together with success in work and recognition, we felt were major reasons inducing certain persons to work after officially retiring.

REFERENCES

Belbin, R. M., and Clark, F. Le Gros. The relationship between retirement patterns and work as revealed by the British Census. *Industrial Gerontology,* 1970, *4,* 12-26.

Cantril, H. *The pattern of human concerns.* New Brunswick, N.J.: Rutgers University Press, 1965.

Clark, F. Le Gros. *Work, age and leisure.* London: Michael Joseph Ltd., 1966.

Donahue, W., Orbach, H. L., and Pollak, O. *Retirement: The emerging social pattern.* In C. Tibbitts, (Ed.), *Handbook of social gerontology: Societal aspects of aging.* Chicago: University of Chicago Press, 1960.

Friedmann, E. A., and Havighurst, R. J. *The meaning of work and retirement.* Chicago: University of Chicago Press, 1954.

Karp, S. A. Field dependence and occupational activity in the aged. *Perceptual & Motor Skills,* 1967, *24,* 603-609.

Palmore, E. B. Differences in the retirement patterns of men and women. *Gerontologist,* 1965, *5,* 4-8.

Simpson, I. H., Back, K. W., and McKinney, J. C. Work and retirement. In I. H. Simpson, and J. C. McKinney, (Eds.), *Social aspects of aging.* Durham: Duke University Press, 1966.

Steiner, P. O., and Dorfman, R. *The economic status of the aged.* Berkeley: Institute of Industrial Relations, University of California Press, 1957.

Wentworth, E. C. *Employment after retirement.* Research Report No. 21. Office of Research and Statistics, Social Security Administration, US Department of Health, Education, and Welfare, 1968.

Wright, C. R., and Hyman, H. H. Voluntary association membership of American adults. *American Sociological Review,* 1958, *23,* 284-294.

Chapter 20

WORK VERSUS LEISURE ROLES: AN INVESTIGATION OF MORALE AMONG EMPLOYED AND RETIRED MEN

GAYLE B. THOMPSON

THERE IS CONSIDERABLE controversy regarding the social-psychological impact of retirement upon American men. One argument is that separation from work at retirement leads or can lead to demoralization because it represents the loss of a culturally dominant social role and the acquisition of a culturally devalued one. According to this position, the leisure or secondary roles available to the retiree are generally not adequate substitutes for the worker role because of a lack of clear-cut and positive norms regulating behavior in these secondary roles (Riley, Foner, Hess, and Toby, 1969). A basic premise of this argument is that work and not leisure is the dominant value in American society and the major source of a man's social status and self-respect. In view of this, retirement is believed to signify to the individual as well as to others that the retiree is old, useless, and no longer a contributing and vital member of the community. The result frequently is the loss of social status and positive role supports from others and, as a result, a decline in self-respect and self-

Reprinted by permission from the *Journal of Gerontology*, 1973, 28, 339-344.

concept (Blau, 1956; Cavan, 1962; Miller, 1965; Phillips, 1957).

At the opposite end of the controversy are those who contend that positive role realignment is possible upon retirement and that leisure and/or citizenship-service roles can replace work roles and provide a sense of usefulness, personal satisfaction, and positive social support (Atchley, 1971; Bultena and Wood, 1969). Streib and Schneider (1971) reached this conclusion after examination of longitudinal data from the Cornell Study of Occupational Retirement revealed that retirement did not precipitate in sharp decline in feelings of usefulness, satisfaction with life, or self-image. Others have demonstrated that retirement can be a pleasant phase of life, given an adequate retirement income (Barfield and Morgan, 1969) and good health (Shanas, Townsend, Wedderburn, Friis, Milhoj, and Stehouwer, 1968).

The purpose of this paper is to examine the merits of these opposing points of view by investigating differences in the morale of retired and employed men and the reasons for any existing differences. For the sake of argument, the position is taken here that work is the primary source of a man's identity and social position and that retirement results in demoralization because it represents the loss of a primary social role and subsequently undermines the individual's social status and the role supports necessary for a positive self-image. It is also assumed that adequate role substitutes are not available to the retiree because they run counter to the dominant social values.

If this position is valid, then one would expect to find that the retired have lower morale than the employed regardless of any physical or socioeconomic differences which may exist between them. Therefore, the *hypothesis* to be examined is: retired men have lower morale than employed men. To be supported, this hypothesis must hold even when consideration is given to other differences existing between the two groups of men, in age, health, and income, for example, which could conceivably account for the variation in morale.

Methods and Materials

The Sample

This paper is based on data obtained in 1968 from personal interviews with a multistage probability sample of 3,996 non-institutionalized men and women sixty-five years of age and older living in the United States, excluding Alaska and Hawaii. The analysis deals only with the 1,589 men in the sample.

Inasmuch as the units in the sample were selected with unequal probabilities, unbiased estimates of distributions of characteristics in the population were achieved through the introduction of weights which were proportional to the inverse of the probability of selection. These weights also included a constant of such magnitude that the sum of the weighted frequencies would approximate the sum of actual frequencies for the total sample. The size of N reported in the remainder of this paper refers to these weighted frequencies.

The Variables

The variables examined are morale, employment status, physical health, age, and income. Morale is the dependent and employment status the independent variable. The remaining variables are treated as controls.

Since it was assumed that morale, physical health, and social relations were multidimensional, each domain was submitted to a factor analysis using Hotelling's Principle Components Analysis (unity rather than a communality estimate was used in the main diagonal of the correlation matrix) and Kaiser's Varimax method of orthogonal rotation to simple structure. Five morale, six social relations, and four health factors containing 39.0 percent, 42.6 percent, and 51.2 percent of the variance in each domain, respectively, were extracted. Rotated factor scores were computed using all items in the domain. For cross-tabulation, individuals were divided into three or more categories of approximately equal size on the basis of their rotated factor scores.

The analysis presented here is restricted to three of the above mentioned factors: age-associated morale, perception of physical health, and functional disability. The following briefly describes these three factors and other variables used in this investigation.

AGE-ASSOCIATED MORALE: This factor reflects reactions to aging. It measures whether the individual has a positive or negative age identification, perceives of himself as getting less useful and less happy with age, and views aging and the future with optimism or pessimism. Items with loadings over .350 were as follows:

Age image (positive vs. negative)	.577
Things keep getting worse as you get older. (yes or no)	.563
You have as much pep as you did last year. (yes or no)	.636
As you grow older, you are less useful. (yes or no)	.668
As you get older, would you say things are better, worse, or the same as you thought they would be?	.398
You are as happy now as when you were younger. (yes or no)	.368
What will life be like for you in a year (happier, the same, not as happy)?	.354
Little things bother you more this year. (yes or no)	.351

PERCEPTION OF PHYSICAL HEALTH: This factor measures the individual's subjective evaluation of his general physical health, whether it was very good or very poor, how it compared to others' health and to his own at age sixty and the extent to which health was believed to restrict his activities or require help from others. The items with factor loadings over .350 were as follows:

In general, would you say that your health today is very good, good fair, or poor?	.727
Would you say that your health is better, about the same, or worse than most people your age?	.643
How is your health today compared to how it was last year? Is it better, about the same, or worse?	.654
Comparing your health today to how it was when you were sixty, is it better, about the same, or worse?	.692
Does bad health, sickness or pain ever stop you from doing things you'd like to be doing? (Never, most of the time, half the time, once in a while)	.582
Length of time R had had any existing medical condition.	.449
How much help do you need for health reasons (none, some a lot)?	.386

FUNCTIONAL DISABILITY: This factor measures functional limitations in the ability to carry out a series of tasks such as gardening, painting furniture, driving a car, and taking short trips. Items with factor loadings over .350 were as follows:

Whether or not you can do them, do you think you would have trouble physically doing any of the following tasks (never, occasionally, frequently, always)?

Fixing appliances in need of minor repair	−.772
Driving a car a short distance	−.739
Taking a train or airplane trip for half a day or longer	−.669
Painting or touching up furniture or parts of the house	−.803
Planting and keeping up a lawn or garden	−.728
Cooking a meal	−.427
How much help do you need for health reasons (none, some, a lot)?	−.413
Would you have trouble doing things about the house without help (never, occasionally, frequently, or always)?	−.398

AGE: The men in this study ranged in age from sixty-five to ninety-eight and over with a mean of seventy-three and a median of seventy-one. Of the 1,568 *Ss* reporting age, 36.4 percent were aged sixty-five to sixty-nine, 29.0 percent were aged seventy to seventy-four, 21.5 percent were aged seventy-five to seventy-nine, and 13.1 percent were eighty years of age and older.

EMPLOYMENT STATUS: Information on employment status was obtained by responses to the following two questions: "Are you employed now?" and if employed, "Are you employed full-time or part-time?" An individual was classified as retired if he had ceased working whether he was seeking employment or not and as employed if he performed full-time or part-time work. Approximately 80 percent of the 1,575 *Ss* answering were retired; the other 20 percent were employed.

INCOME: Income was measured as the sum of money income, as recalled by the respondent, received by the aged person and his or her spouse from all sources except assistance from family members in the twelve months prior to the interview. These income sources were wages, salaries and commissions, professional fees, business profits, rent, insurance payments, interest and dividends, public and private pensions, unemployment benefits, and other sources such as sick benefits. Of those reporting income (N = 1,331), the sample distributed as follows: 7.7 percent under 1,000; 27.1

percent between $1,000 and $1,999; 21.8 percent between $2,000 and $2,999; 23.9 percent between $3,000 and $4,999; 14.5 percent between $5,000 and $9,999; and 5.0 percent at $10,000 and over.

Results

The data in Table 20-I indicate a definite tendency for the retired to experience lower age-associated morale than the employed with 35.3 percent of the retired men and 18.6 percent of the employed men falling in the low morale group. This finding lent tentative support to the main hypothesis.

A preliminary comparison of these two groups of men revealed that the retired were somewhat older, more disabled, more likely to perceive their health in negative terms, and poorer than the employed. It is plausible, therefore, that their lower morale could be the result of these socioeconomic and physical disadvantages and not a retirement itself. To test this, the main hypothesis was reexamined with age, functional disability, perception of health, and income introduced as controls, both separately and in combination. Since the retired and employed did not differ significantly on occupation, education, marital status, or extent of participation in clubs or interaction with friends, it was not necessary to control for the effects of these variables.

TABLE 20-I

AGE - ASSOCIATED MORALE BY
EMPLOYMENT STATUS

Morale	Employed %	Retired %
Low	18.6	35.3
Medium	35.5	33.5
High	45.9	31.2
Total %	100.0	100.0
N	318	1257

Gamma = —.313 $p < .0001$

Functional disability and perception of health, taken separately, did not fully account for the morale differences existing between retired and employed men as the data in Tables 20-II and 20-III demonstrate. This means that the lower morale of the retired cannot be explained solely in terms of their more negative health perceptions nor their functional limitations.

Although health perception did not account for all of the variation in age-associated morale, it is interesting to note that substantial morale differences existed only for those with average health perceptions.

Another interesting phenomenon demonstrated by the data in Table 20-III is that morale steadily declined as health perceptions became more negative. While only 12.5 percent of the retired men with positive health perceptions had low morale, 33.4 percent of those with average and 57.3 percent of those with negative perceptions exhibited low morale. The proportions of employed men with low morale in each of these health groups were 4.9 percent, 16.7 percent, and 55.7 percent, respectively.

These latter two findings suggest that performance of a socially acceptable role, that of worker, may be insufficient to overcome the demoralizing effects of a negative evaluation of health and, further, that positive health perceptions may intervene between role loss and morale. It appears that if retirement has any impact on psychological well-being, its effects are restricted to those whose health perceptions fall in the middle range.

Given the negative cultural value attached to the aging role (Rosow, 1967) and the fact that the retired tend to be older than the employed, it would seem that age by itself could explain a major portion of the variation in morale between the retired and the employed. The data presented in

TABLE 20-II

AGE - ASSOCIATED MORALE BY EMPLOYMENT STATUS CONTROLLED FOR
FUNCTIONAL DISABILITY

			Functional Disability			
	High		Average		Low	
Morale	Employed	Retired	Employed	Retired	Employed	Retired
	%	%	%	%	%	%
Low	40.3	52.8	7.6	25.8	19.5	25.5
Medium	35.5	32.2	37.9	29.2	34.1	39.4
High	24.2	15.0	54.5	45.1	46.3	35.1
Total %	100.0	100.0	100.0	100.1	99.9	100.0
N	62	446	132	407	123	404

Gamma = —.233   Gamma = —.274   Gamma = —.187
N   =   .002 p =   .0008 p =   .017

TABLE 20-III

AGE - ASSOCIATED MORALE BY EMPLOYMENT STATUS CONTROLLED FOR
PERCEPTION OF HEALTH

			Perception of Health			
	Negative		Average		Positive	
Morale	Employed	Retired	Employed	Retired	Employed	Retired
	%	%	%	%	%	%
Low	55.7	57.3	16.7	33.4	4.9	12.5
Medium	29.5	31.3	39.5	39.1	35.7	29.8
High	14.8	11.4	43.8	27.5	59.4	57.7
Total %	100.0	100.0	100.0	100.0	100.0	100.0
N	61	436	114	432	143	389

Gamma = —.049   Gamma = —.343   Gamma = —.090
p =   .363 p <   .0001 p =   .174

Table 20-IV indicate that this is not the case. Regardless of chronological age, the retired tended to have lower morale than the employed. Furthermore, the magnitude of the morale differences, as indicated by the size of Gamma, became larger for each successive age group. This suggests that for the very old, those over the age of seventy, the state of being in retirement may be a more psychologically negative life situation than it is for those seventy years of age and younger and that work may help them overcome negative feelings toward themselves as aging persons.

What about the effect of income? Can

the lower morale of the retired be attributed to financial deprivation rather than to a negative reaction to loss of the worker role? The data in Table 20-V suggest that the lower morale of the retired cannot be explained solely in terms of their financial deprivation relative to the employed group. Regardless of income level, the retired have lower morale than the employed. For example, among those with incomes of less than $3,000 per year, 29.3 percent of the employed compared to 42.4 percent of the retired had low morale.

To say that income does not explain all of the variation between employment

TABLE 20-IV

AGE - ASSOCIATED MORALE BY EMPLOYMENT STATUS CONTROLLED FOR AGE

Morale	65 — 67 Years		68 — 70 Years		71 — 75 Years		76 Years +	
	Employed %	Retired %	Employed %	Retired %	Employed %	Retired %	Employed %	Retired %
Low	21.6	26.2	10.4	25.1	17.6	37.4	25.0	45.6
Medium	33.3	41.7	33.8	25.9	40.5	34.6	33.9	33.0
High	45.0	32.1	55.8	49.0	41.9	28.0	41.1	21.3
Total %	99.0	100.0	100.0	100.0	100.0	100.0	100.0	99.9
N	111	214	77	283	74	352	56	401

Gamma $= -.190$ Gamma $= -.204$ Gamma $= -.342$ Gamma $= -.392$

$p = .028$ $p = .038$ $p = .0006$ $p = .0003$

TABLE 20-V
AGE - ASSOCIATED MORALE BY EMPLOYMENT STATUS CONTROLLED FOR
INCOME

	INCOME					
	$0 — $2,999		*$3,000 — $4,999*		*$5,000 and Over*	
Morale	*Employed*	*Retired*	*Employed*	*Retired*	*Employed*	*Retired*
	%	%	%	%	%	%
Low	29.3	42.4	14.3	27.9	17.8	22.5
Medium	36.4	31.1	38.1	37.9	24.8	31.4
High	34.3	26.5	47.6	34.2	57.4	46.1
Total %	100.0	100.0	100.0	100.0	100.0	100.0
N	99	654	63	254	101	159

| Gamma = —.211 | Gamma = —.285 | Gamma = —.186 |
| p = .009 | p = .009 | p = .049 |

status and morale does not mean, however, that it exerted no influence at all. The fact that only 4.7 percentage points separated the employed and the retired with low morale among those with incomes of $5,000 or more per year (compared to differences of 13.1 and 13.6 among those with incomes of less than $3,000 and between $3,000 and $4,999, respectively) suggests that adequate retirement income may partially compensate for role loss. Furthermore, the substantial increase in the proportion of retired men with low morale with decreases in income suggests that financial deprivation may intensify the psychological effects of retirement.

The findings discussed above indicate that no single factor fully accounts for the morale differences existing between employed and retired men. But what about the combined effects of age, health, and income? In order to answer this question, partial correlations were computed. The results are presented in Table 20-VI.

These partial correlations demonstrate that when the combined effects of perception of health, age, functional disability, and income were controlled, the relationship between employment status and age-associated morale became quite small, although still significant at the .01 level. This means that the variation in morale between retired and employed men was primarily accounted for by the combined effects of differences in perception of health, disability, age, and income. These findings suggest, then, that the retired exhibit lower morale than the employed principally because they are older, functionally more disabled, more likely to view their health in negative terms, and less well off financially and not because of any negative reaction to loss of the worker role.

Summary

The basic thesis underlying this paper is that work is the primary source of a man's social status and self-identity and that, as a result, retirement from the role of worker has negative consequences for psychological adjustment. In order to evaluate this thesis, it was hypothesized that the retired have lower morale than the employed regardless of any differences which might exist between these two groups on other factors related to both employment status and morale.

Investigation of this hypothesis revealed that most of the variation in the morale of retired and employed men was explained

TABLE 20-VI

PARTIAL CORRELATIONS: AGE - ASSOCIATED MORALE WITH EMPLOYMENT
STATUS, CONTROLLED FOR HEALTH, AGE, AND INCOME

Control Variables	Partial	N
Health Perception	—.135**	1575
Functional Disability	—.175**	1575
Income	—.163**	1331
Age	—.168**	1508
Functional Disability and Age	—.158**	1568
Functional Disability and Income	—.149**	1331
Age and Income	—.143**	1331
Health Perception and Functional Disability	—.112**	1575
Health Perception and Age	—.106**	1568
Health Perception and Income	—.118**	1331
Functional Disability, Income, and Age	—.136**	1331
Functional Disability, Income, and Health Perception	—.100**	1331
Functional Disability, Health Perception, and Age	—.093**	1568
Health Perception, Income, and Age	—.095**	1331
Health Perception, Functional Disability, Age, Income	—.085*	1331

$*p<.01$　　　$**p<.001$

Note: The zero-order correleation between employment status and morale was —.194.

in terms of a combination of four variables: perception of health, age, income, and functional disability. The retired exhibited lower morale than the employed principally because they had more negative evaluations of their health, were more functionally disabled, were poorer and were older *and not* simply because they were retired.

These results challenge the thesis on which this analysis was originally based and the theory that work is necessarily the central value in the lives of all older American males. It appears that given relative youth, an optimistic view of health, a lack of functional disability, and an adequate income, the retirement years can be as pleasant as the years of employment for a great many men and that leisure roles can adequately substitute for that of worker.

REFERENCES

Atchley, R. C. Retirement and leisure participation: Continuity or crisis. *Gerontologist,* 1971, *11,* 13-17.

Barfield, R., and Morgan, J. *Early retirement The decision and the experience.* University of Michigan, Institute for Social Research, Ann Arbor, 1969.

Blau, Z. S. Changes in status and age identification. *American Sociological Review,* 1965 *21,* 198-203.

Bultena, G. L., and Wood, V. The American retirement community: Bane or blessing *Journal of Gerontology,* 1969, *24,* 209-218.

Cavan, R. S. Self and role in adjustment during old age. In A. M. Rose (Ed.), *Human behavior and social processes.* Houghton Mifflin, Boston, 1962.

Miller, S. J. The dilemma of a social role fo the aging. Papers in Social Welfare, No. 8 Heller Graduate School, Brandeis Univ. Waltham, Mass., 1965.

Phillips, B. S. A role theory approach to adjustment in old age. *American Sociologica Review,* 1957, *22,* 212-217.

Riley, M. W., Foner, A., Hess, B., and Toby M. L. Socialization for the middle and late years. In D. Goslin (Ed.), *Handbook of soc ialization theory and research.* Rand Mc-Nally, Chicago, 1969.

Rosow, I. *Social integration of the aged.* Free Press, New York, 1967.

Shanas, E., Townsend, P., Wedderburn, D., Friis, H., Milhoj, P., and Stehouwer, J. *Old people in three industrial societies.* Atherton Press, New York, 1968.

Streib, G. F., and Schneider, C. J. *Retirement in American society.* Cornell University Press, Ithaca, NY, 1971.

ATTITUDES TOWARD AGE AND AGING

ALTHOUGH GERONTOLOGY HAS SHOWN an interest in attitudes from its beginnings, research among different age groups began in earnest during the late 1940s and early 1950s. For the most part, these studies involved samples of college students and employed relatively uncomplicated measuring devices. The principal goal of these efforts was to document a number of stereotypes concerning age. On the basis of these populations, a generally negative view of both age and the aged was evidenced (Tuckman and Lorge, 1953; 1954). In addition to the young, however, older individuals were also found to associate age with decay, decline, and disrespect. Their denial of age group membership (Tuckman and Lorge, 1954) as well as their use of unfavorable adjectives to describe older persons (Mason, 1954), convinced many researchers of the reality of these stereotypical views.

Along with attitudes toward age and aging, gerontologists attempted to assess the predispositions of older persons toward a host of factors. Attitudes toward religion, retirement, and death multiplied. Portions of these data were to form the empirical base for theories regarding such issues as morale, adjustment, and life satisfaction. Relatively few efforts were made, however, to relate attitudes to patterns of behavior. On the basis of correlational measures, causal connections were implied rather than stated explicitly. Perhaps the principal exception to this picture occurred in the case of self attitudes. Sharing the heritage of an earlier phenomenology, gerontologists postulated numerous relationships between the self-view of the aged and their subsequent behavior (Mason, 1954).

As one would expect, this research was essentially descriptive in character. Although efforts were made to tap the attitudes of one generation toward another, the results of such study were often limited to the cataloguing and comparison of apparent differences. Few attempts were made to relate given attitudes to specific patterns or styles of behavior. At best, correlational techniques established tentative relationships between the attitudes of the aged and such phenomena as good health, high morale, and retirement adjustment. For the most part, however, attitudes comprised only a tangential element in the theories of the period.

The late 1950s and early 1960s were to see significant advances in both the measurement and understanding of attitudes. Researchers expanded the adjective checklists of the previous era. In addition, use was made of such devices as sentence completion tests (Golde and Kogan, 1959), likert scales, and semantic differential formats (Kogan, 1961). Through the use of several such measures, gerontologists not only compiled information as to age-related attitudes, but were also able to assess the validity and reliability of their instruments.

In addition to considering the relationship between aging and attitudes, attention was focused on the social and psychological circumstances giving rise to such predispositions (Hansen, 1965; Heyman and Jeffers, 1964; Anderson, 1965). High on the list of interest were those factors related to the concept of self (Bloom, 1961; Zola, 1962). Through such efforts, self-views were regarded as intervening elements in the behavioral repertoire of the older adult. With this, a new model of behavior emerged. Social and psychological events became viewed as the precursors of aging attitudes. In turn, these attitudes assumed a dominant role in the behavior of the elderly.

Together with the emphasis upon phenomenological investigation went attempts to relate personality attributes to attitudinal changes (Dean, 1962; Kogan, 1961; Kuhlen, 1964; Slater, 1964). While frequently productive of contradictory outcomes, such efforts succeeded in deepening the gerontologist's appreciation for individual differences. In a similar fashion, the assessment of aging stereotypes questioned seriously the negative findings of the preceding era. These contradictory results were to figure prominently in the development of cross-generational research.

The work of this period, then, moved beyond the realm of description. In addition to seeking the source(s) of attitudes prevalent among the aged, researchers gave full emphasis to the motivational dimensions of each. Such efforts led to a number of theories concerning the behavior of the aged (see Section II). Nevertheless, the greatest contribution to theory formation came as a result of a number of advances in methodology and research design. Along these lines, the longitudinal or panel format rapidly became the most useful and meaningful device relative to theory construction and verification. In the same fashion, statistical advances improved the limited effectiveness of cross-sectional analyses.

Gerontological study in the late 1960s and early 1970s continues to refine attitudinal instruments. Besides adjective checklists (Aaronson, 1966), semantic differential, likert scale, and experimental designs have been enlisted by contemporary scholars (Peters, 1971; Preston and Gudiksen, 1966; Rosencranz and McNevin, 1969). These efforts have cast considerable doubt on a generalized negative view of the aged. Generational studies, for instance, have reported numerous positive judgments with the advancing age of a stimulus person or group (Eisdorfer, 1966; Hickey and Kalish, 1968; Shanas, 1968). Intergenerational research has also shown a lessening of negative affect relative to older respondents (Bortner, 1967; Carp, 1967; Back, 1971; Robin, 1971). Still other studies report a more positive view of self and the future among the aged (Gergen and Back, 1966; Lehr, 1967). It would appear that contemporary social changes have included a more positive view of age and the aged.

Along with the emphasis upon attitudinal measurement and intergeneration-al comparisons have gone renewed attempts to delineate the situations and circumstances giving rise to such attitudes. One result of these efforts has been to place the variables of income, health, and social class in perspective relative to the attitudes of the elderly (Becker and Strauss, 1968). These attitudes have, in turn, been related to several behavioral patterns (e.g. retirement adjustment and social participation). What has emerged is a theory of behavior which holds attitudes to be tempered in their effects by a number of social and psychological factors. Thus, in the contemporary view, attitudes represent only one of several elements influencing the behavior of the aged.

Still another development of the contemporary era has been a willingness to test and modify these theoretical formulations. In so doing, researchers have gone beyond "typical" populations of older persons to include both the ethnic and minority aged (Wylie, 1971). In general, these efforts have combined both longitudinal and cross-sectional formats. The upshot has been to introduce still other intervening factors into the attitude-behavior equation.

The papers which follow are examples of contemporary attitudinal research. For the most part, these works reflect the concern for instrumental improvement. They also illustrate the changing character of aging stereotypes. In addition, they champion interest in the various circumstances and contexts which influence attitude formation. Finally, each paper alludes to probable relationships between attitudes and specific patterns (or styles) of behavior.

The paper by Seltzer and Atchley examines various changes in the attitudes and stereotypes toward the aged by means of an analysis of a sample of children's literature encompassing the period from 1870 to 1960. Given the youth orientation in the culture and an increase in the proportion of older persons in the population, the authors hypothesize that (1) attitudes toward old people or things will have become decreasingly positive over the past century; (2) there will have been a decrease in the number of references to old people or things relative to the number of references to young people or new things; and (3) the more recent children's literature should reveal an increasing variability in the descriptions of old people or things.

The authors observe that while differences are found to exist in terms of the positive or negative references to the aged over this period, these differences for the most part were not statistically significant. On the other hand, while the number of references to old people relative to young became fewer over the period, this decrease followed a curvilinear rather than a linear course. Finally, the findings reveal an increase in the relative proportion of acts having positive value initiated by old compared with younger individuals.

The work of Cryns and Monk represents an exploration of the attitudes of the aged toward the young. The authors point out that attitudinal studies for the most part have failed to consider the fact that, "perceptual processes are shaped not only by the attributes, real or alleged, of the objects of attitudes or perceptions, but also by the subjective frame of mind of the perceiver or attitude carrier himself." As a consequence, this study attempts to test the hypothesis that the aged's attitudes toward the young will be a function of two subjective dimensions, the older person's level of life satisfaction, and the quality of the relationship which prevails, or at one time did prevail, between him and his children.

Data for the study were obtained from fifty-three white elderly male participants of one of four Senior Citizens Centers located in a Western New York urban area. The findings suggest that the attitudinal evaluation of the young is apt to be influenced by the subjective attributes of life satisfaction and quality of filial relationship. Aged persons with high life satisfaction and good filial relationships tend to demonstrate a significantly more favorable attitude toward the young than do those of low life satisfaction and with poor filial relationships.

Ahammer and Baltes examine the question of age attitudes more comprehensively. Specifically, the authors focus attention not only on how the old and young perceive each other, but also consider how each respective age group views itself. Their purpose is to investigate both objective and perceived age differences in four personality dimensions across a wide age range. The imposition of both an objective and subjective measure of age differences permits an examination of the generation gap phenomenon.

To determine whether misperceptions exist not only between adolescents and adults but also between adults and their parent generation, the authors include three age groups in their study—adolescents (15–18), adults (34–40), and older people (64–74). Information representing the behavioral areas of affiliation, achievement, autonomy, and nurturance was obtained by means of the Jackson Personality Form.

The authors observe that on two dimensions (autonomy and nurturance) perceived and actual age differences did not coincide. Nevertheless, adolescents and adults perceived older people as judging nurturance as more and autonomy as less desirable, and adults perceived adolescents as valuing autonomy higher than they actually did. The results of this study make it apparent that if self-reports are taken as the criterion on some dimension, age groups do in fact misperceive each other.

The final paper in this section concerns the relationship between chronological age and reported attitudinal judgments. The authors observe that much of the current literature regarding perceptual evaluations stems essentially from survey methodologies. These methodologies rarely consider both sides of the generational picture. In addition, they focus upon hypothetical "older" or "younger" individuals to whom are assigned a group of descriptive adjectives or attributes. The present paper, however, employs not only a different research design (i.e. an experimental format), but uses the "nominal" services of a stimulus person with respect to two different age groupings.

The data reveal a slight but nonsignificant tendency for younger subjects to rate the older stimulus person more positively than do the older subjects. "In the case of actual age judgments, however, all subjects, regardless of age, reflect a tendency . . . to rate the younger stimulus person more positively than the older individual. In and of itself, chronological age appears insufficient to control strongly a pattern of judgment relative to a stimulus person." The authors suggest their findings call into question (1) the employment of chronological categories in assessing age-related attitudes, and (2) that research which reports the predominately negative character of such responses.

REFERENCES

Aaronson, B. S. Personality stereotypes of aging. *Journal of Gerontology*, 1966, *21*, 458-462.

Anderson, N. N. Institutionalization, interaction, and self conception in aging. In A. M. Rose and W. A. Peterson (Eds.), *Older people and their social world*. Philadelphia: F. A. Davis, 1965.

Back, K. W. Transition to aging and the self image. *Aging and Human Development*, 1971, *2*, 296-304.

Becker, H. S., and Strauss, A. Careers, personality, and adult socialization. In B. L. Neugarten (Ed.), *Middle age and aging*. Chicago: University of Chicago Press, 1968.

Bloom, K. L. Age and self concept. *American Journal of Psychiatry*, 1961, *118*, 534-538.

Bortner, R. W. Personality and social psychology in the study of aging. *Gerontologist*, 1967, *7*, 23-36.

Carp, F. M. Attitudes of old persons toward themselves and toward others. *Journal of Gerontology*, 1967, *22*, 308-312.

Dean, L. R. Aging and the decline of affect. *Journal of Gerontology*, 1962, *17*, 440-446.

Eisdorfer, C. Attitudes toward old people: a re-analysis of the item validity of the stereotype scale. *Journal of Gerontology*, 1966, *21*, 455-462.

Gergen, K. J., and Back, K. W. Cognitive constriction in aging and attitudes toward international issues. In I. H. Simpson and J. C. McKinney (Eds.), *Social aspects of aging*. Durham, North Carolina: Duke University Press, 1966.

Golde, P., and Kogan, N. A sentence completion procedure for assessing attitudes toward old people. *Journal of Gerontology*, 1959, *14*, 355-363.

Hansen, G. D., Yoshioka, S., Taves, M. J., and Caro, F. Older people in the midwest: conditions and attitudes. In A. M. Rose and W. A. Peterson (Eds.), *Older people and their social world*. Philadelphia: F. A. Davis, 1965.

Heyman, D. K., and Jeffers, F. C. Study of the relative influence of race and socio-economic status upon the activities and attitudes of a southern aged population. *Journal of Gerontology*, 1964, *19*, 225-229.

Hickey, T. and Kalish, R. A. Young peoples' perceptions of adults. *Journal of Gerontology*, 1968, *23*, 215-219.

Kogan, N. Attitude toward old people in an old sample. *Journal of Social Psychology*, 1961, *62*, 616-622.

Kogan, N., and Wallach, M. A. Age changes in values and attitudes. *Journal of Gerontology*, 1961, *16*, 272-280.

Kuhlen, R. G. Personality change with age. In P. Worchel and D. Byrne (Eds.), *Personality change*. New York: John Wiley, 1964.

Lehr, U. Attitudes toward the future in old age. *Human Development*, 1967, *10*, 230-238.

Mason, E. Some correlates of self-judgments of the aged. *Journal of Gerontology*, 1954, *9*, 324-337.

Peters, G. R. Self conceptions of the aged, age identification, and aging. *Gerontologist*, 1971, *11*, 69-73.

Preston, C. E., and Gudiksen, K. S. A measure of self perception among older people.

Journal of Gerontology, 1966, *21,* 63-71.

Robin, E. P. Discontinuities in attitudes and behaviors of older age groups. *Gerontologist,* 1971, *11,* 79-84.

Rosencranz, H. A., and McNevin, T. E. A factor analysis of attitudes toward the aged. *Gerontologist,* 1969, *9,* 55-59.

Shanas, E. A note on restriction of life space: attitudes of age cohorts. *Journal of Health and Social Behavior,* 1968, *9,* 86-90.

Slater, P. E., and Scarr, H. A. Personality in old age. *Genetic Psychology Monographs,* 1964, *70,* 229-269.

Tuckman, J., and Lorge, I. Attitudes toward old people. *Journal of Social Psychology,* 1953, 7, 249-260.

Tuckman, J., and Lorge, I. Classification of the self as young, middle-aged, or old. *Geriatrics,* 1954, *9,* 534-536.

Wylie, R. W. Attitudes toward aging and the aged among black Americans: some historical perspectives. *Aging and Human Development,* 1971, *2,* 66-70.

Zola, I. K. Feelings about age among older people. *Journal of Gerontology,* 1962, *17,* 65-68.

Chapter 21

THE CONCEPT OF OLD: CHANGING ATTITUDES AND STEREOTYPES

MILDRED M. SELTZER AND
ROBERT C. ATCHLEY

ONE OF THE CENTRAL tenets of the symbolic interactionist approach to social psychology is that the mental constructs which go to form what we call the mind intervene between stimulus and response and influence both. It is widely held that what we think about a person influences how we will perceive him, and how we perceive him influences how we will behave toward him.

Two particularly important types of mental constructs involved in this process are attitudes and stereotypes. Attitudes are predispositions to respond toward a person or thing in either a positive or a negative way. Stereotypes are sets of beliefs which purport to describe typical members of a category of people, objects, or ideas. These beliefs are then acted upon as if they were true, regardless of the empirical facts. Those mental constructs which influence our perceptions and behavior are thought to be *learned,* either by trial and error or by the somewhat more conscious and often subtle teaching processes of socialization.

Since attitudes and stereotypes are felt to have a strong influence on perception and behavior, those who study human aging have devoted considerable attention

Reprinted by permission from the *Gerontologist,*
1971, *11,* 226-230.

to research on attitudes and stereotypes concerning old people. (Calhoun and Gottesman, 1963; Eisdorfer and Wilkie, 1967; Golde and Kogan, 1959; Hickey and Kalish, 1968; Kogan, 1961; Tuckman, 1958; Tuckman and Lorge, 1953.) However, the processes people go through to acquire these attitudes and stereotypes have not been studied in any detail. It has been assumed that many attitudes and stereotypes, including those concerning old people, are learned early in life. Such concepts may be relatively enduring and have consequences for both the behavior others direct *toward* older people and the development of one's self-concept *as* an older person. Hence, the knowledge of the means by which children learn their concepts about the old and of the changes that may have occurred in the concepts being presented through these means would appear to be necessary for an adequate understanding of attitudes and stereotypes concerning the old. The rationale for this is that changes in attitudes and stereotypes should be reflected in their means of transmission.

The present research sought to examine changes in attitudes and stereotypes concerning old people and things as presented in children's books during the period from 1870 to 1960. Several hypotheses were advanced based on two general historical trends in American society during this period.

The first trend was the increasing youth-orientation of American culture. While this is not the place to go into the genesis of this trend, perhaps it can be said that various structural changes in American society have gradually produced a situation in which the prospective contributions of the young receive greater attention and have greater influence than the past contributions of the old. As a concomitant of this trend it was expected that (H:1) attitudes toward old people or things would have become decreasingly positive over the past century; and that (H:2) there would have been a decrease in the number of references to old people or things relative to the number of references to young people or new things.

The second trend was the increase in the size of the population of older people in the United States since the Civil War. Based on the proposition that as the population increases, variations of and deviations from the norms increase (Mott, 1965), it was expected that (H:3) the more recent children's literature would reveal an increased variability in the descriptions of old people or things.

Materials and Methods

While support for the three hypotheses could be sought in any of a number of sources, it was sought in children's literature published since 1870. The decision to use this source was based on the assumption that such literature serves as a major agent of socialization and culture transmission, at least for the middle and upper social classes. It provides a particularly rich source of data for assessing changes through time in both the language and the concepts used by society.

The sample of children's literature to be analyzed was selected from four time periods spaced thirty years apart, beginning with the first census following the Civil War (e.g. 1870, 1900, 1930, and 1960). By using thirty-year intervals it was anticipated that any changes in time and direction could be easily observed.

The specific sample of books and pages was randomly selected from a universe consisting of a well-known collection of children's books, the E. W. King Collection, housed at Miami University, plus selected

issues of *The Horn Book*. Forty books were used, ten from each of the four time periods studied. These books were a diverse selection including various kinds of literature and levels of reading ability. The use of an unstructured reading sample avoided the formality, structure, and regional biases particularly for the earlier time periods that make classroom readers and textbooks less desirable sources. Unstructured reading was also considered more characteristic of an individual's natural reading experiences.

Three separate but interrelated methods of analysis were used: semantic differential, content analysis, and frequency count.

The first hypothesis, that attitudes toward old people or things would have become decreasingly positive over the past century, was tested by means of the semantic differential. The original semantic differential technique developed by Osgood, Succi, and Tannenbaum (1965) was modified by subdividing each of the three semantic dimensions of evaluation, activity, and potency into three levels: psychological, social, and physical. Eighteen bipolar adjectives were assigned to the three dimensions and three levels of semantic space each set being used twice, once for the dimension and once for the level. A nineteenth set, old-young (or old-new) was used as a check on the original selection of characters and articles in relation to their age.

From the original sample of forty books, twenty-eight were selected for semantic differential analysis, seven from each of the four time periods. These twenty-eight books contained the most complete data for making comparisons between old and young characters. Semantic differential booklets of eight pages each were developed for each of the twenty-eight books. Con cept headings were individual old and young characters and old and new objects from the books, the book or selections from it, and control characters.

Two groups of readers, seven married housewives and seven graduate students read these books and completed the appropriate semantic differential booklets. A housewife and a graduate student were both assigned to one book from each of the four time periods. Immediately after reading each book, the reader was asked to complete the semantic differential booklet developed for that specific book. The data obtained in this manner were then used to test changes in meaning over time, particularly on the evaluation dimension, as an indication of changes and variability in descriptions of characters, both over time and within time periods.

Rater reliability for each pair of raters was computed. With the exception of one pair whose inter-rater reliability was 2.6, reliability ranged from .56 to .77. While one would have preferred greater rater reliability, these were greater than chance correlations.

Semantic differential data were also used to test the third hypothesis that the more recent children's literature would reveal an increased variability in the descriptions of old people or things. For testing purposes, this hypothesis was broken down into three components: (1) there are significant differences between personality descriptions of old and young characters both within and across time periods, (2) there are significant differences between activities initiated by old and by young characters within and across time periods, and (3) there are significant differences in actions directed toward or upon old people and things compared with young people or new things within and over time periods.

Frequency count technique involved the simple enumeration of all age-related words and the total number of words on sample pages in the original sample of forty books. These data provided information on the total number of words, the total number of age-related words, and the breakdown of these into young and old words. The percentages and ratios obtained in this manner provided information on trends in age-grading in children's literature over the past century. Data obtained in this way were used to test the hypothesis that there would have been a decrease in the number of references to old people or things relative to the number of references to young people or new things. Pooled rater reliability for frequency count enumerators was .97.

Content analysis judges coded the same sample data used for the frequency count. These sentences containing any kind of age referent constituted the basic unit of analysis. Judges classified sentence content with reference to five categories: the age of the referent (old or young), sex of the referent, whether the referent were animate or inanimate, whether the referent were an initiator or recipient of action, and the valence of the action. All content analysis data were coded by two judges. When differences in categorizing occurred, a third judge made the final coding decision. Judges' reliability ranged from .75 to .89.

Results

In testing the first hypothesis, that attitudes toward old people or things would have become decreasingly positive over the past century, statistically significant changes in the evaluation dimension of semantic differential data were used as evidence of attitude change. Interestingly enough, while the raw data showed the means of the evaluation dimension almost consistently lower for old compared with young characters, the differences between means for old and young characters on this dimension were not statistically significant except for the period 1870.

The second hypothesis predicted a decrease in the number of references to old people or things relative to the number of references to young people or new things. Frequency count data supported this hypothesis. Again there was a particularly interesting twist in that this decrease followed a curvilinear rather than an expected linear decrease so that the 1960 proportions were similar to those found in 1870 (Table 21-I).

Both content analysis and semantic differential data were to test the third hypothesis that the more recent children's literature would reveal an increased variability in the descriptions of old people and things. As noted previously, this hypothesis was broken down into three component parts.

Semantic differential data were used to test the first subhypothesis that there are significant differences between personality descriptions of old and young characters within and across time periods. Personality was operationally defined as the mean scores on the three semantic dimensions and the three levels of semantic analysis. Significant *t*-statistics were considered evidence of differences in personality descriptions within time periods. From Table 21-II it is apparent that, particularly in 1870 and 1900, there were some significant differences between the descriptions of old and young characters. In 1870 differences were found on the dimensions of activity and evaluation and on the physical level: in 1900, only on the activity dimension and on the physical level. The lack of more statistically significant differences is perhaps the most significant piece of datum in testing this hypothesis.

An analysis of variance design was used to test for differences across time periods. It was found that the two factors, time and age, were significant in accounting for some of the differences in personality descriptions. Time, for example, was significant for all three semantic dimensions and for the physical level. Age accounted for differ-

TABLE 21-I
RELATIONSHIP OF OLD WORDS TO ALL AGE - ORIENTED WORDS
BY TIME PERIOD

Words	Time Period				
	1870	1900	1930	1960	Total
Old	174	244	105	263	786
% old of all age-related words	20.74	41.50	41.67	31.76	31.35
Young	665	344	147	565	1,721
% young of all age-related words	79.26	58.50	58.33	68.24	68.65
Total	839	588	252	828	2,507

$\chi^2 = 83.78$
$df = 3$

$p < 0.001$ (indicates significant difference between the old and young subjects at the .001 level of probability. A difference this large would occur by chance alone only once in 1000 times).

TABLE 21-II
T - TEST SCORES FOR PERSONALITY
CHARACTERISTICS OF OLD AND YOUNG CHARACTERS BY DIMENSION,
LEVEL, AND TIME PERIOD

Dimension and Level	Time Period			
	1870	1900	1930	1960
Dimension				
Activity	3.75*	2.15*	1.75	1.11
Potency	.48	.44	.48	.23
Evaluation	2.44***	1.16	1.79	.48
Level				
Psychological	1.45	.66	.46	.22
Social	1.79	.41	.53	.50
Physical	2.49**	2.95*	2.05	.98****

*significant $p<0.01$ (a difference this large would occur by chance only once in 100 times).

**significant $p<0.02$ (a difference this large would occur by chance only once in 200 times).

***significant $p<0.05$ (a difference this large would occur by chance only once in 500 times).

****This finding, while statistically not significant, should be noted because in 1960 there was a marked break in the pattern found on this level of analysis. For the three preceding time periods (1930 — 2.05 missed .05 level of significance by .01) there were significant differences between old and young characters on the physical level. In 1960 there was not. This raised the question of whether at present fewer distinctions are made between descriptions of old and young characters with reference to physical characteristics than were in the past.

nces in the dimensions of activity and evaluation on the physical level. There were no significant interactions between time and age. The lack of effects from the interaction of time and age indicated that whatever significant changes in descriptions had occurred could be accounted for by the age of the category being described or by the passage of time, but those changes did not occur as the result of descriptions consistently changing over time.

The next two subhypotheses predicted significant differences between activities initiated by old and by young characters both within and across time; and, significant differences in actions directed toward or upon old people and things compared with young people or new things both within and over time periods. Difference in activities was operationalized as valence of acts: positive, negative or neutral. The χ^2 statistic was used to test for significance. There

was statistical support for the predicted differences between activities performed by old and young characters across time. Such differences were both qualitative and quantitative in that over time there had been an increase in the proportion of acts initiated by old compared with young characters. There had also been an increase in the relative proportion of acts having positive valence initiated by old compared with young characters. A similar pattern was observed with reference to the initiation of acts having neutral and negative valence. While the finding was that over time older characters increased the proportion of activity they initiated relative to young characters within any given time period, the young were proportionately more often the initiators of activity. The only exception to this finding was for the most recent time period sampled, 1960. Here one analysis showed that the proportion of old male

TABLE 21-III
ANIMATE INITIATORS: OLD AND YOUNG: MALE AND FEMALE

Animate Male and Female Initiators	Time Period				
	1870	*1900*	*1930*	*1960*	*Total*
Old	49	83	35	108	275
% of all animate male and female initiators	15.81	35.32	43.75	50.00	32.70
Young	261	152	45	108	566
% of all animate male and female initiators	84.19	64.68	56.25	50.00	67.30
Total	310	235	80	216	841

$\chi^2 = 74.74$
$df = 3$

$p < 0.001$ (indicates a significant difference between the old and young subjects at the .001 level of probability. A difference this large would occur by chance alone only once in 1000 times).

and female initiators of action equaled that of young male and female initiators (Table 21-III).

The predicted significant differences between activities performed toward or upon old compared with those performed toward or upon young (or new) people (or things) was also strongly supported. Differences were again operationalized in terms of valence and it was found that the young in relation to the old were the recipients not only of proportionally more acts but these acts were more often acts having positive valence, neutral valence, and interestingly enough, negative valence.

Discussion

The findings did not support a generally negative picture about older people and things. For the most part, there were both fewer and less strong negative patterns than had been expected. Not only was this found to be the case, but an expected linear relationship between the increased proportion and numbers of old people on the one hand and a corresponding increase in nega-

tive attitudes and stereotypes toward them on the other hand failed to materialize. There were some anticipated differences but these were for specific time periods and limited to specific semantic dimensions and levels rather than across-the-board generally negative changes. An interaction between the age of a referent and the meaning of age over time, which could logically have been expected, did not materialize in any statistically measurable way.

Despite these caveats and shortcomings the authors believe this general area of study is a fruitful one. They would suggest a replication of the study using children's literature of various types or examining other means of informal socialization, such as television programs, advertising, comic books, or preretirement literature.

REFERENCES

Calhoun, N., and Gottesman, L. Stereotypes of old age in two samples. Paper read at the Midwestern Psychological Association, 1963.
Eisdorfer, C., and Wilkie, F. Attitudes toward older people: A semantic analysis. Pape

presented at the annual meeting of the Gerontological Society. St. Petersburg. Fla., 1967 (prepublished copy: Mimeographed).

Golde, P., and Kogan, N. A sentence completion procedure for assessing attitudes toward old people. *Journal of Gerontology*, 1959, *14*, 355-363.

Heise, D. Semantic differential profiles for 1,000 most frequent English words. *Psychological Monographs*, 1965, *79*, 1-31.

Hickey, T., and Kalish, R. Perceptions of adults. *Journal of Gerontology*, 1968, *23*, 215-220.

Kogan, N. Attitudes toward old people: The development of a scale and an examination of correlates. *Journal of Abnormal & Social Psychology*, 1961, *62*, 44-54.

Kogan, N. Attitude toward old people in an old sample. *Journal of Social Psychology*, 1961, *62*, 616-622.

Mott, P. *The organization of society.* New York: Prentice-Hall, 1965.

Osgood, C., Succi, G., and Tannenbaum, P. *The measurement of meaning.* Urbana: University of Illinois Press, 1965.

Tuckman, J. The projection of personal symptoms into stereotypes about aging. *Journal of Gerontology*, 1958, *13*, 70-73.

Tuckman, J., and Lorge, I. Attitudes toward old people. *Journal of Social Psychology.* 1953, *7*, 249-260.

Chapter 22

ATTITUDES OF THE AGED TOWARD THE YOUNG: A MULTIVARI-ATE STUDY IN INTER-GENERATIONAL PERCEPTION

ARTHUR G. CRYNS AND ABRAHAM MONK

THE FOLLOWING IS AN empirical study of the attitudinal and perceptual orientation of the aged toward the young. In this time of heightened interest in intergenerational dynamics, review of the relevant gerontological literature discloses an interesting anomaly: research on the reciprocal attitudes of age groups has developed quite unevenly. Substantial attention has been given to the attitudes of the young (i.e. adolescents and young adults) to the old (Axelrod and Eisdorfer, 1961; Drake, 1957; Golde and Kogan, 1959; Kogan and Shelton, 1962; Tuckman and Lorge, 1958). However, little, if any, empirical effort has been directed toward the measurement of senescent images of the young. It is in this particular area of gerontological inquiry that this study wishes to make a contribution.

This investigation is based upon the implicit assumption that attitudinal and perceptual processes are shaped not only by the attributes, real or alleged, of the ob-

Reprinted by permission from the *Journal of Gerontology*, 1972, 27, 107-112.

jects of attitudes or of perception, but also by the subjective frame of mind of the perceiver or attitude carrier himself. This study attempts to test the specific hypotheses that the attitudes of the old toward present-day youth are a function, *inter alia*, of the aged individual's level of life satisfaction as well as of the socioemotive quality of the relationship that prevails, or at one time did prevail, between him and his own child or children. Or, expressed more concretely, that aged individuals of relatively high levels of life satisfaction and with good relationships with their own offspring tend to be more favorably inclined toward today's young than are those aged of low life satisfaction and with poor filial relationships. The basic rationale for these assumptions, to be elaborated upon later, is that individuals, having derived reasonable satisfactions from their own lives, may be more accepting and tolerant of others by virtue of the fact that their need to release frustration-instigated aggressions against others is significantly lower than for those of low life satisfaction. Also, those aged with good relationships with their "own young" may generalize the resulting positive feelings and attitudes toward the latter to projectively include all, or most, other young people.

Method

The Sample

The *Ss* of this study were fifty-three well-doing, white elderly males who were either married, divorced, or widowed. They ranged in age from sixty through sixty-nine years with a mean age of 65.41 years. Sixty-five percent of them were fully retired from work, while the remainder considered themselves still active vocationally, either on a full- time or on a part-time basis. Socioeconomically, the *Ss* were drawn from the upper-low through the upper-middle classes. Vocationally, twenty-seven were, or had been, skilled laborers, fourteen small businessmen, and twelve came from a managerial or professional background. The average number of living children per *S* was 2.04. The fifty-three participants in this study were selected from an incidental sample of sixty-seven elderly males participating in a more extensive survey of senescent attitudes and opinions. All were active members of one of four Senior Citizen Centers located in a Western New York urban area. Interviews and tests were administered in these centers and participation in the study was on a voluntary basis. The fourteen *Ss* removed from the original sample were screened out on the basis of their having no offspring of their own, and, as such, of not possessing one of the *S* attributes manipulated as an independent variable in this study.

Measuring Instruments

The following measuring devices were used in this study:

LIFE-SATISFACTION INDEX A (LSIA): This index is a test of life satisfaction or morale developed by Neugarten, Havighurst, and Tobin (1961). Its purpose was to differentiate the aged *Ss* of this study into low and high life-satisfaction subgroups with the median score as the dividing point between the two categories.

SEMANTIC DIFFERENTIAL (SD): In order to measure the connotative evaluation by the aged of today's young this study employed the Rosencranz-McNevin (1969) Semantic Differential. The *Ss* were requested to rate three categories of young people: *today's young people; our boys in Vietnam; college students,* on the same thirty-two scales of bipolar adjective pairs.

The test was chosen primarily because of its known factorial content as well as of its successful prior use in the field of intergenerational perception. Rosencranz and McNevin identify three main connotative factor loadings in the twenty-three adjective pairs: Factor I—*Instrumental-Ineffective* (I-I): nine adjective pairs denoting adjustive-maladjustive person-attributes, such as level of effective goal orientation; adaptability and energy-output; Factor II—*Autonomous-Dependent* (A-D): nine adjective pairs indicating a person's rated level of personal autonomy or dependency upon others; Factor III—*Personal Acceptability-Unacceptability* (PA-U): fourteen adjective pairs describing a person's perceived acceptability or unacceptability to the rater.

The choice of the three concepts to be semantically evaluated was based upon the assumption that the first one (*today's young people*) would constitute a generic assessment of present-day youth in general; the second one (*our boys in Vietnam*) an evaluation of a youth subgroup with a high degree of perceived "ideology congruence" with the adult world; the third one (*college students*) an attitudinal judgment of a reputedly dissenting youth group.

MEASURE OF FILIAL RELATIONSHIP: The quality of relationship with own offspring was inferred from a cluster of five questions which were part of a more extensive, focused interview designed by the second author of this article. These questions dealt with the individual's locus of interpersonal trust; whether he has a trusting and confiding relationship with his own child(ren); what the frequency of contact (face-to-face and other) is with his child(ren); how customary it is for the child(ren) to seek the advice of respondent. The *S* responses to these questions were content-analyzed and used to differentiate them into two subgroups: those with good and those with poor relationships with their own offspring.

Research Design

In order to test the hypotheses formulated above, these researchers developed a 2 × 2 factorial design with life-satisfaction and filial relationships as the independent variables and S SD-scores as the dependent ones. The respondents in this study were divided into a high and a low life-satisfaction group as well as into a group with good relationships with their own children and a group with poor relationships. As for life satisfaction, those with below median scores in the LSIA (Mdn = 13.41) were operationally defined as manifesting low life-satisfaction; those with above median scores as being of high life satisfaction. Those of the respondents, who admitted of the father-child relationship that it was largely without intimacy, trust, and affective rapport were categorized as having poor relationships with their own children; those who intimated that either party or both vested some trust and empathy in that relationship were identified as having good relationships with their offspring. In order to reduce rater bias, the Ss were divided into good and poor filial relationship groups prior to the calculation of their SD-scores.

The above S differentiations having been made, the fifty-three participants in this study were appropriately distributed over the four-cell matrix of the resulting 2 × 2 design.

All of the Ss completed the Rosencranz-McNevin SD for each of the three concepts mentioned above: *today's young people, our boys in Vietnam, college students.* In addition to a general search for overall significant intergroup differences in SD-scores for the three concepts rated, the data were subjected to a two-way, fixed effects multivariate analysis of variance in the manner prescribed by Bock (1963) and Finn (1968). Scores on the three SD's were treated as multiple dependent variables. Finally, a univariate analysis of variance was performed on the data yielded by each of the three SDs separately. The units of analysis were the mean item scores for Factors I, II, and III of the SD.

Results

The results obtained in this study are given in Tables 22-I and 22-II. They contain the mean item scores for the concepts rated, differentiated by connotative factor.

Overall Differences in Concept Ratings

In assessing the overall appreciation by the aged of the three youth groups specified above, it was found that our Ss are most positive in their attitudes toward the boys in Vietnam and that they are less positive in their evaluations of young people and least positive toward college students. Table 22-I indicates that the respondents

TABLE 22-I

MEAN ITEM SCORES SD - FACTORS FOR YOUTH GROUPS RATED (N = 53)

Rosencranz - McNevin *SD - Factors*	*Concepts Rated*		
	Boys *Vietnam*	*Young* *People*	*Coll.* *Students*
I: Instrumental - Ineffective	2.41	3.00	3.01
II: Autonomous - Dependent	2.47	3.26	3.53
III: Personal Acceptability - Unacceptability	2.39	3.63	4.11

Note: Theoretical score range is 1 (very favorable) to 7 (very unfavorable).

TABLE 22-II

MEAN ITEM SCORES SEMANTIC DIFFERENTIAL FACTORS FOR LEVELS OF LIFE
SATISFACTION AND QUALITY OF FILIAL RELATIONSHIPS

	High				*Low*		
SD-Factor	*Boys Vietnam*	*Young People*	*Coll. Stud.*	*SD-Factor*	*Boys Vietnam*	*Young People*	*Coll. Stud.*
		Good Relations with Children					
I: I-I	1.83	1.71	1.55	I: I-I	2.61	2.71	2.40
II: A-D	2.06	2.26	2.04	II: A-D	2.71	2.74	2.79
III: PA-U	1.71	2.40	2.25	III: PA-U	2.64	3.16	3.43
			n = 16				n = 10
		Poor Relations with Children					
I: I-I	2.49	3.11	3.44	I: I-I	2.69	4.36	4.65
II: A-D	2.63	3.36	4.13	II: A-D	2.46	4.69	5.12
III: PA-U	2.53	4.15	5.15	III: PA-U	2.66	4.82	5.62
			n = 19				n = 8

perceive the boys in Vietnam as being better adjusted, more self-directive or autonomous, as well as more acceptable to them than the two other groups rated. The mean item scores on the three SD-factors denote rather sizeable differences in attitudinal appreciation of the three youth groups.

The results of a repeated measures ANOVA on the interconcept differences in mean rating did indicate that the difference between each adjoining pair of means across rows is significant at $p < 0.01$ except for the italicized one: the rated adjustment levels (Factor I) of young people today and of college students were found to be practically identical.

Analysis of Variance (Multivariate and Univariate)

Table 22-II gives the SD responses of the Ss in this study cross-tabulated over the two independent variables of this research design: *(life-satisfaction and filial relationships)*.

The multivariate ANOVA is based upon the psychometric assumption that the three dependent variable measures of this design: ratings of: (1) young people today,

(2) boys Vietnam, (3) college students, are interdependent and are to be treated simultaneously, as a set. As Table 22-III indicates, the multivariate test of life satisfaction × filial relationship interaction, eliminating main effects, failed to reach significance at $p < 0.05$. The multivariate test of life-satisfaction main effect, eliminating quality of filial relationships, was found to be significant at $p < 0.01$ for all three SD-factors. So was the multivariate test of filial relationship main effect, eliminating life satisfaction; this proved to be highly significant for all three SD factors at $p < 0.001$.

The preceding data indicate that the mean differences for the three youth group ratings considered as a multiple set are a function of both life-satisfaction and of quality of relationship with one's own offspring. Both life-satisfaction and filial relationship did affect the semantic evaluation of the young by the aged Ss of this study: those of high life satisfaction and those with good filial relationships manifest significantly more positive attitudes toward the young than do those of low life satisfaction and those with poor filial relationships.

Concretely, the former perceive the young as better adjusted, more autonomous, and as more acceptable to them than do the *Ss* in the latter categories. These findings confirm the hypotheses formulated above.

TABLE 22-III

MULTIVARIATE F - RATIOS OF THREE COMBINED CONCEPT RATINGS DIFFERENTIATED BY FACTORIAL CONNOTATION

SD-Factor	Source of Variance	F
I: I-I	Life satisfaction	6.96*
I: I-I	Filial relation	20.08*
I: I-I	Interaction (life × fil.)	1.16
II: A-D	Life satisfaction	3.77*
II: A-D	Filial relation	25.73*
II: A-D	Interaction (life × fil.)	2.40
III: PA-U	Life satisfaction	3.97*
III: PA-U	Filial relation	26.85*
III: PA-U	Interaction (life × fil.)	1.62

*Significant $p < 0.05$ for 3 and 47 degrees of freedom.

Subsequent to the multivariate analysis, a univariate ANOVA was performed on the same SD data. The latter method treats each of the dependent variables of a design as separate, discrete measures. In refining the observations yielded by the multivariate ANOVA, it established that life satisfaction and quality of filial relationship did particularly influence the evaluation by the aged of young people today and of college students, but to a lesser extent the one of our boys in Vietnam. Of the six univariate ANOVAS performed to test the two main effects on the perception of the boys in Vietnam, only two yielded significant F-ratios, in contrast to the two other concepts rated where, in each case, all six F-ratios were found to be significant.

Discussion

The most salient finding of this study appears to be its confirmation of the hypo-thesis that the attitudinal-perceptual evalu-ation of others is apt to be influenced by *S* attributes as life satisfaction and quality of filial relationship. The tendency of our aged *Ss* to be more positive in their evalua-tion of today's youth to the extent that they themselves manifest higher life satisfaction and more favorable relationships with their own offspring is clearly indicated by the data enumerated above.

The existing literature on intergenera-tional dynamics, young as it is, provides few, if any, clues as to the reason for these findings. These authors speculate that senescent life satisfaction may be related to acceptance of today's young by virtue of the fact that those of reasonably high satis-faction levels are sufficiently fulfilled in their own lives as not to require them to displace their own dissatisfactions and frus-tration-induced aggressions upon others. By definition, they are individuals of low emo-tional disaffection and, thus, less in need of expressing negative sentiments in intoler-ant behavior and attitudes toward others. The relationship between personal disen-chantment and interpersonal intolerance has been reasonably well-documented by modern psychological research (Adorno 1950; Berkowitz, 1962; Kirscht and Dille-hay, 1967).

A second interesting finding is that the aged *Ss* of this study have rather diversified perceptions of the three categories of youth rated. There is a marked tendency on their part to perceive the young military in Viet-nam significantly more favorably than they do college students or the generalized young. These authors believe that the most important variable effecting this outcome may have been the perceived congruence of the first group with the ideologically modal position of society at large and the reputed deviation from same of the other two groups. "Our boys in Vietnam" denotes a

outh group that is most intimately identi-
ied with societally accepted valences such
s love of country, loyalty to authority,
ense of responsibility, etc. They may well
e perceived as the youthful ideological
llies of their cross-generational counterparts in the adult and the senescent age-co-
norts. Conversely, semantic concepts as
"young people today" and "college students" tend to evoke images of youthful re-
ellion and dissidence, which may cause
hose groups to be perceived as ideological
postates from adult and senescent norms.

Summary

Utilizing a 2 × 2 factorial design, this
tudy explores the social attitudes of elder-
y males toward three present-day youth
roups. It was found that the aged *S's* se-
nantic evaluation of today's young is a
unction of his level of life satisfaction and
f the quality of relationship he has with
is own offspring. Aged of high life-satis-
action and with good filial relationships
end to demonstrate a significantly more
avorable attitude toward the young than
lo those of low life satisfaction and with
oor filial relationships. No interaction
ffects were found between life satisfaction
nd filial relationship. There is some evi-
lence to suggest that the above *S* attributes
lid affect particularly the senescent ratings
f college students and of young people in
eneral, but, to a lesser degree, their ratings
f the young military in Vietnam. It was
urther observed that the aged *Ss* of this
tudy are significantly more positively in-
lined toward the latter group than they
re toward the generalized young or to col-
ege students.

REFERENCES

Adorno, T. W. *The authoriarian personality.*
New York: Harper 1950.

Axelrod, S., and Eisdorfer, C. Attitudes toward
old people: An empirical analysis of the
stimulus group validity of the Tuckman-
Lorge questionnaire. *Journal of Gerontology*, 1961, *16*, 75-80.

Berkowitz, L. *Aggression: A social-psychological
analysis.* New York: McGraw-Hill, 1962.

Bock, R., Programming univariate and multivariate analysis of variance. *Technometrics*,
1963, *5*, 95-117.

Drake, J. T. Some factors influencing students'
attitudes toward old people. *Social Forces*,
1957, *35*, 266-271.

Finn, J. *Multivarance-univariate and multivariate analysis of variance, covariance and
regression: A Fortran IV program.* Buffalo:
State University of New York at Buffalo
1968.

Golde, P., and Kogan, N. A sentence completion procedure for assessing attitudes
toward old people. *Journal of Gerontology*,
1959, *14*, 355-363.

Kirscht, J. P., and Dillehay, R. C. *Dimensions
of authoritarianism: A review of research
and theory.* Lexington: University of Kentucky Press, 1967.

Kogan, N., and Shelton, F. C. Beliefs about old
people: A comparative study of older and
younger samples. *Journal of Genetic Psychology*, 1962, *100*, 93-111.

Neugarten, B. L., Havighurst, R. J., and
Tobin, S. S. The measurement of life satisfaction. *Journal of Gerontology*, 1961, *16*,
134-143.

Rosencranz, H. A., and McNevin, T. E. A
factor analysis of attitudes toward the aged.
Gerontologist, 1969, *9*, 55-59.

Tuckman, J., and Lorge, I. Attitudes toward
aging of individuals with experiences with
the aged. *Journal of Genetic Psychology*,
1958, *92*, 199-204.

Chapter 23

OBJECTIVE VERSUS PERCEIVED AGE DIFFERENCES IN PERSONALITY: HOW DO ADOLESCENTS, ADULTS, AND OLDER PEOPLE VIEW THEMSELVES AND EACH OTHER?

INGE M. AHAMMER AND PAUL B. BALTES

I N RECENT PAPERS, a number of authors pointed to the importance of investigating perceived (subjective) age differences in addition to actual (objective) age differences (Ahammer, 1970; Baltes and Goulet, 1971; Bengtson and Kuypers, 1970; Labouvie and Baltes, 1971; Riegel, 1971; Thomae, 1970). Thomae (1970), for example, argued that perceived rather than objectively occurring environmental change is often an antecedent for behavioral change. Similarly, Bühler (1961) reported that perceived age change (perceived decline or nondecline) was more critical for adjustment in old age than functional change. Furthermore, Ahammer (1970) and Bengtson and Kuypers (1970) suggested that perceived rather than actual age differences are of prime significance in determining interage and intergenerational actions.

In our view, the surge of concern with

Reprinted by permission from the *Journal of Gerontology*, 1972, 27, 46-51.

perceived age changes and age structures reflects a number of significant research perspectives. On the one hand, and perhaps most importantly, the study of perceived age change implies a revival of the phenomonological approach delegating a major role to perceptual aspects of behavior (Riegel, 1971). In this context, then, research on perceived age changes is interesting in its own right by providing the data for the conceptualization of a phenomenologically oriented developmental theory, thus supplementing existing theoretical frameworks which are primarily based on actual (objective) age differences. On the other hand, perceived age changes and age structures are significant in that they might contain important information about developmental antecedents for the patterning and directionality of ontogenetic change sequences (Thomae, 1970).

Thus far, research on perceived age related characteristics has centered on the elderly. Quite a few studies, for example, examined how younger age groups perceive older people (Aaronson, 1966; Axelrod and Eisdorfer, 1961; Golde and Kogan, 1959; Hickey and Kalish, 1968; Kogan and Shelton, 1962; Kogan and Wallach, 1961; Tuckman and Lorge, 1952; 1953; 1958). However, these studies almost exclusively focused on older persons as the perceived target group and younger persons as the perceiving group. There appear to be no published studies which systematically varied the age of both the perceiving and the perceived groups. Moreover, none of the studies incorporated the systematic comparison of perceived with actual age differences. Such comparisons, if at all considered, were typically based on extraexperimental information.

The purpose of the present study was to investigate perceived age differences in some personality dimensions across a wide age range. In contrast to earlier research, both the age of the perceiving and the age of the perceived groups were varied. In addition, perceived age differences were compared to actual age differences. The latter comparison of perceived with the actual age differences was also included because of its implications for the study of the generation gap. Recent discussions of the generation gap bear out the notion that many of its features might be contrived rather than real (Kalish, 1970). Thus, in studies in which actual age differences in value systems are compared, these differences turn out to be relatively small, especially if within-family comparisons are performed (Bengtson, 1969; Keniston, 1968; Thomas, 1969). Nevertheless, a large percentage of Ss from different age groups or generations admit the existence of a generation gap (Bengtson and Kuypers, 1970). These apparently contradictory findings can be easily explained within the above-mentioned phenomenological framework. Thus, at least in some areas, the generation gap may be conceptualized in terms of misperceptions rather than in terms of actual differences between age and/or generation groups. In other words, it is hypothesized that Ss of different ages exhibit highly similar (self-reported) behavior but perceive each other as being different.

Method

Subjects

To test the concept that misperceptions exist not only between adolescents and adults but also between adults and their parent generation (Kalish, 1969), three age (or generation) groups were included in the present study: adolescents (age 15—18), adults (34—40), and older people (64—74). Forty Ss, twenty male and twenty female, were selected from each age range.

All Ss came from New York City and were white and middle to upper middle class (as determined by the Hollingshead Two-Factor-Index of Social Position; Hollingshead, 1965). The various age groups did not differ significantly with respect to social class. Ss for the older two age groups were sampled from an apartment complex in Manhattan (New York) consisting of 11,000 apartment units. A random sample of Ss was selected from the telephone directory of this apartment complex, and 53 percent of the Ss contacted were willing to participate. Ss for the adolescent age group came from a New York high school close to Manhattan. The parents of all adolescents had telephone listings and all Ss were volunteers.

Questionnaire

Items representing the behavioral areas of Affiliation, Achievement, Autonomy, and Nurturance were selected from the Jackson Personality Research Form (PRF; Jackson, 1967). These four dimensions were selected, since they were assumed to exhibit age differences (although no evidence with the PRF is available), and since these dimensions indicate areas which appear to be of considerable significance for interage and intercohort relationships.

Ten items from each scale were chosen at random and collated as a forty-item questionnaire. Desirability judgments, obtained using a nine-point rating scale ranging from extremely undesirable (1) through neutral (5) to extremely desirable (9), were the basis for assessing values.

Instructions

Different instructions were presented to each of four independent groups of Ss in each age group, (1) *Personal Desirability:* Ss were asked to indicate how desirable or undesirable they personally consider a given behavior; (2) *Cohort-Desirability: Ss* were instructed to judge how desirable or undesirable they thought individuals of their own age and sex would consider a given behavior; and (3) *Age-Desirability: Ss* were asked to indicate how desirable or undesirable they thought individuals of a specified target age (15—18, or 34—40, or 64—74) would consider a given behavior. Independent samples of each age group judged one of the two remaining target ages considered (i.e. separate groups of adolescents rated either adults or old people, and separate groups of adults rated either adolescents or old people, etc.). The fact that two independent samples from each age group rated two target ages resulted in two levels for the Age-Desirability condition. Thus, a total of four instructional sets was included in the data analysis.

Whereas the Personal Desirability (PD) instruction was intended to indicate objective age differences, Age-Desirability (AD) was assumed to measure perceived age differences. Cohort-Desirability (CD) was included primarily as a control instruction in order to explore a potential method effect associated with other-perception conditions. Note that both the Cohort-Desirability and Age-Desirability instructions involve the evaluation of other people's behavior.

Design

Five male and five female *Ss* of each age group were randomly assigned to each of the instruction levels. For each *S* a sum score (across 10 items) was obtained for each of the four scales. The data were analyzed by ANOVA. The design was three-factorial with the factors age (3), sex (2), and instruction (4). Separate analyses of variance were computed for each behavioral dimension.

Results and Discussion

A summary of the mean desirability scale values (neglecting the sex component) is presented in Table 23-I. In addition, the significant F-values from the analyses of variance are contained in Table 23-II.

Affiliation

Considering the behavioral area of Affiliation it should be noted first that over all it is the most valued dimension ($\overline{X} = 6.6$). Statistically significant main-effects for age ($p < 0.05$) and sex ($p < 0.01$) were obtained. Multiple comparisons (Newman Keuls; Winer, 1962) regarding the age effect indicated that both adolescents ($\overline{X} = 6.9$) and older people ($\overline{X} = 6.7$) obtained higher desirability values for affiliation than adults ($\overline{X} = 6.4$). Since no significant

TABLE 23-I

MEAN DESIRABILITY SCALE VALUES FOR EACH DIMENSION AND EACH TARGET AGE

Instruction	15 - 18				Target Age 34 - 40 Dimension[1]				64 - 74			
	Aff	Ach	Aut	Nur	Aff	Ach	Aut	Nur	Aff	Ach	Aut	Nur
Personal desirability	7.04	5.96	4.38	5.76	5.91	6.13	4.58	5.83	6.40	6.27	4.38	5.87
Cohort desirability	6.90	5.35	4.29	5.97	6.69	6.87	4.78	6.31	6.26	6.52	4.28	5.70
Age desirability												
By 15 — 18					6.25	6.38	4.34	5.86	7.16	5.92	3.67	7.13
By 34 — 40	6.78	6.75	5.37	6.50					6.87	6.92	3.60	7.01
By 64 — 74	6.90	5.40	4.10	5.83	6.68	5.95	4.84	6.46				

Aff = Affiliation, *Ach* = Achievement, *Aut* = Autonomy, *Nur* = Nurturance.

Age by Instruction interaction resulted, this outcome can be generalized across all instructional sets. These age differences are in agreement with previous studies in which adolescents were reported to show high social interests (Campbell, 1969; Douvan and Adelson, 1966), while adults were reported to place more emphasis on professional aims than personal ties (Campbell, 1969). The finding that older people assign such high desirability values to affiliation is surprising in light of Cumming and Henry's (1961) disengagement theory which is often interpreted as implying that older people withdraw voluntarily from social contacts (see, however, Maddox, 1964). This outcome, however, receives support from a study by Golde and Kogan (1959) showing that older people describe their own age group as highly affiliation oriented.

The main effect of sex indicates, in agreement with most research findings, that female *Ss* ($\overline{X} = 6.9$) evaluate affiliation as more desirable than do male *Ss* ($\overline{X} = 6.4$). Again, this sex difference held true for all age levels and all instructional sets.

Achievement

The achievement domain received the second highest overall mean desirability value ($\overline{X} = 6.2$), although barely different from the value for Nurturance. The only effect that reached statistical significance ($p < 0.01$) was the main effect of age indicating that adolescents ($\overline{X} = 5.9$) showed significantly smaller desirability values than adults ($\overline{X} = 6.3$) and older people ($\overline{X} = 6.4$), even though the mean desirability value adolescents obtained for Achievement was still above the neutral point. This finding is partly supported by Cole-

TABLE 23-II

SIGNIFICANT F - VALUES FROM THE ANALYSES OF VARIANCE FOR EACH DIMENSION

| Source | df | Dimension | | | |
		Affiliation	Achievement	Autonomy	Nurturance
Age (A)	2	4.43*	5.61**	6.46**	
Sex (S)	1	10.02*			
Instruction (I)	3				3.48*
A × S	2				
A × I	6			3.14**	2.28*
S × I	3				
A × S × I	6				
Error	96				

*p<0.05
**p<0.01

With regard to Affiliation then, contrary to prediction, perceived age or generation differences did not represent an overaccentuation of objective age differences (see also Kogan and Shelton, 1962). On the contrary, if self-descriptions are taken as criterion, all age groups perceived each other accurately.

man (1961) and Douvan and Adelson (1966), who reported that adolescents do not consider achievement a very important class of behavior. Again, as was the case with Affiliation, contrary to prediction the objective age differences were not different from the age differences obtained under Cohort- and Age-Desirability instructions.

This finding is surprising, also in light of a study by Golde and Kogan (1959), in which older *Ss* were perceived by college students as considering work and success as less important than indicated by the self-perceptions of older people (Kogan and Shelton, 1962).

Autonomy

Considering Autonomy, the overall desirability value ($\overline{X} = 4.4$) was slightly in the unfavorable direction and the lowest of the four dimensions considered. Both the Age main-effect and the Age by Instruction interaction reached statistical significance ($p < 0.01$). Multiple comparisons showed that the age groups did not differ under Personal and Cohort-Desirability but did differ under the Age-Desirability condition. Thus, using conventional self-reports as indicators, no age or generation differences resulted.

The Age by Instruction interaction is illustrated in Figure 23-I, which shows the relationships separately for two age groups each. It can be seen that adults perceived adolescents as valuing autonomy higher than they actually did ($p < 0.05$). Furthermore, both adolescents and adults perceived older people as evaluating autonomy as significantly less desirable than older people viewed their own age group or described themselves ($p < 0.05$). Thus, adolescents were misperceived by adults in the direction of being more autonomy-oriented, and older people were misperceived by adolescents and adults as placing less value on autonomy behavior. Again, part of these data is in agreement with an earlier study (Golde and Kogan, 1959) which showed that college students perceive older *Ss* as being dependent, although the older *Ss* did not describe themselves as such. Since the age groups did not differ under Personal and Cohort-Desirability instructions, the results support the proposition that perceived age differences may exist even though no actual age differences are obtained when self-reports or descriptions of one's own peer groups are considered.

NURTURANCE: With Nurturance ($\overline{X} = 6.2$) as the behavioral dimension a similar outcome was obtained. A significant instruction main-effect indicated different desirability judgments for the various instructional conditions. Multiple comparisons of the significant Age by Instruction interaction ($p < 0.05$) showed that these differences are a reflection of the oldest age group only. Older people were perceived by both adolescents and adults as judging Nurturance more desirable than older people actually did in self-reports ($p < 0.05$). Furthermore, adolescents perceived older people as judging Nurturance to be significantly more desirable than adolescents did in the personal instruction (Fig. 23-2). Older people, on the other hand, accurately perceived the two younger age groups. Again, since none of the instructions (Personal Desirability, Cohort-Desirability) aimed at describing one's own age level produced age differences, these data support the hypothesis that, in some areas, age or generation differences are perceived to exist even though such developmental

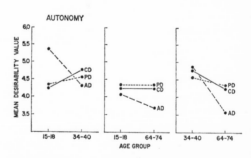

Figure 23-1. Personal Desirability (PD), Cohort-Desirability (CD), and Age-Desirability (AD) of Autonomy. Each segment of the graph shows the relationship between two age groups.

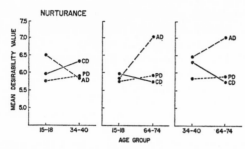

Figure 23-2. Personal Desirability (PD), Cohort-Desirability (CD), and Age-Desirability (AD) of Nurturance. Each segment of the graph shows the relationships between two age groups.

differences are absent if self-reports are taken as comparison standard.

Conclusions

The present study, in general, confirmed the proposition that the study of perceived age and/or generation differences is useful for the understanding of developmental phenomena. As to the specific objective of the study, the examination of the reality status of the age or the generation gap, it was shown that some of the generation differences are indeed of a "perceived" type. In other words, when the dimensions of Autonomy and Nurturance are considered, perceived and actual age differences did not coincide. This finding suggests that on some dimensions, if self-reports are taken as criterion, age groups do in fact misperceive each other.

At the same time, however, the present data suggest that the relationship between actual and perceived change is not a simple one but needs to be specific in terms of the age levels and behavioral dimensions involved. Thus, in the present study, misperceptions were observed only in instances where no actual age differences existed (Autonomy, Nurturance), and not in cases where the age groups differed in

self-descriptions. Since only four dimensions were investigated, it is not clear to what extent such a finding can be generalized to other personality areas. Similar restrictions, of course, apply to the age levels included in the present study.

The relationship among the age levels offers additional evidence of interest for the study of interage or intergenerational actions. Note, for example, that the adult age group was never misperceived, since the results of all instructions coincided for that target age. Older people, however, represented the group which was always misperceived (by both adolescents and adults) on those dimensions (Autonomy, Nurturance) where misperceptions occurred, whereas adolescents were misperceived (by adults) on Autonomy only. Further, the adult age group (although never misperceived) was, in all cases of misperceptions, among those that misperceived.

Summary

Independent groups of adolescents (N = 40, age 15–18), adults (N = 40, age 34–40), and older people (N = 40, age 64–74) were asked to indicate the desirability of forty behavioral items representing four personality dimensions (Affiliation, Achievement, Autonomy, Nurturance), either for themselves (personal desirability), for their peers (cohort-desirability) or for the two remaining age groups (age-desirability). Personal desirability judgments were assumed to reflect objective age differences, whereas age-desirability judgments were assumed to reflect perceived age differences, with cohort-desirability judgments being a control instruction.

ANOVAs showed that objective and perceived age differences did not coincide on Autonomy and Nurturance. Although no objective age differences existed on the two latter dimensions, adolescents and adults perceived older people as judging Nurturance as more and Autonomy as less desirable, and adults perceived adolescents as valuing Autonomy higher than they actually did.

REFERENCES

Aaronson, B. S. Personality stereotypes of aging. *Journal of Gerontology*, 1966, *21*, 458-462.

Ahammer, I. M. Alternative strategies for the investigation of age differences. Paper presented at the Regional Meeting of the Southeastern Conference of the Society for Research in Child Development, Athens, 1970.

Axelrod, S., and Eisdorfer, C. Attitudes toward old people: An empirical analysis of the stimulus-group validity of the Tuckman-Lorge Questionnaire. *Journal of Gerontology*, 1961, *16*, 75-80.

Baltes, P. B., and Goulet, L. R. Exploration of developmental variables by manipulation and simulation of age differences in behavior. *Human Development*, 1971, *14*, 149-173.

Bengtson, V. L. The "generation gap": Differences by generation and by sex in perception of parent-child relations. Paper presented at the meeting of the Pacific Psychological Association, Seattle, 1969.

Bengtson, V. L., and Kuypers, J. A. The drama of generational difference: Perception, reality, and the developmental stake. Paper presented at the Meeting of the American Psychological Association, Miami, 1970.

Bühler, C. Meaningful living in the mature years. In R. W. Kleemeier (Ed.), *Aging and leisure*. New York: Oxford University Press, 1961.

Coleman, J. S. *The adolescent society*. New York: Free Press of Glencoe, 1961.

Cumming, M. E., and Henry, W. E. (Eds.), *Growing old: The process of disengagement*. New York: Basic Books, 1961.

Douvan, E. and Adelson, J. *The adolescent experience*. New York: Wiley, 1966.

Golde, P., and Kogan, N. A sentence completion procedure for assessing attitudes toward old people. *Journal of Gerontology*, 1959, *14*, 355-363.

Hickey, T., and Kalish, R. A. Young people's perceptions of adults. *Journal of Gerontology*, 1968, *23*, 215-219.

Hollingshead, A. B. *Two factor index of social position*. New Haven: Unpublished manuscript, Yale Station, 1965.

Jackson, D. M. *Personality research form manual*. Goshen, NY: Research Psychologists Press, 1967.

Kalish, R. A. The old and the young as generation gap allies. *Gerontologist*, 1969, *9*, 83-89.

Kalish, R. A. (Chm.) The generation gap: Real or contrived? Symposium presented at the Meeting of the American Psychological Association, Miami, Sept., 1970.

Keniston, K. *Young radicals*. New York: Harcourt, Brace & World, 1968.

Kogan, N., and Shelton, F. C. Beliefs about "old" people: A comparative study of older and younger samples. *Journal of Genetic Psychology*, 1962, *100*, 93-111.

Kogan, N. and Wallach, M. A. Age changes in values and attitudes. *Journal of Gerontology*, 1961, *16*, 272-280.

Labouvie, G. V., and Baltes, P. B. Adolescents' perceptions of adolescent change in personality and intelligence. Unpublished manuscript, West Virginia University, 1971.

Maddox, G. L. Disengagement theory: A critical evaluation. *Gerontologist*, 1964, *4*, 80-82.

Riegel, K. F. Time and change in the development of the individual and society. Unpublished manuscript, University of Michigan, 1971.

Thomae, H. Theory of aging and cognitive theory of personality. *Human Development*, 1970, *13*, 1-16.

Thomas, L. E. Family congruence on political orientations in politically active parents and their college-age children. Paper presented at the 8th International Congress of Gerontology, Washington, D.C., Aug., 1969.

Tuckman, J., and Lorge, I. Attitudes toward older workers. *Journal of Applied Psychology*, 1952, *36*, 149-153.

Tuckman, J., and Lorge, I. "When aging begins" and stereotypes about aging. *Journal of Gerontology,* 1953, *8,* 489-492.

Tuckman, J., and Lorge, I. Attitudes toward aging of individuals with experiences with the aged. *Journal of Genetic Psychology,* 1958. *92,* 199-204.

Winer, B. J. *Statistical principles in experimental design.* New York: McGraw-Hill, 1962.

Chapter 24

CHRONOLOGICAL AGE IN RELATION TO ATTITUDINAL JUDGMENTS: AN EXPERIMENTAL ANALYSIS

BILL D. BELL AND GARY G. STANFIELD

CULTURAL ATTITUDES toward older people have long been of interest to social gerontologists (Axelrod and Eisdorfer, 1961; Kogan, 1961; Slater, 1963; Tuckman and Lorge, 1952a, b). Nevertheless, serious research in this area has been of relatively recent origin. The researches of Tuckman and Lorge (1952a, b; 1953a, b; 1954; 1958), for example, signaled the beginnings of an empirical thrust in this direction. In this regard, many early findings suggested old age to be a period marked by failing physical and mental powers, economic insecurity, and resistance to change. These factors, often in combination, have supposedly fostered a negative stereotype toward older adults in general.

Subsequent research has done little to either challenge or alter the above suggestions. For the most part, research attention has been focused on the development of various instruments for assessing age-stereotypical information. Axelrod and Eisdorfer (1961) and Eisdorfer (1966), for example, have attempted to shorten as well as to increase the validity of the Tuckman-Lorge

Reprinted by permission from the *Journal of Gerontology*, 1973, *28*, 491-496.

scale. Generally speaking, however, these efforts have not proven fruitful. Besides scalar modifications, other techniques and devices have enjoyed popularity. Eisdorfer and Altrocchi (1961), for instance, prefer the use of the semantic differential, whereas Kogan (1961) favors a Likert scaling procedure. Aaronson (1966) and Golde and Kogan (1959), on the other hand, utilize attitude checklists and sentence completion instruments, respectively. In all instances, however, negative attitudes are observed with respect to older age groupings (Ginzberg, 1952; Slater, 1963).

The present research suggests the need for a new look at attitudes toward age. This suggestion is based on both theoretical and empirical considerations. Theoretically speaking, cultural attitudes, like cultural values, seldom remain static (McKee, 1969). The social movements of the late sixties (e.g. women's liberation, gay liberation, etc.) have done much to focus attention on different value perspectives. As a consequence, a new tolerance has arisen relative to various "minority groupings" (Toby, 1971). To some extent, the aged fall within this category. From an empirical standpoint, on the other hand, local, state, and federal programs for the elderly have had an influence on the ideas and values of the young with respect to their older age counterparts. In a series of researches yet to be published, for instance, the authors observed significant shifts in the value perspectives of both young and old respondents following exposure to an extension course on aging. As a consequence of these and other observations, it seems probable that many of the previously-referenced attitudes toward age may have undergone significant changes in the last ten years.

The most immediate reason for renewed concern involves the methodological considerations of previous research. In this regard, it is clear that the major portion of this work has been conducted in the university setting. As such, the sample survey has proven the most utilized methodological tool. For the most part, subjects are asked to evaluate certain age categories (e.g. 50—64, 65–74, 75–84, etc.) with respect to a number of personal and social characteristics. Although an "efficient" procedure for gathering data, such an approach tends to ignore such problems as response-set biases as well as errors of central tendency (Eisdorfer, 1966). In addition, a "knowledge bias" is probable. That is, a subject's reported judgment relative to a given grouping may reflect assumed "knowledge" of what is held culturally in this regard rather than any *personal* feelings relative to the group(s) in question. To the extent that such factors are or have been operative in previous methodologies, the entire issue of attitudes toward age invites a more contemporary reexamination.

The following research is an extension of an earlier study of attitudes toward age which employed an experimental format (Bell and Stanfield, 1973). This previous investigation was conducted within a college-age population (N = 280). The methodology reported below is essentially the same with the exception of the measurement device employed and the consideration of a contrasting context. In the initial study of the college sample, two scales were utilized: (1) a modified Tuckman-Lorge scale, and (2) an aging semantic differential (Rosencranz and McNevin, 1969). Although the students involved in Experiment One below are the same as those previously reported, the present research concerns itself with those findings associated with the Rosencranz and McNevin instrument. In addition, the experimental procedure has been adapted to a second setting, a sample

of older retired adults (N = 96). In the latter context, only the Rosencranz and McNevin device was employed.

Experiment One
Methodology

The experiment was performed in four sections of an undergraduate sociology course at the University of Missouri, Columbia. Of the 280 individuals comprising the sample, 136 were male; 144 were female. The mean age of the sample was nineteen years. In each of the classes the experimenter prefaced a recorded discussion by a previously unknown stimulus person (SP) with the following explanation:

> Mr. Stanfield and I are interested in the different ways and manners by which one individual forms an impression of another. To examine this process more closely we have devised the following study. We will shortly play for you a recording made by a Mr. John Cross. Mr. Cross is a real person and additional information about him appears on the booklets you will be receiving presently. Following his discussion we will ask you to give us your impressions of him utilizing the format in the impression booklet. We will pass out the booklets now and you can familiarize yourself with them before we play the recording. PLEASE READ OVER THESE TO YOURSELVES AND DON'T TALK ABOUT THIS AMONG YOURSELVES UNTIL WE HAVE COLLECTED ALL PAPERS AT THE END OF THE STUDY.

In the experimental classes (n's = 126, 80, and 32), two kinds of information were distributed. The forms were identical except that in one the SP was described as being "twenty-five years old"; in the other, the phrase "sixty-five years old" was used. These descriptions reference the SP as "young" and "old," respectively.

Both young and old versions were distributed randomly within each of the experimental groups, in such a manner that no one was aware that discrepant information was being dispersed. In the control group (n = 42), no indication of age was provided. All subsequent information, however, remained the same. The experimenter then played for each class a fifteen-minute recording on the topic of ecology.

The subjects then rated the SP on the thirty-two-item Rosencranz and McNevin semantic differential. This scale is arrayed in a seven-choice response format. An additional bipolar pair (young-old) was included as a check on the age manipulation. The point biserial correlation between experimental treatments and actual judgment proved significant at the .001 level. The analysis to follow employs the point biserial statistic instead of the t-test, since the former technique measures both level of significance and strength of association (Ferguson, 1966). The alpha level utilized was .05 or less.

The Findings

As the differences in the ratings produced by the young-old variable were consistent from one experimental section to the other, the data were combined by equating means (the SD's were essentially identical) and the results subjected to final analysis. Column two of Table 24-I illustrates the differential ratings of the SP by subjects receiving "young" or "old" preinformation.

It will be noted that only six of the adjectives in the original scale are significantly associated with the type of preinformation presented. This was one less than observed with the use of the Tuckman-Lorge instrument (Bell and Stanfield, 1973). Contrary to the expectations of previous writers, the associations reflect a *positive* bias

toward the *older* SP. That is, those subjects given "old" preinformation tended to rate the SP as significantly more progressive, strong, active, friendly, aggressive, and exciting, than those provided with "young" descriptions. In the case of the Tuckman-Lorge scale, the older person was seen to possess a better memory, be less cranky, and have less respect for tradition. His younger counterpart, on the other hand, was viewed as having more friends, being more productive, worrying less about unimportant things, and in a better position from which to marry (Bell and Stanfield, 1973). In both instances, however, these relationships, although significant, were quite weak. The strongest association in the present research, for example, accounted for only 2 percent of the variance in the dependent variable. For the Tuckman-Lorge measure, the strongest relationship explained only 3 percent of the variance. Under these circumstances, it was not possible in either instance to conclude a definite pattern of attitudinal judgment from the data. Nevertheless, it is interesting to note the trend toward a more *positive* evaluation of the SP on the part of those receiving "old" as opposed to "young" preinformation.

Column three of Table 24-I presents the correlation of each scale item with the subject's independent judgment of age. Although nonparametric sign tests indicated a significant tendency for subjects to favor the younger SP in this condition, the associations in question are decidedly weak. In only four instances did these associations prove significant. This is in contrast to the fourteen significant relationships noted with the Tuckman-Lorge measure (Bell and Stanfield, 1973). In the latter instance, the tendency again was to evaluate the "old" SP more favorably than his younger counterpart. Once again, however, it should be pointed out that the degree of associ-

TABLE 24-I

RELATIONSHIP BETWEEN ADJECTIVE RATINGS AND EACH INDEPENDENT
VARIABLE IN THE YOUNGER SAMPLE

High End of Scale	Low End of Scale	Age Indication vs. No Age Indication[a] (N = 280)	Pre-information Young — Old[b] (N = 238)	Actual Judgment Young — Old[c] (N = 280)
		I	II	III
Progressive	Old-fashioned	—.04	—.12*	.06
Consistent	Inconsistent	—.08	.09	.04
Independent	Dependent	—.08	—.07	—.02
Rich	Poor	—.04	—.10	—.21**
Generous	Selfish	—.03	—.04	—.01
Productive	Unproductive	.06	—.09	—.04
Busy	Idle	.02	—.06	.02
Secure	Insecure	—.03	—.05	—.06
Strong	Weak	—.08	—.12*	.04
Healthy	Unhealthy	.03	.02	.14**
Active	Passive	.01	—.15**	.03
Handsome	Ugly	—.09	—.04	.14**
Cooperative	Uncooperative	—.00	—.08	—.03
Optimistic	Pessimistic	—.15**	.02	.09
Satisfied	Dissatisfied	—.07	—.02	.03
Expectant	Resigned	—.07	.04	.09
Flexible	Inflexible	—.02	—.08	.05
Hopeful	Dejected	—.08	—.05	.02
Organized	Disorganized	—.02	—.07	.02
Happy	Sad	—.03	—.04	—.02
Friendly	Unfriendly	.05	—.11*	.05
Neat	Untidy	.00	.10	.02
Trustful	Suspicious	—.10*	.08	.00
Self-reliant	Dependent	.00	—.05	—.04
Liberal	Conservative	.02	—.03	.09
Certain	Uncertain	—.09	—.01	—.02
Tolerant	Intolerant	—.06	—.07	—.03
Pleasant	Unpleasant	.04	—.09	.05
Ordinary	Eccentric	.09	.09	.07
Aggressive	Defensive	—.02	—.12*	.08
Exciting	Dull	—.06	—.15**	.17**
Decisive	Indecisive	—.03	.03	.07

[a]A positive correlation indicates a higher score for those subjects receiving no age informaation.

[b]A positive correlation indicates a higher score for those subjects receiving "young" preinformation.

[c]A positive correlation indicates a higher score for those subjects responding with "young" judgments.

*p = <.05.   ** = p<.01.

ation between young and old impressions varied with each dimension of perception tapped. This fact argues against a "halo effect" interpretation of the findings. The young-old variable appears to be related to some scale items more than others.

The employment of a control group made possible an examination of the effect of no preinformation as well as "young-old" preinformation on the impressions formed. Column one of Table 24-I indicates the differential effects of preinformation-no preinformation on scale ratings. As can be seen, those subjects receiving age information generally tended to rate the SP higher on the scales in question. The same finding was observed in the case of the Tuckman-Lorge measure (Bell and Stanfield, 1973). In the present study, significant relationships were noted in only two instances (optimistic and trustful). In the former, only three significant associations were observed (should marry; never a nuisance to others; has great potential). On the whole, however, these associations were not frequent or strong enough to warrant interpretation.

Ratings by experimental and control groups showed a weak pattern of more favorable ratings of the older SP. This tendency proved significant in six instances. On the other hand, in the case of actual age judgments, a more favorable evaluation of the *younger* SP was evidenced. Associations in this instance, however, were notably weak. Only three of the twenty-one correlations favoring younger age proved statistically significant. It is apparent from the data, therefore, that age indications *per se* are not sufficient to control strongly either positive or negative judgments of the type called for in the present research.

Experiment Two

Methodology and Findings

This experiment was performed on a sample of older adults representing retirement organizations in fifteen counties in central Missouri. The meeting in question was held for the purpose of discussing the implications of the 1971 White House Conference on Aging. Thirty-two of the subjects were male; sixty-four were female. The mean age of the group was sixty-six years. Essentially the same research format was employed. On the basis of the previous analysis, however, no control group was utilized. Column one of Table 24-II illustrates the differential ratings of the SP by subjects receiving "young" or "old" preinformation.

It will be noted that none of the adjectives in the original scale are significantly associated with the type of preinformation presented. That is, there is no significant pattern of attitudinal judgment reflected in the data. This is true for those receiving "old" as well as "young" descriptions of the SP. On the other hand, there seems a slight tendency for the present sample to rate the "younger" SP somewhat higher on the aging semantic differential scales than was the case in the college-age sample. Again, however, this finding is only suggestive and far from significant.

Column two of Table 24-II gives the correlation of each scale item with the subject's independent judgment of age. Again, although nonparametric sign tests indicated a significant tendency for subjects to favor the younger SP in this condition, the associations in question were quite weak. In only four instances did these associations prove significant. Specifically, the younger

TABLE 24-II

RELATIONSHIP BETWEEN ADJECTIVE RATINGS AND EACH INDEPENDENT
VARIABLE IN THE OLDER SAMPLE

High End of Scale	Low End of Scale	Preinformation: Young — Old[a] (N = 96) I	Actual Judgment: Young — Old[b] (N = 96) II
Progressive	Old-fashioned	.10	.34**
Consistent	Inconsistent	—.12	—.09
Independent	Dependent	.00	.03
Rich	Poor	.12	.03
Productive	Unproductive	.10	.08
Busy	Idle	.09	.07
Secure	Insecure	—.04	—.01
Strong	Weak	.05	.08
Generous[c]	Selfish	.07	.13
Healthy[c]	Unhealthy	—.04	.02
Active	Passive	—.16	.02
Handsome	Ugly	.13	.36**
Cooperative	Uncooperative	.05	.09
Optimistic[c]	Pessimistic	.17	.13
Satisfied	Dissatisfied	.01	—.05
Expectant	Resigned	—.16	.03
Flexible	Inflexible	.14	.22*
Hopeful	Dejected	.19	.09
Organized	Disorganized	—.10	—.03
Happy	Sad	.04	.09
Friendly[c]	Unfriendly	.14	.16
Neat	Untidy	—.06	.01
Trustful	Suspicious	.14	.17
Self-reliant[c]	Dependent	.01	—.07
Liberal	Conservative	.07	.12
Certain	Uncertain	.04	.09
Tolerant	Intolerant	.17	.09
Pleasant[c]	Unpleasant	.17	.17
Ordinary	Eccentric	.10	.02
Aggressive	Defensive	—.07	.09
Exciting	Dull	.11	.33**
Decisive	Indecisive	—.07	.11

[a]A positive correlation indicates a higher score for those subjects receiving "young" preinformation.

[b]A positive correlation indicates a higher score for those subjects responding with "young" judgments.

[c]These scales were reversed when presented to the subjects.

*$p = <.05$.   **$p = <.01$.

SP was seen as significantly more progressive, handsome, exciting, and flexible. While the general pattern is not statistically significant, the present sample does tend toward a more positive rating of the *younger* SP than was the case in the college groupings.

Discussion

A number of things are suggested by the present study. First of all, the data do not clearly demonstrate a social change effect. While the tendency among younger age groups to rate the *older* SP higher on the aging scales is apparent, it is not reflected to the same extent among the older respondents. To the contrary, the older respondents tended to rate the younger more favorably. In addition, both young and old subjects tended to rate the younger SP more favorably in those instances where an actual judgment of age was made. Although the biserial r's are seldom significant in either instance, the trend in evaluation reversal is clear. It should be noted in this instance that these findings were consistent across the age and sex categories of both groups of subjects.

The apparent contradictions between preinformation set and actual age judgments may be endemic to the present methodology. As the manipulation of age and impression utilized a tape recorded conversation, it seems certain that in addition to the explicit information given on age, the implicit information conveyed by tone of voice, professional attainment, expressive style, etc. may have acted to influence the research findings. The tendency, for example, to rate the younger SP more favorably in instances of actual age judgments is consistent with the tendency of controls to rate the SP somewhat younger than experimental groups. It may also be

the case that the age attributed to the voice in the "old age" condition may not actually have been old enough. There may very well be a point when a marked shift in attitude toward older adults occurs, and this point quite possibly is after age sixty-five. As for the higher ratings of the older SP in the younger sample, it may be that a sixty-five-year-old journalist, still employed, is viewed as considerably more prestigious than a younger journalist. Consequently, prestige rather than age designations may be determinative of present judgments.

Summary

The present study utilized an experimental format to examine the influence of age designations upon differential rating of a stimulus person. Two experiments were conducted one in a college-age population (N = 280); the other in a grouping of older, retired adults (N = 96). In both settings, subjects heard a recorded discussion by a SP described as being either twenty-five or sixty-five years of age. Ratings were made on the thirty-two-item Rosencranz and McNevin aging semantic differential. The data reveal a slight but nonsignificant tendency for younger subjects to rate an older SP more positively on the scales in question than do the older subjects. In the case of actual age judgments, however, all subjects, regardless of age, reflect a tendency (again, not statistically significant) to rate the younger SP more positively than the older individual. In and of itself, chronological age appeared insufficient to control strongly a pattern of judgment relative to a SP. These findings call to question (1) the employment of chronological categories in assessing age related attitudes, and (2) that research which reports the predominately negative character of such responses.

REFERENCES

Aaronson, B. S. Personality stereotypes of aging. *Journal of Gerontology*, 1966, *21*, 458-462.

Axelrod, S., and Eisdorfer, C. Attitudes toward old people: An empirical analysis of the stimulus-group validity of the Tuckman-Lorge Questionnaire. *Journal of Gerontology*, 1961, *16*, 75-80.

Bell, B. D., and Stanfield, G. G. The aging stereotype in experimental perspective. *Gerontologist*, 1973, *13*, 341-344.

Eisdorfer, C., and Altrocchi, J. A comparison of attitudes toward old age and mental illness. *Journal of Gerontology*, 1961, *16*, 340-343.

Eisdorfer, C. Attitudes toward old people: A re-analysis of the item-validity of the stereotype scale. *Journal of Gerontology*, 1966, *21*, 455-462.

Ferguson, G. A. *Statistical analysis in psychology and education*. McGraw-Hill, New York, 1966.

Ginzberg, R. The negative attitude toward the elderly. *Geriatrics*, 1952, 7, 297-302.

Golde, P., and Kogan, N. A. A sentence completion procedure for assessing attitudes toward old people. *Journal of Gerontology*, 1959, *14*, 355-363.

Kogan, N. A., and Wallach, M. A. Age changes in values and attitudes. *Journal of Gerontology*, 1961, *16*, 272-280.

Kogan, N. A. Attitudes toward old people: The development of a scale and an examination of correlates. *Journal of Abnormal Social Psychology*, 1961, *62*, 44-54.

Labovitz, S. Some observations on measurement and statistics. *Social Forces*, 1967, *46*, 151-160.

McKee, J. B. *Introduction to sociology*. Holt, Rinehart & Winston, New York, 1969.

Rosencranz, H. A., and McNevin, T. E. A factor analysis of attitudes toward the aged. *Gerontologist*, 1969, *9*, 55-59.

Slater, P. E. Cultural attitudes toward the aged. *Geriatrics*, 1963, *18*, 308-314.

Toby, J. *Contemporary society: An introduction to sociology*. John Wiley & Sons, New York, 1971.

Tuckman, J., and Lorge, I. The effect of institutionalization on attitudes toward old people. *Journal of Abnormal Social Psychology*, 1952, *47*, 337-344. (a)

Tuckman, J., and Lorge, I. The influence of a course in the psychology of the adult on attitudes toward old people and older workers. *Journal of Educational Psychology*, 1952, *43*, 400-407. (b)

Tuckman, J., and Lorge, I. Attitudes toward old people. *Journal of Social Psychology*, 1953, *37*, 249-260. (a)

Tuckman, J., and Lorge, I. When does old age begin and a worker become old? *Journal of Gerontology*, 1953, *8*, 483-488 (b).

Tuckman, J., and Lorge, I. The influence of changed directions on stereotypes about aging: Before and after instruction. *Educational Psychological Measurements*, 1954, *14*, 128-132.

Tuckman, J., and Lorge, I. Attitude toward aging of individuals with experiences with the aged. *Journal of Genetic Psychology*, 1958, *92*, 199-204.

Section VI

FAMILY ROLES AND SOCIAL RELATIONS

Perhaps no area has received more attention in gerontology than the social relations of the aged. For the most part, these efforts have focused on later life and, particularly, on the relationships associated with retirement and similar transitions in the life span. In this regard, the family arena has commanded considerable interest. This setting became a focal point of research in the 1930s and early 1950s. During this period of time the family was considered both as an institution and as a refuge for the older adult.

As was true of many subareas in gerontology, research in this domain gave precedence to the aged male. Principal changes in family structure and relations were held to be closely related to the status changes attendant upon the male member of the family. The family's patterns of social behavior, their internal unit relations, and the members' personal morale and adjustment potential were closely associated with the employment status, income, and health of the family head. By and large, the "success" of family interaction was viewed as a reflection of the male's activities in the larger society.

During this period of time, particular attention was given to the informal and formal participation of the aged (Mayo, 1951; Dotson, 1951; Webber, 1954). Age, retirement, and such factors as income and health were seen to significantly affect these patterns of behavior. Over time, the aged seemed to "drop out" of formal and/or voluntary organizations. On the other hand, their informal relationships with friends, neighbors, and family members were seen to remain stable or increase slightly. The status transitions of the older male (e.g. retirement) again provided a plausible explanation for these observations. In this regard, the individual was felt to lose personal and social status with the relinquishment of the work role. As much of his participation was linked to his occupational endeavors (Mayo, 1951), this status loss became reflected not only in the makeup of organizational structures, but also in the nonverbal reactions of other participants. As a consequence, the individual's participation declined because of perceived as well as institutionalized impediments.

Another factor considered important was the primary relationship. These intimate relations were held to provide the individual with a sense of self worth and personal identity. The fact that such associations were no longer as readily

233

available in formal settings led many researchers to regard the desire for such relations as the principal motivation for expanded informal behavior (Smith *et al.,* 1954; Dotson, 1951). An anomaly in this regard, however, was the rather persistent religious involvement of the elderly. Although representing a formal organization in the strict sense of the term, gerontologists pointed to the traditional character of the church and its potential for primary relations as the explanation for this behavior (Smith *et al.,* 1954). Accordingly, the general character of their explanation remained unchanged.

Along with the above explanation went a desire to delineate the variables and conditions affecting these relationships. While most of this research was guided by cross-sectional designs and correlational techniques, it succeeded in placing participation in a class perspective. The nature of such resources as income, health, and education made clear the fact that more was involved in the social behavior of the aged than a desire for primary relations. One needed also to consider a host of class-related factors.

Within the family, gerontologists gave consideration to the quality of social relations. As expected, family relationships proved closely related to the health, income, and occupational status of the participants, especially the male. Illness or disability, for example, could add to the burden of status loss and prevent the playing out of newly-assigned roles (e.g. grandparenthood). In addition, the quality of these relationships were seen to affect the morale and adjustment of family members (see Section VII). Probably the only facet of the family left unexplored during this period was the area of sexual behavior. On the other hand, this aspect of family life was to see development in a related discipline (Kinsey, 1948; 1953).

In general, then, the period made a significant contribution to the knowledge base of gerontology. Although most of these efforts were atheoretical and descriptive in nature, they served to establish several relationships later to figure prominently in a number of aging theories. In addition, these efforts emphasized the quality of family relations and the influence of such interaction on both individual and social adjustment.

Research in the late 1950s and early 1960s continued to emphasize the role of family and friends in the personal adjustment and morale of the older person (Axelrod, 1960; Bell and Boat, 1957; Rosow, 1965). To the focus of income, health, and community setting was added the concept of the family life cycle (Lansing and Kish, 1957; Wilensky, 1961). This variable provided a context for the interaction associated with such phenomena as religious participation (Lazerwitz, 1961; Wilensky, 1961), kinship interaction (Cavan, 1962; Cumming and Schneider, 1961), and sexual relations (Neuman and Nichols, 1960; Rubin, 1965; Thompson and Streib, 1961). With respect to the latter variable, the sexual relations of the aged became less a curiosity and assumed considerable significance in such issues as morale and marital stability (Rubin, 1965).

In addition to expanding earlier discussions of social participation, gerontologists sought to incorporate these observations within theoretical frameworks. Many of the formulations of the period make explicit the character and function of these relations for older adults. For the most part, each orientation specifies the conditions and circumstances calling for differential behaviors. In addition, longitudinal methodologies served as the most appropriate means of theory construction and verification. These developments were bolstered by significant advances in statistical techniques.

In essence, the family remained a significant source of role behavior for the older person. In much the same manner as before, gerontologists described the family and peer group as refuges and support devices to cushion the shock of status loss (Taietz, 1961). Nevertheless, the influence of external situations on the frequency and quality of family relations could not be ignored. Accordingly, the traditional variables of health, income, and status were incorporated in most theories. In addition, family behavior was seen as influenced both by and through interactions external to the family. This was especially the case with religious behavior (Albrecht, 1958; O'Reilly, 1957; Wright and Hyman, 1958). In this instance, family solidarity played a prominent role in the religious behavior of the aged.

This total view of family and social relations included a renewed emphasis on intergenerational matters. These efforts frequently included assessments of attitudes as well as behavior. In this regard, the role of grandparent received special attention. In addition, an increase in the number of "one member families" (i.e. widows) forced consideration of the effects of marital loss on personal morale and adjustment, as well as upon residential arrangements and patterns of behavior within the kin network. Such research added an additional dimension to the study of the "generation gap."

The emphasis on empiricism and theoretical development has continued through the late 1960s and early 1970s. Such efforts have led to a new conceptualization of family. Along with the potential for refuge and support, the family can and often does constitute a threat to the older person. That is, the status loss characteristic of societal withdrawal may not be ameliorated by family relations (Brody, 1966; Riley and Foner, 1968; Troll, 1971; Deutscher, 1969). As a consequence, status changes external to the family sphere may serve to exacerbate latent conflicts and misunderstandings. One result of this contemporary view has been to place the friendship and peer group in a position of greater importance relative to the morale and adjustment of the aged (Lawton and Simon, 1968; Rubenstein, 1971; Jacobs, 1969). On the other hand, however, the effects indicated above appear less marked among rural than urban respondents (Britton and Britton, 1967; Townsend, 1968).

Interest in the sexual and religious behavior of the aged has continued apace. No longer considered a curiosity or a tangential element in family relations, sexual behavior and its significance have become part and parcel of aging theories in general. This is particularly true of those theories dealing with marital stability (Masters and Johnson, 1966; Berezin, 1969; Pfeiffer, 1969). By the same token, religious behavior has been explored both as a function of the quality of family relationships and as a major influence upon them as well (Ailor, 1969; Bahr, 1970). The findings from these as well as cross-cultural studies suggest both dimensions critical to an understanding of the family and social relations of the aged.

Another facet of contemporary research has been a closer look at role structures through the life cycle. Generally, this has meant a concentration on the roles of grandparenthood as well as others influencing intergenerational behavior (Kahana and Kahana, 1971). A spin off from this approach has been to give serious attention to the factors of disability and loss of spouse. Still another aspect of this picture has been to connect the quality and frequency of intergenerational ties to such issues as morale and life satisfaction. To some extent, perceived success of offspring has been linked to marital solidarity and personal adjustment. This finding suggests a new dimension to be explored in subsequent research.

It is apparent that contemporary gerontologists have provided both breadth and depth relative to the family and social relations of the aged. They have succeeded in delineating the role relationships of age and in providing a context from which to examine them. Such efforts have placed a number of variables in theoretical perspective and have challenged the once-pessimistic views of generational phenomena. For the most part, researchers have placed a rigid emphasis on empiricism and made frequent use of cross-sectional, longitudinal, and cross-cultural methodologies. The results of this work have yet to be fully evaluated. In general, however, the social behavior of the aged continues to be one of the most rapidly advancing areas of gerontological interest.

The papers which follow present two outlines of contemporary research in this area. In most instances, there is a strong emphasis on the role of the friendship or peer group as well as the family. Besides focusing upon those factors related to interaction in these settings, the authors discuss the function of such relations for the older adult. In addition, this behavior is cast within a conceptual framework (i.e. the family life cycle). Such a device permits the reader a context from which to view the nature and development of these relationships.

The paper by Bultena examines age-grading in the social interaction patterns of elderly men. Reviewing the literature regarding the emergence of an aged subculture, the author hypothesizes that, (1) older persons should interact more with each other than with persons of a younger generation, and (2) advancing age should be associated with an increased prominence of horizontal as opposed to vertical, social ties in extended family, kinship, and community groups.

Data were obtained from interviews with 434 noninstitutionalized retired men living in Wisconsin. The findings are such as to confirm the first hypothesis. Bultena reports elderly male respondents to have a substantially greater amount of face-to-face contact with age mates than with younger individuals. On the other hand, "advancing age was associated with a diminished, rather than increased degree of confinement of social interactions to age peers. The respondents aged 80 and older had both a greater number of contacts with younger persons and a higher proportion of their total interaction within the younger age categories than did their counterparts aged 65 to 79 years."

The paper by Rosenberg focuses upon the friendship ties of the aged and the social context within which these relationships take place. For the author, the neighborhood is the primary social setting for friendship interaction among the working class aged. In this regard, neighborhood characteristics are seen as limiting the likelihood of a given individual making friends within its confines. For the most part, these limitations are built around the extent to which this environment is rich in status-similars. That is, neighborhoods which are similar in socioeconomic characteristics (i.e. consonant neighborhoods) should be more conducive to the establishment of friendship ties than settings where the individual's social characteristics differ significantly from those of his neighbors (i.e. dissonant neighborhoods).

In testing these hypotheses, data were obtained from 1596 white, working class residents of a large eastern city. Rosenberg observes that contextural dissonance accounts for isolation from friends among males over age sixty-five, but not for those under sixty-five. Older men living in neighborhoods where their socioeconomic characteristics differ from that of other local residents tend to be more isolated from their friends. "While this pattern of affiliation holds for both poor and solvent old men, it is the solvent who are more strongly affected by, and the poor who are less responsive to, such class-linked neighborhood contexts in terms of friendship."

The writer's paper constitutes an exploration of the formal and informal social participation patterns of older adults within the framework of the family life cycle. This variable constitutes a methodological tool for examining how an aged individual's social relationships change over time both internally (in relation to the family context) and externally (with respect to his relationships in the larger society).

Data for the study were obtained from interviews with a stratified random sample of sixty white, male respondents representative of the white collar population of a large protestant church in central Kansas. Three samples of twenty persons each were drawn from each of three designated life cycle stages. The findings indicate no significant differences between the family life cycle stages with regard to either the number of formal organizational memberships or the frequency of participation in such groupings. By the same token, a significant difference does not obtain between the different stages with respect to the number of informal social contacts or the frequency of participation with such individuals. The writer argues the social participation of the aged to be a function of the interrelationship between primary relational needs and contextual availability.

The work of Wingrove and Alston focuses upon yet another dimension of the social relations of older adults, the area of church attendance. The authors observe little consensus in the literature regarding the relation between church attendance and the processes of aging. By and large, what information is available is frequently contradictory and often an artifact of different methodological strategies and cross-sectional designs. As a consequence, the authors' task becomes one of employing an alternative methodology (i.e. cohort analysis) in an effort to assess the relationship of age and aging to church attendance. In the process, this technique permits an evaluation of four frequently used models for categorizing the relationship in question, the traditional, stability, family cycle, and disengagement models.

Data for the study were obtained from Gallup Poll surveys taken between 1939 and 1969. While church attendance is found to be related to age, the findings of the study reveal no consistent pattern in this relationship for age cohorts. That is, "each cohort manifests its own peculiar church attendance profile as reflected both by absolute rates of attendance and by variation in attendance by age." As a result, no one of the four explanatory models receives convincing support on the basis of the data.

The final paper in this section concerns an area of family and social relations frequently omitted in the literature, the sexual behavior of older adults. In this exposition, Pfeiffer reviews the history of those studies involving the sexual relations of the aged and points to some of the factors responsible for the scarcity of research in this area. In this regard, he examines the nature of the taboo against sex in old age and finds the taboo prevalent among the younger as well as older segments of the population. In addition, he cites the research efforts of Kinsey as well as Masters and Johnson in resolving some of the sexual stereotypes regarding the aged. Finally, he references the findings of the Duke longitudinal studies to provide a more contemporary framework for observing the changes in sexual relations with age.

REFERENCES

Ailor, J. W. The church provides for the elderly. In R. R. Boyd and C. G. Oakes (Eds.), *Foundations of practical gerontology.* Columbia, South Carolina: University of South Carolina Press, 1969.

Albrecht, R. E. The meaning of religion to older people—the social aspect. In D. L. Scudder (Ed.), *Organized religion and the older person.* Gainesville, Florida: University of Florida Press, 1958.

Axelrod, L. L. Personal adjustments in the post-parental period. *Marriage and Family Living,* 1960, *22,* 66-70.

Bahr, H. M. Aging and religious disaffiliation. *Social Forces,* 1970, *49,* 60-71.

Bell, W., and Boat, M. Urban neighborhoods and informal social relations. *American Journal of Sociology,* 1957, *62,* 391-398.

Berezin, M. A. Sex and old age: a review of the literature. *Journal of Geriatric Psychiatry,* 1969, *2,* 131-149.

Britton, J. H., and Britton, J. O. The middle-aged and older rural person and his family. In E. G. Youmans (Ed.), *Older rural Americans.* Lexington, Kentucky: University of Kentucky Press, 1967.

Brody, E. M. The aging family. *Gerontologist,* 1966, *6,* 201-206.

Cavan, R. S. Family tensions between the old and the middle-aged. In R. F. Winch, R. McGinnis, and H. R. Barringer (Eds.), *Selected studies in marriage and the family.* New York: Holt, Rinehart & Winston, 1962.

Cumming, E., and Schneider, D. Sibling solidarity: a property of American kinship. *American Anthropologist,* 1961, *63,* 498-507.

Deutscher, I. Socialization for post parental life. In J. K. Hadden and M. L. Borgatta (Eds.), *Marriage and the family.* Itasca, Illinois: Peacock Publishers, 1969.

Dotson, F. Patterns of voluntary association among urban working class families. *American Sociological Review*, 1951, *16*, 64-69.

Jacobs, R. H. The friendship club: a case study of the segregated aged. *Gerontologist*, 1969, *9*, 276-280.

Kahana, E., and Kahana, B. Theoretical and research perspectives on grandparenthood. *Aging and Human Development*, 1971, *2*, 261-268.

Kinsey, A. C., Pomeroy, W. B., and Martin, C. R. *Sexual behavior in the human male.* Philadelphia: Saunders, 1948.

Kinsey, A. C., Pomeroy, and Martin, C. R. *Sexual behavior in the human female.* Philadelphia: Saunders, 1953.

Lansing, J. B., and Kish, L. Family life cycle as an independent variable. *American Sociological Review*, 1957, *22*, 512-518.

Lawton, M. P., and Simon, B. The ecology of social relationships in housing for the elderly. *Gerontologist*, 1968, *8*, 108-115.

Lazerwitz, B. Some factors associated with variation in church attendance. *Social Forces*, 1961, *39*, 301-309.

Masters, W. A., and Johnson, V. E. *Human sexual response.* Boston: Little, Brown, 1966.

Mayo, S. C. Social participation among the older population in revival areas of Wake County, North Carolina. *Social Forces*, 1951, *30*, 53-59.

Newman, G., and Nichols, C. R. Sexual activities and attitudes in older persons. *Journal of American Medical Association*, 1960, *173*, 33-35.

O'Reilly, C. T. Religious practice and personal adjustment of older people. *Sociology and Social Research*, 1957, *42*, 119-121.

Pfeiffer, E., Verwoerdt, A., and Wang, H. S. The natural history of sexual behavior in a biologically advantaged group of aged individuals. *Journal of Gerontology*, 1969, *24*, 193-198.

Riley, M. W., and Foner, A. *Aging and society, Vol. I: an inventory and research findings.* New York: Russell Sage Foundation, 1968.

Rosow, I. The aged, family and friends. *Social Security Bulletin*, 1965, *28*, 18-20.

Rubenstein, D. An examination of social participation found among a national sample of black and white elderly. *Aging and Human Development*, 1971, *2*, 172-188.

Rubin, I. Sexual life after sixty. New York: Basic Books, 1965.

Smith, J., Form, W., and Stone, G. Local intimacy in a middlesized city. *American Journal of Sociology*, 1954, *60*, 276-284.

Taietz, P., and Larson, O. F. Social participation and old age. *Rural Sociology*, 1961, *21*, 229-238.

Thompson, W. E., and Streib, G. F. Meaningful activity in a family context. In R. W. Kleemeier (Ed.), *Aging and leisure.* New York: Oxford University Press, 1961.

Townsend, P. Problems in the cross-national study of old people in the family: segregation versus integration. In E. Shanas and J. Madge (Eds.), *Methodology problems in cross-national studies in aging.* New York: S. Karger, 1968.

Troll, L. E. The family of later life: a decade review. *Journal of Marriage and the Family*, 1971, *33*, 263-290.

Webber, I. L. The organized social life of the retired in two Florida communities. *American Journal of Sociology*, 1954, *59*, 340-346.

Wilensky, H. L. Life cycle, work situation, and participation in formal associations. In R. W. Kleemeier (Ed.), *Aging and leisure.* New York: Oxford University Press, 1961.

Wright, C. R., and Hyman, H. H. Voluntary association memberships of American adults: evidence from national surveys. *American Sociological Review*, 1958, *23*, 284-294.

Chapter 25

AGE-GRADING IN THE SOCIAL INTERACTION OF AN ELDERLY MALE POPULATION

Gordon L. Bultena

It recently has been suggested (Rose, 1965) that a distinct subculture is emerging among the aged in American society. Fundamental to this view is the observation that, ". . . the elderly tend to interact with each other increasingly as they grow older, and with younger persons decreasingly." The argument for an emergent aged subculture, however, rests on other propositions as well (see Anderson, 1967).

Cultural trends provide considerable justification for suggesting that the frequency of contact between the aged population and younger persons is diminishing and that the aged thereby are coming to constitute a subculture. However, the extent to which the interaction of older persons is age-graded has received little empirical study.

Findings are reported here from a study in which two hypotheses central to the theory of an aged subculture were tested. The first hypothesis is that older persons interact more with each other than with persons of a younger generation; the second, that advancing age among the elderly brings an increased prominence of horizontal, as *vis-à-vis* vertical, social ties in ex-

Reprinted by permission from the *Journal of Gerontology*, 1968, *23*, 539-543.

tended family, kinship, and community groups.

Theoretical Considerations

Critical to the conceptualization of an aged subculture is the observation of a growing isolation between the aged and individuals in younger age groups. As such, it has been suggested that the social integration of the aged may hinge increasingly in the future on solidarity among age-mates rather than on intergenerational relationships (Cumming and Schneider, 1961; Hawkinson, 1965; Rosow, 1967).

The deterioration which is noted in the vertical social ties of the aged is commonly attributed to changes in family and kinship patterns precipitated by urban-industrial trends. Of importance in this regard is an increase in the physical isolation of the aged from younger age groups as a result of greater independence from children in living arrangements, high rates of residential mobility among children, and a growth in the number of older persons living in retirement communities and congregate-care facilities. The sizable increase in recent decades in the aged population in small towns similarly has resulted in greater age-homogeneity in many communities, and diminished opportunity for contact with younger persons.

A number of social changes, in addition to physical factors, can be identified as having altered the traditional position and relationships of the aged within the social structure. First, there is evidence of a general devaluation, and social rejection, of the aged by younger persons. Second, the institutionalization of retirement has diminished the opportunities of older persons to interact with younger coworkers. Third, the emergence of organizations and groups catering exclusively to the elderly, such as community centers, "Golden Age Clubs," and age-segregated religious activities, has facilitated interaction among agemates and in addition has served to isolate them from contact with other generations. Fourth, the necessity in modern society of reconciling economic achievement motives with the more particularistic obligations and expectations of kin-family systems has undermined the traditional functioning of these social units. Fifth, the rapidity of social and economic change in American society has precipitated a growing "communication gap" between the generations, with younger persons often evidencing a reluctance to interact with the aged, given their generally divergent perspectives, activities and problems.

These physical and social changes have been identified as instrumental in reducing the level of contact which is believed to have obtained at an earlier period between the aged population and younger persons. This is not to say that vertical social relationships are inconsequential today for the aged, but rather that from a historical perspective the prevalence of such relationships relative to all social ties appears to have diminished.

In addition to the historical or cultural changes which are altering the interactional patterns of the aged, the aging process itself becomes relevant to the issue of social isolation and age-grading. It has been found in previous research that advancing age is associated with a loss of social roles, diminished group membership and decreased social interaction (Cumming and Henry, 1961). An increased confinement of social relationships within the older age group has been suggested as one important consequence of this process of withdrawal (Anderson, 1967; Rose, 1965).

Materials and Methods

SUBJECTS: The data were taken from interviews in 1967 with 434 retired men in Wisconsin. The respondents comprised a random sample of all retired males in six communities, which ranged in size from a small rural community to a city of 170,000 population. The samples in the five smaller communities (all of which were under 10,000 population) were drawn randomly from lists of retired persons in these places, as determined in door-to-door enumerations. Area-probability techniques were employed in obtaining a qualified sample in the largest place. The sample did not include persons in congregate-care facilities such as retirement units or nursing homes.

SOCIAL INTERACTION: Information was obtained on the frequency of each respondent's face-to-face contact with a spouse, children, grandchildren, siblings, relatives, and friends. The data reported here are based only on those persons reported as seen regularly during the week. Family members, relatives, and friends seen less often than on a weekly basis, as well as casual acquaintances and persons seen irregularly, were not included in the analysis.

In addition to ascertaining the frequency of interaction, a determination was made of the age of each of the interactants. Thus, not only was information available on the number of persons seen regularly, but also as to whether these contacts were with other elderly persons or were directed to younger age groups. For purposes of the analysis, persons age sixty or older were defined as in the same age cohort as the respondents.

A determination also was made of the number of organizations or formal groups (such as church, civic, fraternal, and social groups) which the respondents attended on a monthly or more frequent basis. The extent to which each of these groups was age-graded (i.e. whether all, most, half, few, or none of the members were retired) was ascertained in the interviews.

χ^2 tests were used to test the statistical significance of differences between age groups. All differences which are reported were significant at the .05 level of confidence.

Results

INTERACTION: It was found, in accordance with the first hypothesis, that the majority of the daily and weekly contacts of these retirees were with older persons.

The 434 respondents saw a total of 684 persons regularly on a daily basis (an average of 1.6 contacts) and 1,475 different persons one or more times a week (3.4 contacts). Sixty-seven percent of the daily contacts were with persons age sixty or older, as were 59 percent of the weekly contacts (Table 25-I).

In addition to assessing the extent of age-grading, as reflected in the contacts of the total sample, a determination was made of the proportion of each respondent's daily and weekly contacts which were with older persons. Only 16 percent of the retirees were found not to have regular daily contact with an elderly person. Conversely, the daily interaction for 59 percent was confined exclusively to age-mates, and 80 percent saw as many, or more, older persons during the day as younger persons.

An analysis of interaction patterns during the period of a week revealed that the proportion of respondents seeing a younger person increases, although the majority (68%) still saw as many, or more, older persons as those who were younger. The weekly interaction of 33 percent of the respondents was confined exclusively to older persons.

The data reported in Table 25-I provide further evidence as to the interaction patterns of the respondents. The most significant source of daily and weekly contact was with a spouse (72% saw a spouse daily). (The remaining one-fourth of the retirees were either widowed, separated from their spouses, or had never married.) In addition, 25 percent saw at least one child daily,

TABLE 25-I

NUMBER AND PROPORTION OF RESPONDENTS HAVING DAILY AND WEEKLY CONTACT WITH SPECIFIED PERSONS

Person Interacted With	Seen Daily		Seen One or More Times a Week	
	Number	%	Number	%
Spouse	315	72	315	72
Child	108	25	218	50
Grandchild	16	4	37	8
Sibling	24	6	86	20
Other relative	32	7	77	18
Friend	74	17	192	44
No contact	41	9	10	2
Total number of contacts	684		1475	
Proportion that older persons comprise of all contacts	67		59	

and 50 percent interacted with a particular child one or more times a week. Forty-four percent had contact during each week with a specific friend, 20 percent saw a sibling, and 18 percent interacted with a relative. Less than one tenth of the respondents (9%) indicated that they did not see a particular person on a daily basis, and only 2 percent had no weekly contact (Table 25-I).

Interaction with relatives and friends was predominantly with age-mates, with 60 percent of those seeing a relative during the week having contact exclusively with older persons. Similarly, 60 percent of those seeing a friend interacted only with persons their own age; 78 percent reported as many, or more, older friends as they did younger friends. Only 15 percent of the respondents drew their friends solely from a younger age group.

The intergenerational contacts of the respondents were confined largely to family members rather than directed to younger relatives and friends (72% of the total weekly contacts with younger persons were with children and adult grandchildren). Thus, from a historical perspective, the increased geographical mobility of children that has accompanied the urban-industrial growth of American society would appear to be critical to the continued emergence of an aged subculture. While many (60%) of the respondents with children had at least one child located nearby (i.e. in the household or community), the majority (57%) of the children had migrated from their home county and were physically unavailable for frequent interaction. Residential mobility was particularly pronounced in the rural communities, with upward of two thirds of the children in these places having left their home county. The migration of children also precluded frequent contact with grandchildren, thus further diminishing the possibility of viable linkages emerging between the generations.

To test the second hypothesis, a comparative analysis was made of the interaction patterns of the younger segment of the sample (age 65 to 79) and those who are very old (age 80 or older). These findings, based on a cross-sectional analysis, do not support the argument that advancing age is associated with a greater confinement of social relationships to age-mates. On the contrary, the "very-old" retirees, while averaging fewer daily and weekly contacts, had a greater proportion of their social contacts crossing generational lines than did their younger counterparts. Whereas 71 percent of the daily contacts, and 63 percent of the weekly contacts, of those under age eighty were with older persons, 57 percent and 47 percent, respectively, of the contacts of the older retirees were within their own age group (Table 25-II). Looking at age-grading from the standpoint of the interaction of individual respondents, it was found that whereas 62 percent of the younger retirees interacted on a daily basis exclusively with age-mates, 51 percent of the oldest group did so. The corresponding proportions for weekly contacts were 38 percent and 18 percent, respectively. Over three times as many of the very old respondents (20%) compared to the younger retirees (6%) had their weekly interaction confined entirely to members of a younger generation.

Not only did the proportion of all contacts which were with younger persons increase with age, but the absolute number of contacts increased as well (those 65–79 years old averaged 1.3 weekly contacts with younger persons as compared to 1.7 contacts for those 80 or older). Thus, while advancing age brings disengagement or withdrawal from social relationships with

TABLE 25-II

PROPORTION OF RESPONDENTS HAVING CONTACT WITH SPECIFIED PERSONS,
BY AGE[a]

	Age			
	65 — 79		80 or Older	
Persons Interacted With	*Daily Contact*	*Weekly Contact*	*Daily Contact*	*Weekly Contact*
Spouse	77*	77*	58	58
Child	23	44	31	68*
Grandchild	2	6	8*	16*
Sibling	6	22*	4	11
Other relative	6	19	12*	15
Same age	4	13	5	8
Younger	2	7	8*	8
Friend	16	47	19	37
Same age	13	40	15	33
Younger	7	19	4	13
No contact	8	2	14	4
Total number of contacts	517	1130	167	345
Proportion that older persons comprise of all contacts	71	63	57	47

[a]These proportions are based on an N of 328 for those sixty-five to seventy-nine, and 106 for those eighty or older. Differences in the proportions of the two age groups having daily and weekly contact which are statistically significant at the .05 level of confidence are indicated by an asterisk (e.g. a significantly higher proportion of those 65 — 79 than those 80 or older have weekly contact with a spouse and one or more siblings).

age-mates, it also brings a greater amount of contact with persons who are younger.

Data are presented in Table 25-II which point up in greater detail the differential nature of the interaction patterns of the two age groups. It was found that the proportion of respondents seeing a spouse declined with age, as did the proportion seeing a sibling. On the other hand, a significantly higher proportion of the very old reported daily or weekly contact with a child, grandchild, and younger relative.

Advancing age brings an increased likelihood that one's spouse will be decreased, thus cutting the individual off from an important source of contact within his age group. The reduced mobility of the very old also works against their maintaining frequent contact with elderly friends in the community. Also, older relatives and friends increasingly pass from the scene as the individual ages. Thus, the opportunity for interaction with age-mates is diminished, rather than enhanced, with the aging process. On the other hand, there is a greater likelihood of the older person having a child in the household, or being seen regularly by children and grandchildren living nearby. This undoubtedly reflects a greater concern and possible obligation by children for the welfare of an aged parent if he is living alone than if both parents are present.

ORGANIZATIONAL PARTICIPATION: Another dimension of age-grading in interaction, in addition to informal contact with family members, kin and friends, is through participation in formal organizations or groups. A growth in the number of organizations which are composed of older persons is deemed a salient factor in the emergence of an aged subculture in American society.

To assess the extent to which the participation of the respondents was directed to age-graded organizations, an analysis was made of the number of formal groups, exclusive of church services, attended at least once a month, and the extent to which the membership of these groups was made up of aged persons.

Consistent with "disengagement theory," the proportion of respondents participating in groups declined with age (42% of those 65–79 attended one or more formal groups as compared to 20% of those 80 or older). However, no difference was found in the extent to which the membership of the organizations attended by the respondents was characterized by extensive age-grading (44% of these organizations were reported as having one-half or more of their membership composed of retired or elderly persons, 21% drew most or all of their members from the older age groups) .

Summary

Two hypotheses drawn from Rose's theory of an emergent aged subculture were tested in this study: first, that older persons interact more with age-mates than with younger persons; second, that the prominence of horizontal, as *vis-à-vis* vertical, social ties increases with the advancing age of the elderly.

The first hypothesis was supported by our data. Elderly male respondents had a substantially greater amount of face-to-face contact with age mates than with younger persons.

Contrary to theoretical expectations, however, advancing age was associated with a diminished, rather than increased, degree of confinement of social interaction to age peers. The respondents aged eighty and older had both a greater number of contacts with younger persons and a higher proportion of their total interaction within the younger age categories than did their counterparts aged sixty-five to seventy-nine years.

While advancing age was associated with a diminished level of participation in formal groups, there was no difference in the relative proportion that age-graded groups made up of all formal groups attended by older and younger retirees.

REFERENCES

Anderson, N.: The significance of age categories for older persons. *Gerontologist, 7:* 164-167, 1967.

Cumming, E., and W. E. Henry: *Growing old.* Basic Books, Inc., New York, 1961.

Cumming, E., and D. Schneider: Sibling solidarity; a property of American kinship. *Amer. Anthrop., 63:*498-507, 1961.

Hawkinson, W.: Wish, expectancy, and practice in the interaction of generations. *In:* A. Rose and W. Peterson (Editors), *Older People and Their Social World.* F. A. Davis Co., Philadelphia, 1965.

Rose, A.: The subculture of the aging; a framework for research in social gerontology. *In:* A. Rose and W. Peterson (Editors), *Older People and Their Social World.* F. A. Davis Co., Philadelphia, 1965.

Rosow, I.: *Social integration of the aged.* The Free Press, New York, 1967.

Chapter 26

AGE, POVERTY, AND ISOLATION FROM FRIENDS IN THE UR-BAN WORKING CLASS

GEORGE S. ROSENBERG

T HIS INVESTIGATION attempts to explore the relationship between poverty and old age on the one hand and social isolation from friends on the other. A general proposition which can be extracted from studies of class patterns of social interaction (Bell, 1957; Bell and Boat, 1957; Smith, Form, and Stone, 1954) and of interaction of the aged with friends (Langford, 1962; Rosow, 1967) is that the more the neighborhood is populated by others with social characteristics similar to his, the more a working class individual is led to associate with others in the local area. And the more a neighborhood is populated by others with dissimilar social characteristics, the more he is led to withdraw from local association. The neighborhood, then, is the social context of working class friendship interaction. It serves to limit the likelihood of a given individual making friends within its confines according to whether it provides an environment rich in status-similars. This notion has been formalized (Rosenberg, 1962) in the concepts of "contextual dissonance" and "consonance." When the individual's social characteristics differ from the social characteristics of

Reprinted by permission from the *Journal of Gerontology*, 1968, *23*, 533-538.

others in his neighborhood, the *relationship* between the individual and his surrounding social environment is dissonant, and when there is similarity between individual and social environment the relationship is termed consonant. These concepts will be employed to elucidate the relationship between a variety of characteristics of neighborhoods and the isolation from friends of a sample of aged working class males some of whom are poor and some of whom are solvent. The expectation is that dissonant neighborhood contexts will tend to increase the level of isolation from friends and consonant neighborhood contexts to minimize the level of social isolation.

Materials and Methods

SUBJECTS: The *Ss* of study were the white, working class people of a large eastern city, Philadelphia, Pennsylvania, who were between the ages of forty-five and eighty. Poverty was defined for purposes of this study by a variable family income criterion, depending upon family size. Virtually all of the respondents termed poor in our sample had less than $3,000 per year family income from all sources. All those considered solvent had family income exceeding this figure, but below $7,500 per year, which is the income ceiling imposed on this sample. Furthermore, the sample was restricted to those presently employed as blue-collar workers, or who, if retired, had worked for most of their lives in blue-collar jobs. Spouses of eligible heads of households were included in the sample, however. Approximately 43 percent of the respondents were males.

Since a critical variable of this study was the respondent's neighborhood, a sample of city blocks in Philadelphia was drawn in a manner insuring that all types of neighborhoods would be represented in the study. The almost 14,000 blocks within the city limits were arrayed by Census Tract and ordered geographically in a serpentine manner. From a random start, every thirty-fourth block was selected. In the second stage of the sampling, a census of households was conducted in the blocks selected. It had a dual purpose: to screen eligible respondents according to the study criteria and to describe the block by the social characteristics of the remaining, ineligible persons. On completion of the screening, 230 of the 405 sample blocks were found to contain eligible respondents. These numbered 1596 respondents, of whom 668 were aged sixty-five or more. The 1596 respondents who were interviewed represented a 70 percent completion rate of eligible respondents. Since the uninterviewed were randomly distributed over the 230 sample blocks, with no large clusters in any one block, it was assumed that no inherent bias was introduced in the sampling. The blocks on which the respondents lived were composed almost exclusively of row houses.

INTERVIEW SCHEDULES: The interview schedule, which took an average of about two hours to complete, was designed to elicit information about a large number of variables. In this report, we will focus on the ones most relevant to our expectation that contextual dissonance will isolate people from friends. Accordingly, the following six characteristics of neighborhoods (blocks) were examined in order to assess their relationship to the friendship patterns of the respondents: mean yearly family income of the neighborhood, number of blue-collar workers over age forty-four in the neighborhood, proportion of Negro households in the neighborhood, mean age of the residents of the neighborhood, proportion of neighbors sixty-five years old or more, and proportion of neighbors who were married.

Results

INCOME LEVEL: First, consider the proportion of poor and of solvent men, aged sixty-five to eighty, who were isolated from friends in neighborhoods with different levels of wealth. The mean yearly family income of the residents of the block was the indicator of neighborhood wealth.

TABLE 26-I

FRIENDSHIP PATTERNS OF POOR AND SOLVENT MALES, AGED 65 OR MORE, BY NEIGHBORHOOD ECONOMIC LEVEL (IN PERCENTAGES)[a]

Friendship Patterns	Poor			Solvent		
	Mean Yearly Family Income of Neighborhood					
	$4,000 or Less (N=41)	$4,001 to 5,000 (N=54)	$5,001 or More (N=57)	$4,000 or Less (N=22)	$4,001 to 5,000 (N=77)	$5,001 or More (N=74)
Isolates	26.8	33.3	40.4	54.5	45.5	29.7
Friends beyond the neighborhood	9.8	18.5	21.1	18.2	26.0	17.6
Friends within the neighborhood	63.4	48.1	38.6	27.3	28.6	52.7
Total	100.0	100.0	100.0	100.0	100.0	100.0

*Percentages may not add to 100 because of rounding.

TABLE 26-II

FRIENDSHIP PATTERNS OF POOR AND SOLVENT MALES, AGED 65 OR MORE, BY
NUMBER OF BLUE-COLLAR WORKERS OVER AGE 44 IN THE NEIGHBORHOOD
(IN PERCENTAGES)

| Friendship Patterns | Number of Blue-Collar Workers Over Age 44 in the Neighborhood | | | |
| | 0 — 15 | | 16 or More | |
	Poor (N = 73)	Solvent (N = 90)	Poor (N = 79)	Solvent (N = 83)
Isolates	41.1	52.2	27.8	26.5
Friends beyond the neighborhood	15.1	15.6	19.0	27.7
Friends within the neighborhood	43.8	32.2	53.2	45.8
Total	100.0	100.0	100.0	100.0

Table 26-I shows that the proportion of isolates among poor old men increases regularly with neighborhood wealth, from 27 to 40 percent, poor people in rich neighborhoods being in dissonant contexts. (Unless otherwise stated, all differences between proportions are significant at the $P = 0.05$ level using χ^2.) But also, as expected on the contextual dissonance principle, the proportion of isolates among solvent old men *decreases* from 55 to 30 percent as the wealth of the neighborhood goes up. It is important to note that this change in proportion of isolates among the solvent is considerably greater than among the poor; 25 percent in contrast to 13 percent. That is to say, the poor old men seem to be less responsive to a neighborhood context related to socioeconomic status than the solvent old men.

WORKER STATUS: An additional socioeconomic characteristic of neighborhoods is the extent to which they contain blue-collar workers. An opposite measure here is the number of blue-collar workers over age forty-four who reside on the respondent's block. Since all the male respondents in the sample are or have been for most of their working lives blue-collar workers themselves, increasing numbers of blue-collar neighbors should decrease the level

of social isolation for poor and solvent old men alike, for neighborhood contextual dissonance is reduced also in such circumstances. And this indeed is the case. In Table 26-II, among the poor the proportion of isolates drops from 41 percent to 28 percent as the number of blue-collar neighbors rises; and among the solvent the proportion of isolates drops from 52 to 26 percent. However, note that again the poor were less responsive to the socioeconomic neighborhood context: living among larger numbers of blue-collar neighbors reduced their isolation by 13 percent, while the effect on the solvent of the same neighborhood characteristic was to reduce their isolation by 26 percent.

RACIAL INTEGRATION: A third socioeconomic characteristic of neighborhoods is the extent of racial integration, measured here by the proportion of Negro households on the respondents' block. As expected, the contextual dissonance created by the presence of Negro households in a neighborhood is associated with increased isolation for both men and women who are poor and solvent. However, as Table 26-III shows, the magnitude of these differences is considerably greater for the solvent than for the poor. The proportion of poor old people isolated from friends in segregated neighborhoods is 29 percent. In the most heavily integrated neighborhoods the proportion of isolates rises to 48 percent, an increase of 19 percent. But the proportion of isolated solvent old people rises from 34 to 64 percent in neighborhoods one-half or less integrated, an increase of 30 percent. In the most heavily integrated neighborhoods, the isolation of solvent old people is somewhat reduced. But the increase in proportion of isolates in these neighborhoods still exceeds that of the poor old people. The impact of racial integration of the neighborhood falls most heavily, then, upon the solvent old people. The aged poor are relatively nonresponsive. Racial contextual dissonance affects them to a lesser extent than the solvent. Not only are fewer of the poor isolated, but in heavily Negro neighborhoods they have proportionately more friends than solvent old people and proportionately fewer of them maintain active friendships beyond the confines of the neighborhood.

AGE STRUCTURE OF THE NEIGHBORHOOD: Turning to aspects of the neighborhood less closely related to socioeconomic factors, we find a contrasting pattern of isolation

from friends. Consider the age of a neighborhood, as measured by the mean age of the residents of the block. For poor old men, as expected on the hypothesis that contextual consonance lessens isolation from friends, the higher the mean age of the neighborhood the smaller the proportion who are isolated. In Table 26-IV, 41 percent of them have no friends in neighborhoods where the mean age is thirty-four years or less and 27 percent have no friends where the mean age is forty-five years or more. But the proportion of solvent old men with no friends rises from 32 to 39 percent under the same neighborhood conditions. As far as the age structure of the neighborhood is concerned then, we find a reversal of the pattern heretofore encountered, now the poor are more responsive than the solvent old men when we deal with a contextual factor not linked to social class.

But the mean age of the neighborhood is only one possible measure of neighborhood age context. The proportion of persons in the respondents' block who are sixty-five years old or more permits a direct focus on the presence of age peers in the

TABLE 26-III

FRIENDSHIP PATTERNS OF THE POOR AND SOLVENT, AGE 65 OR MORE, BY PROPORTION OF NEGRO HOUSEHOLDS IN THE NEIGHBORHOOD
(IN PERCENTAGES)[a]

Friendship Patterns	Poor			Solvent		
	Proportion Negro Households in Neighborhood					
	0	.01 — .50	.51 — .99	0	.01 — .50	.51 — .99
	(N = 249)	(N = 76)	(N = 44)	(N = 234)	(N = 42)	(N = 23)
Isolates	28.5	46.0	47.7	33.8	64.3	56.5
Friends beyond the neighborhood	17.3	7.9	6.8	20.9	9.5	26.1
Friends within the neighborhood	54.2	46.0	45.5	45.3	26.2	17.4
Total	100.0	100.0	100.0	100.0	100.0	100.0

[a]Percentages may not add to 100 because of rounding.

TABLE 26-IV

FRIENDSHIP PATTERNS OF POOR AND SOLVENT MALES, AGE 65 OR MORE, BY
MEAN AGE OF NEIGHOBORHOOD (IN PERCENTAGES)[a]

Friendship Patterns	*Poor*			*Solvent*		
	Mean Age of Neighborhood					
	0 — 34 Years (N = 61)	*35 — 44 Years (N = 58)*	*45 or More Years (N = 33)*	*0 — 34 Years (N = 73)*	*35 — 44 Years (N = 69)*	*45 or More Years (N = 31)*
Isolates	41.0	31.0	27.3	31.5	49.3	38.7
Friends beyond the neighborhood	24.6	15.5	6.1	19.2	20.3	29.0
Friends within the neighborhood	34.4	53.4	66.7	49.3	30.4	32.3
Total	100.0	100.0	100.0	100.0	100.0	100.0

[a]Percentages may not add to 100 because of rounding.

local area. For, in neighborhoods where a high probability exists for contact with age peers, old people, both poor and solvent, may exhibit lower rates of isolation from friends by virtue of the increased availability of age-status similars. However, a pattern emerges which is similar in most respects to what obtains when we use mean age of neighborhood as an indicator of the neighborhood age context. Table 26-V shows that as the proportion of our respondents' neighbors who are sixty-five or over increases, the isolation of poor old men drops from 37 to 17 percent and that of the solvent old men rises slightly from 38 to 46 percent. And when the neighborhood concentration of old people reaches an extremely high level, 40 percent or more of the inhabitants of the block, the isolation of the poor old men rises to 45 percent, which is more than what it was in the youngest neighborhood. The isolation of the solvent old men falls back to about what it was in the youngest neighborhood.

These findings with respect to age contexts are not a function of income level,

TABLE 26-V

FRIENDSHIP PATTERNS OF POOR AND SOLVENT MALES, AGE 65 OR MORE, BY
PROPORTION OF PERSONS IN THE NEIGHBORHOOD WHO ARE 65 YEARS OLD
OR MORE (IN PERCENTAGES)

Friendship Patterns	*Poor*			*Solvent*		
	Proportion of Neighborhood 65 Years Old or More					
	0 — .19 (N = 105)	*.20 — .39 (N = 29)*	*.40 or More (N = 18)*	*0 — .19 (N = 117)*	*.20 — .39 (N = 46)*	*.40 or More (N = 10)*
Isolates	37.1	17.2	44.4	37.6	45.7	40.0
Friends beyond the neighborhood	20.0	13.8	5.6	19.7	23.9	30.0
Friends within the neighborhood	42.9	69.0	60.0	42.7	30.4	30.0
Total	100.0	100.0	100.0	100.0	100.0	100.0

TABLE 26-VI

FRIENDSHIP PATTERNS OF THE POOR AND SOLVENT, AGE 65 OR MORE, BY AGE - INCOME COMPOSITION OF THE NEIGHBORHOOD[a] (IN PERCENTAGES)

Friendship Patterns	Age - Income Composition of the Neighborhood							
	Old-Poor		Old-Wealthy		Young-Poor		Young-Wealthy	
	Poor (N=181)	Solvent (N=141)	Poor (N=43)	Solvent (N=36)	Poor (N=59)	Solvent (N=30)	Poor (N=86)	Solvent (N=92)
Isolates	30.4	44.7	30.2	38.9	39.0	36.7	41.9	33.7
Friends beyond the neighborhood	9.4	21.3	18.6	22.2	18.6	13.3	18.6	18.5
Friends within the neighborhood	60.2	34.0	51.2	38.9	42.4	50.0	39.5	47.8
Total	100.0	100.0	100.0	100.0	100.0	100.0	100.0	100.0

[a]An old neighborhood is here defined as one in which the mean neighborhood age is thirty-five years or more, and a young neighborhood as one in which it is thirty-four years or less. A poor neighborhood is defined as one in which the mean family income per annum is $5,000 or less, and a rich neighborhood as one in which it is $5,001 or more.

older neighborhoods tending also to be poorer neighborhoods, and the increasing isolation of the solvent old people in such neighborhoods possibly being a function of wealth rather than age composition of the block. Quite the contrary, Table 26-VI shows that the age level of the neighborhood has an independent relationship to friendship patterns and isolation from friends. For if it is the poverty of neighbors which most affects the solvent people's friendships even though the neighborhood is populated by relatively many others who are old like themselves, then we should observe the following. In neighborhoods which are both old and relatively wealthy, a larger proportion of the solvent, aged respondents should have local friends than in neighborhoods which are old but relatively poor. However, Table 26-VI renders little support for the idea that age is spuriously related to friendship patterns. The difference in local friendship among solvent old people in old-poor and old-wealthy neighborhoods is slight. The age level of the neighborhood has, then, an independent relationship to friendship patterns, for both the poor and solvent and also as far as both local friendships and isolation are concerned.

MARITAL STATUS: Another contextual variable unrelated to socioeconomic factors is the presence of married people in the neighborhood. The variation in rates of isolation from friends in blocks with increasing proportions of the population who are married again reveals the greater responsiveness of poor old people. In Table 26-VII, the effect of increasing proportions of married neighbors is to increase the proportion of isolates among poor old people from 31 percent to 49 percent. But about the same proportions of the solvent old people, around 40 percent, are isolated from friends in all kinds of marital contexts. These findings are not a function of the marital status of the respondents themselves. At each income level both the married and those of our respondents who are not presently married, the men as well as the women, display the same patterns of isolation from friends. Therefore, it is not the companionship of a spouse which insulates people from loneliness and leads them to ignore the neighborhood as a source of friendships.

Discussion

The younger people in this sample who were under age sixty-five have not been

TABLE 26-VII

FRIENDSHIP PATTERNS OF THE POOR AND SOLVENT, AGE 65 OR MORE, BY PROPORTION OF PERSONS IN THE NEIGHBORHOOD WHO ARE MARRIED (IN PERCENTAGES)

	Poor			Solvent		
	Proportion in Neighborhood Who Are Married					
Friendship Patterns		*.82*				*.82*
	0 — .67	*.68 — .81*	*or More*	*0 — .67*	*.68 — .81*	*or More*
	(N = 142)	*(N = 140)*	*(N = 87)*	*(N = 98)*	*(N = 122)*	*(N = 79)*
Isolates	30.9	28.6	49.4	43.9	36.9	39.2
Friends beyond the neighborhood	10.6	16.4	16.1	19.4	20.5	19.0
Friends within the neighborhood	58.5	55.0	34.5	36.7	42.6	41.8
Total	100.0	100.0	100.0	100.0	100.0	100.0

mentioned so far. This is because the neighborhood context in most cases exerts no effects on their isolation from friends or very weak effects at best. Thus, these findings may be interpreted by considering the simple notion of the activation of a latent role. In old age, the companionship of fellow employees, whether it was negligible or significant before, is absent. A man's time is spent at or near home, and he is exposed to neighbors more than before. Thus, he becomes more vulnerable to the influence of neighborhood contexts; he is no longer a neighbor on weekends only. At this point social class factors become more rather than less potent in influencing friendship relations in the neighborhood. Not that they were absent in the past, but rather they were not operative upon the man under sixty-five for as much of his time nor for as large a sector of his role set. That is, the transition to retirement is misconceived if it is thought of as a change to a condition lacking a central role. The role of neighbor becomes activated and replaces that of worker. And as the preceding has suggested, this involves the governance of friendship relations by such class-related structures as the income, occupational and racial contexts of the neighborhood. Thus, the cessation of economic constraints on behavior does not occur in old age and retirement. This is a period of life, in the working class, in which class-related factors loom large in the lives of men. A central role of old age is as inexorably linked to the economy as the working role of earlier years. We might well divest ourselves, then, of the idea of old age in the working class as a social limbo, of retirement as a beginning of an ineluctable separation of the aging man from society in the sense of the influence of his socioeconomic environment.

But also, the notion might be discarded that there are social costs or social deprivations associated with poverty in old age which deny the poor, as compared with those not poor, companionship because they are poor, and because they are surrounded by affluence. What the findings on contextual dissonance do suggest is that aged poor people who have held blue-collar jobs for most of their lives cope more successfully with the absence of their occupational peers and integrate themselves more thoroughly into informal social networks in the presence of their occupational peers than do solvent blue-collar men. And where their neighbors differ in income standing, fewer of them tend to become isolated and more of them than their solvent counterparts manage to find friends. Proportionately more of the aged poor than the solvent have the ability, apparently, to integrate themselves into socioeconomically dissonant neighborhood contexts. Proportionately more of the poor than the solvent turn neighborhoods to their advantage in terms of local friendships.

Summary

To determine the relation between poverty, aging, and isolation from friends in an urban setting, a sample of white, working class people aged forty-five to eighty was drawn in Philadelphia, Pennsylvania. Income limitation for sample eligibility was established at a maximum of $7,500 per year from all sources, and a division of the sample was made into poor and solvent people on a variable family income criterion depending on family size. In screening systematically selected city blocks for eligible respondents, data also were obtained on the characteristics of all the neighbors in the 230 blocks which contained the *Ss* of this study.

Neighborhood contextual dissonance was found to account for isolation from friends among males over age sixty-five, but not for those under sixty-five. Old men living in neighborhoods where their wealth, occupation, or race differs from that of other local residents tend to be isolated from friends. While this pattern of affiliation holds for both poor and solvent old men, it is the solvent who are more strongly affected by, and the poor who are less responsive to, such class-linked neighborhood contexts in terms of friendship. However, the poor, aged males tend to be more responsive than their solvent peers to the isolating effects of dissonant neighborhood age structure and to the presence of married neighbors.

These findings suggest that in the working class the role of neighbor becomes more salient after retirement and that patterns of friendship in the neighborhood become more closely linked than before to class-related factors in the neighborhood environment.

REFERENCES

Bell, W.: Anomie, social isolation and the class structure. *Sociometry, 20:*105-116, 1957.

Bell, W., and M. Boat: Urban neighborhoods and informal social relations. *Amer. J. Sociol., 62:*391-398, 1957.

Langford, M.: *Community aspects of housing for the aged.* Center for Hous. & Environm. Stud., Cornell Univ., Ithaca, 1962, Res. Rep. No. 5, 49 pp.

Rosenberg, M.: The dissonant religious context and emotional disturbance. *Amer. J. Sociol., 68:*1-10, 1962.

Rosow, I.: *Social integration of the aged.* Free Press, New York, 1967, 354 pp.

Smith, J., W. Form, and G. Stone: Local intimacy in a middlesized city. *Amer. J. Sociol., 60:*276-284, 1954.

Chapter 27

THE FAMILY LIFE CYCLE, PRIMARY RELATIONSHIPS, AND SOCIAL PARTICIPATION PATTERNS

BILL D. BELL

A Meaningful Conceptual Approach

A considerable literature exists regarding the social participation of older adults (Dotson, 1951; Mayo and Marsh, 1951; Taietz and Larson, 1961; Wright and Hyman, 1958). This research has tended to view participation patterns from a chronological age perspective. The result has been a series of impressive correlations with few attempts at casual explanation. The elderly are observed to diminish their formal participation patterns and to increase their personal investment in informal social relationships (Beyer and Woods, 1963; Hansen, Yoshioka, Taves, and Caro, 1965). Aside from correlations with social class, marital status, health, etc. the biological factor of chronological age has remained the chief variable in much of this research.

The present research emphasizes the social rather than the biological character of participation patterns. The Family Life Cycle (FLC) is proposed as an alternative variable for illustrating variations in individual social behavior. Lansing and Kish

Reprinted by permission from the *Gerontologist*, 1973, *13*, 78-81.

(1957) have argued that many of the changes that occur in people's attitudes and behavior as they grow older "may be associated less with the biological processes of aging than with the influence of age up on the individual's family memberships.' Similarly, Wilensky (1961) speaks of the fluctuations in individual participation patterns as participation "careers." He sees these fluctuations as a function of inter locking cycles of family, work, and con sumption. By applying a life-cycle perspec tive to the question of participation, we are illustrating how an individual's patterns of participation can be, as Thompson and Streib (1961) suggest, "determined, facili tated, or limited by (a) social setting." The FLC concept, then, suggests a methodo logical tool for examining how an individu al's social relationships change over time both internally (in relation to the family context) and externally (with respect to his relationships in the larger society).

Criteria for Subject Selection

The data come from interviews with a stratified random sample of sixty male re spondents representative of the white-collar population of the First United Methodist Church of Manhattan, Kansas (c. 2800 members), in the spring of 1970. The Dun can Socio-Economic Index (Blau and Dun can, 1967) was employed to differentiate white-collar respondents. This index com putes SES scores and assigns decile rankings to occupational categories. The present sample was drawn from those whose occu pations had at least a 38.5 SES score and a corresponding decile rank between seven and ten. A total of 236 individuals met all criteria for the study.

In addition to the above, stratification criteria demanded that all respondents be: (a) United Methodists, (b) married and living with their spouse, (c) in relatively good health (e.g. not confined to their homes because of illness or physical disability, able to be out and about town with little difficulty; able to go shopping, conduct their business and go on occasional pleasure outings; able to negotiate the steps leading to the church without help or assistance; and able to mow their own lawns or take care of odd chores about the house), and (d) owning or having access to appropriate means of transportation. Three samples (n's = 20, respectively) from each of three designated life cycle stages were subsequently chosen for study. In addition to the interview procedure, information was obtained by a self-scoring technique relative to their formal and informal social participation. All interviews were conducted in the homes of the respondents.

Major Research Variables

FAMILY LIFE CYCLE: The FLC was defined as, "the span of time from the beginning of a family with the marriage of a young couple, the bearing, rearing, and marrying of their children, through the time when they are again alone together, until the ultimate death of one or both of them" (Deutscher, 1969). The FLC is a way of conceptualizing the expansion and contraction of the human family as it passes through various stages or phases of development. These stages were delineated by significant transitions in role relationships or behavioral expectations of the adult male.

Three of the later stages of the FLC were focused upon (Wilensky, 1961). These included: (1) *the stage of late maturity* (approximate age range 45-54 years) where older children (15 years of age and older) are still present in the home but are beginning to move toward an existence independent of the family group; (2) *the stage*

of preretirement (approximate age-range 55-64 years) or the so-called empty nest phase where children are gone from the home, independently established on their own, and the family is once again a two-person group; and (3) *the stage of retirement* (approximate age range 65-74 years) where the male is no longer employed but is still living with his spouse in a two-person family arrangement.

FORMAL SOCIAL PARTICIPATION: Formal participation refers to the extent of the respondent's involvement in formally recognized organizational groupings (e.g. the American Legion, Lions Club, Chamber of Commerce, fraternal organizations, etc.). Formal participation involves both the number of formal memberships as well as the frequency of participation (i.e. attendance) in these groupings. Respondents were asked to list the names of the organizations, clubs, and associations in the community in which they currently held memberships. Second, using a six-point attendance indicator ranging from "I do not participate in any meetings (0%)," to "I participate in all meetings (100%)," they indicated their participatory behavior relative to these organizations. A subsequent Formal Social Participation Index was constructed employing both types of information.

INFORMAL SOCIAL PARTICIPATION: Informal participation refers to the extent of involvement in informal social relationships, such as those between friends, neighbors, and relatives. Operationally, a *close friend* was considered to be someone the respondent could confide in; whom he liked very much; whom he could trust with personal property; and from whom he could borrow money. A *neighbor* was considered to be someone living in the immediate vicinity to the respondent's home with whom he would at least occasionally "visit over the back fence," borrow various items, play cards, watch television, or have a cookout. A *relative* was considered to be anyone (with the exception of his wife) related to the respondent through blood or marriage ties.

Respondents were asked to list numerically their friends, neighbors, and relatives living in the study community. Second, using a five-response visitation indicator ranging from visitation frequencies of "I never visit them" to "I visit them on the average of two or more times a week," they indicated their participatory behavior relative to these three groupings. The final construction of the informal participation index involved a weighting and summing process. The three indices taken together made up the respondent's informal social participation index.

Hypotheses Tested

In line with suggestions from the aforementioned literature, the following research hypotheses were formulated.

1. *A Significant Decline Will Be Evidenced in Formal Social Participation Toward the Latter Stages of the Family Life Cycle.*

2. *A Significant Increase Will Be Evidenced in Informal Social Relationships Toward the Latter Stages of the Family Life Cycle.*

Results of Analysis

An analysis-of-variance was carried out with regard to both formal and informal participation patterns. The findings indicate no significant differences between the FLC stages in terms of either the number of formal organizational memberships or the frequency of participation in such groupings. Subsequent analysis also failed to demonstrate a significant difference between the different stages with respect to the number of informal social contacts as well as the frequency of participation with such individuals. It would appear that the respondents in the present sample are similarly active in both the formal and informal social arenas. It is apparent, then, that neither research hypothesis has been substantiated by the available data.

Discussion of Relevant Findings

To explain the rather paradoxical findings of this research it should be kept in mind that an important factor in all forms of social activity is the primary relationship. Broom and Selznick (1958) and Chinoy (1967) have argued that such relationships, because they involve the "whole" person, contribute directly to the personal security and well-being of the individual. Cavan (1962) and Thompson and Streib (1961) have also pointed out the continuing significance of these relationships throughout the life of the individual. Further, research has revealed the potential for primary relationships in a variety of social settings (Bates and Babchuk, 1961; Davis, 1948; Faris, 1932). It would appear consistent with this literature to suggest that as primary relationships appear of continuing importance to the individual and the potential for such relationships exists in a variety of social settings, the loss or denial of these relations in one or more contexts should lead one to seek them elsewhere. It would also seem reasonable to conclude that if these types of relational needs are satisfied in one social setting there will be little need to seek them in another. For example, if participation in formal organizations remains high, there should be no need to turn in later years to informal social outlets for primary relational needs; hence, informal social participation should remain relatively stable over time.

From the perspective of the present research, no significant differences were observed in formal social participation patterns between all groups. Subsequent analysis of the data, however, revealed a significant correlation between the number of primary contacts in formal organizational settings and participation scores. While these correlations are not high, they are, such as to suggest the utility of our theoretical framework.

The low correlation between primary contacts and participation in stage three compared with stages one and two may reflect significant generational differences (i.e. the sample being of a cross-sectional nature). Stages one and two could, in terms of Riesman's (1961) typology, be representative of the "other-directed" character type who views participation as an opportunity for peer direction, approval, and support. Those individuals in stage three may be more "inner-directed" and value peer association in a formal context somewhat less. If Riesman is correct, the patterns of participation evidenced by stages one and two might be typical of generations of older adults yet to come.

Research Suggestions

In line with the present theoretical suggestions it would be well to propose an hypothesis for further study: *In Those Instances Where Formal Social Participation Remains High Over the FLC, We Would Expect no Significant Changes in Informal Social Participation Patterns; However, in Those Cases Where Formal Social Participation Is Seen to Decline Over the FLC, a Subsequent and Significant Increase in Informal Social Participation Patterns Should Be Observed.* Indeed, primary relationships might also be pursued as a factor partially accounting for the rather persistent participation of older adults in religious institu-

tions in the absence of formal organizational ties. In the final analysis, primary relational needs may prove a more satisfactory predictor of adult participation patterns than either chronological age or the family life cycle.

REFERENCES

Bates, A. P., and Babchuk, N. The primary group: A reappraisal. *Sociological Quarterly*, 1961, *3*, 181-191.

Beyer, G. H., and Woods, M. E. *Living and activity patterns of the aged.* New York: Center for Housing and Environmental Studies, Research Report No. 6, 1963.

Blau, P. M., and Duncan, O. D. *The American occupational structure.* New York: John Wiley, 1967.

Broom, L., and Selznick, P. *Sociology.* Evanston, Ill.: Row, Peterson, 1958.

Cavan, R. S. Family tensions between the old and the middle-aged. In R. F. Winch, R. McGinnis, and H. R. Barringer (Eds.), *Selected studies in marriage and the family.* New York: Holt, Rinehart & Winston, 1962.

Chinoy, E. *Society: an introduction to sociology.* New York: Random House, 1967.

Davis, K. *Human society.* New York: Macmillan Press, 1948.

Deutscher, I. Socialization for post parental life. In J. K. Hadden and M. L. Borgatta (Eds.), *Marriage and the family.* Itasca, Ill.: Peacock Publishers, 1969.

Dotson, F. Patterns of voluntary association among urban working-class families. *American Sociological Review*, 1951, *16*, 64-69.

Faris, E. The primary group: essence and accident. *American Journal of Sociology*, 1932, *37*, 41-50.

Hansen, G. D., Yoshioka, S., Taves, M., and Caro, F. Older people in the midwest: conditions and attitudes. In A. M. Rose and W. A. Peterson (Eds.), *Older people and their social world.* Philadelphia: F. A. Davis, 1965.

Lansing, J. B., and Kish, L. Family life cycle as an independent variable. *American Sociological Review*, 1957, *22*, 512-518.

Mayo, S. C., and Marsh, C. P. Social participation in the rural community. *American Journal of Sociology*, 1951, *57*, 243-248.

Riesman, D. *The lonely crowd.* New Haven: Yale University Press, 1961.

Taietz, P., and Larson, O. F. Social participation and old age. *Rural Sociology*, 1961, *21*, 229-238.

Thompson, W. E., and Streib, G. Meaningful activity in a family context. In R. W. Kleemeier (Ed.), *Aging and leisure.* New York: Oxford University Press, 1961.

Wilensky, H. L. Life cycle, work situation, and participation in formal associations. In F W. Kleemeier (Ed.), *Aging and leisure.* Ne York: Oxford University Press, 1961.

Wright, C. R., and Hyman, H. H. Voluntary association memberships of America adults: evidence from national survey *American Sociological Review*, 1958, *2* 284-294.

Chapter 28

AGE, AGING, AND CHURCH ATTENDANCE

C. RAY WINGROVE AND JON P. ALSTON

O NE OF THE MORE prolific research areas which brings together the fields of sociology of religion and gerontology is the question of church attendance as related to aging. Argyle (1959) has suggested that one of the better measures of religiosity and religious behavior is church attendance. However, there exists little consensus concerning the relation between church attendance and the process of aging *per se*. That is, little is known of how attendance changes, if at all, during a person's life cycle, nor have researchers completely resolved the questions of the relationship between church attendance and such factors as sex, age, aging, and socioeconomic characteristics. In addition, what is available is often contradictory. This paper will attempt to survey and summarize the relevant literature, in addition to presenting more recent data being developed by the current authors.

Our basic measure is the positive answer to the question "Did you, yourself, happen to attend church in the last seven days;" only the white population was included in the sample. A national representative sample of the white population conducted by the Gallup (AIPO) Organization (Poll #784. July, 1969) found that females were more active attenders (46%)

Reprinted by permission from the *Gerontologist*, 1971, *11*, 356-358.

than males (36%), that Catholics were higher in attendance (64%) than Protestants (35%), and that white-collar workers were higher (46%) than blue-collar workers (38%) (Alston, 1971). In addition, females aged thirty to thirty-nine and fifty to fifty-nine were more likely to be church goers than males in those same age groups (Alston and Wingrove, 1971).

In relation to the question of aging and church attendance, Riley and Foner (1968) suggest that attendance decreases as a person ages. This pattern of decreasing attendance has also been reported by Barron (1958, 1961) and Orbach (1961). Other surveys (*Catholic Digest*, 1953) show no difference in attendance when age is controlled (see also Lazerwitz, 1961).

Four Models Categorizing Relationship Between Aging and Church Attendance

Bahr (1970) describes four models *traditional, stability, family-cycle, and disengagement,* which categorize the relationship between aging and church attendance [for a more complete discussion of studies in this area, see Moberg (1965) and also Orbach (1961)]. In the traditional model, church attendance reaches a low during the ages of thirty and thirty-five, then gradually increases until old age. The research of Cauter and Downham (1954), Fichter (1952, 1954), Glock, Ringer, and Bobbie (1967), O'Reilly (1957), and Smith (1966), as well as the writing of Argyle (1959) support this traditional model. The stability model views church attendance and age as being unrelated, i.e. all groups are perceived as fairly constant in attendance throughout life. This model is advocated by the findings of *Catholic Digest* (1953), Lazerwitz (1961), Orbach (1961), and to some extent by those of Streib (1965). The family-cycle model stresses the importance of the marriage and child-rearing stages. Especially helpful in explaining female attendance patterns, this model suggests that the presence of children among young parents encourages high attendance rates until the last child reaches his teens. Age of the respondent is only significant in that generally younger parents are those with young children for whom they act as models. When the children are assumed to have completed their religious instructions and established their habits, the parents become less conscientious in attending as their behavior is no longer considered a necessary model for socialization. Albrecht (1958) seems to be the chief exponent of the family life-cycle model, although Lazerwitz (1961) did find increased regularity of church attendance among Protestants with children five years old and older. The disengagement model suggests that attendance is relatively high when a person is young and that religious behavior gradually declines as the individual passes through middle and old age. Church-related activities are assumed to be included among those behavior patterns no longer considered appropriate or necessary for those defined by society as aged. The disengagement model finds support from the works of Barron (1958, 1961), Catholic Charities of St. Louis (1955), Hunter and Maurice (1953), Mayo (1951), and McCann (1955).

Methodological Strategies

A major source of contradiction arises from the fact that different authors have used different methodological strategies. With the exception of a few limited longitudinal studies (Streib, 1965), most researchers have depended on crosssectional or retrospective data. Cross-sectional studies are static and better denote differences due

to age at a specific moment than differences due to the aging process itself. Cross-sectional analyses are forced to assume that the activity of the young reflects behavior patterns of older persons when they were younger. This assumption necessitates ignoring such factors as generational differences and generation-specific experience. For example, the generation which experienced the depression years or a World War obviously experienced different social conditions as they were maturing than those born after 1946. Nor do we know who took part or why in the postwar religious revival, when church attendance increased for roughly two decades. In essence the cross-sectional model is a static one and relatively unreliable when investigating respondents in a changing society. It is dangerous to impose dynamic qualities onto a static model. The retrospective approach rests upon the assumption that the life-cycle patterns in church attendance can be recreated from the memories of respondents. This great dependence upon memories seems an unreliable strategy at best, and an inherent bias is suggested by the fact that most retrospective data support the disengagement model (Bahr, 1970).

Cohort Analysis

In an effort to surmount some of the obvious weaknesses of the cross-sectional and retrospective approaches, the present authors are conducting a cohort analysis of church attendance with the use of data collected by the Gallup Poll 1939 through 1969. These data span a thirty-year interval and represent the church attendance patterns of five white cohorts by viewing their rates of attendance at six specific points in time (1939, 1950, 1955, 1960, 1965, and 1969) (see Wingrove and Alston (1971) for details). Church attendance is again measured by the question "Did you, your-self, happen to attend church or synagogue in the last seven days." Cohort analysis in the area has been advocated repeatedly by such scholars in the field as Glenn and Zody (1970), Hammond, (1969), Orbach (1961), and Riley (1968), as the most viable methodological alternative to the cross-sectional and retrospective approaches.

Although church attendance appears related to age, the findings from our study thus far indicate no consistent pattern in this relationship for cohorts. No one of the four models set forth by Bahr receives convincing support, but rather, first one and then another seemed to apply to the successive cohorts. In other words, each cohort manifests its own peculiar church attendance profile as reflected both by absolute rates of attendance and by variation in attendance by age. However, several similarities do appear among the cohorts in our analysis. First, females in each cohort manifest higher church attendance than males at nearly all ages. Second, all cohorts experienced their peaks in attendance during the ten-year interval from 1950 to 1960, which some have referred to as the period of religious revival in the United States. Furthermore, all cohorts show a decline in attendance after 1965 regardless of their ages at the time. These findings suggest the impact of social environment and the mood of the times on church attendance for any age group. Earlier studies, for example that of Webber (1954) and some cited by Barron (1961), have also noted this influence of social climate on church attendance.

Thus, we conclude that even though variation in church attendance is related to age, no single model applies to every cohort. Many additional factors must be taken into consideration. Our research indicates that among these should be included sex, specific cohort membership, and general societal environment.

REFERENCES

Albrecht, R. E. The meaning of religion to older people—the social aspect. In D. L. Scudder (Ed.), *Organized religion and the older person.* Gainesville, Fla.: University of Florida Press, 1958.

Alston, J. P. *Social variables associated with church attendance,* 1971. (In preparation)

Alston, J. P., and Wingrove, C. R. Age, sex, education and church attendance 1971., *Journal of Pastoral Care,* 1971. (forthcoming)

Argyle, M. *Religious Behaviour.* Glencoe, Ill.: Free Press, 1959.

Bahr, H. M. Aging and religous disaffiliation. *Social Forces,* 1970, *49,* 60-71.

Barron, M. L. Role of religion and religious institutions in creating the milieu of older people. In D. L. Scudder (Ed.), *Organized religion and the older person.* Gainesville, Fla.: University of Florida Press, 1958.

Barron, M. L. *The aging American: An introduction to social gerontology and geriatrics.* New York: Crowell, 1961.

Cauter, T., and Downham, J. S. *The communication of ideas.* London: Chatto & Winders, 1954.

Catholic Charities of St. Louis. *Older people in the family, the parish and the neighborhood.* St. Louis: Catholic Churches of St. Louis, 1955.

Catholic Digest. How important religion is to Americans, 1953, *17,* 7-12.

Fichter, J. H. The profile of Catholic religious life. *American Journal of Sociology,* 1952, *58,* 145-150.

Fichter, J. H. *Social relations in the urban parish.* Chicago: University of Chicago Press, 1954.

Fichter, J. H. The Americanization of Catholicism. In T. T. McAvoy (Ed.), *Roman Catholicism and the American way of life.* Notre Dame, Ind.: University of Notre Dame Press, 1960.

Glenn, N. D., and Zody, R. E. Cohort analysis with national survey data. *Gerontologist,*

1970, *10*, 233-240.

Glock, C. Y., Ringer, B. B., and Bobbie, E. R. *To comfort and challenge.* Berkeley: University of California Press, 1967.

Hammond, P. E. Aging and the ministry. In M. W. Riley, and A. Foner (Eds.), *Aging and society,* Vol. II, *Aging and the professions.* New York: Russell Sage Foundation, 1969.

Hunter, W. W., and Maurice, H. *Older people tell their story.* Ann Arbor: Institute for Human Adjustment, Division of Gerontology, University of Michigan, 1953.

Lazerwitz, B. Some factors associated with variation in church attendance. *Social Forces,* 1961, *39*, 301-309.

Mayo, S. C. Social participation among the older population in revival areas of Wake County, North Carolina. *Social Forces,* 1951, *30*, 53-59.

McCann, C. W. *Long Beach senior citizens' survey.* Long Beach, Calif.: Community Welfare Council, 1955.

Moberg, D. O. Religiosity in old age. *Gerontologist,* 1965, *5*, 78-87.

Orbach, H. L. Aging and religion: A study of church attendance in the Detroit metropolitan area. *Geriatrics,* 1961, *16*, 530-540.

O'Reilly, C. T. Religious practice and personal adjustment of older people. *Sociology & Social Research,* 1957, *42*, 119-121.

Riley, M. W., and Foner, A. *Aging and society,* Vol. 1: *An inventory of research findings.* New York: Russell Sage Foundation, 1968.

Smith, J. The narrowing social world of the aged. In I. H. Simpson and J. E. McKinney (Eds.), *Social aspects of aging.* Durham, NC: Duke University Press, 1966.

Streib, G. *Longitudinal study of retirement,* Final report to the Social Security Administration, Washington, DC, 1965.

Webber, I. L. The organized social life of the retired in two Florida communities. *American Journal of Sociology,* 1954, *59*, 340-346.

Wingrove, C. R., and Alston, J. P. *Cohort analysis and church attendance, 1939-1969,* 1971. (In preparation) chapter **29**

SEXUAL BEHAVIOR IN OLD AGE

ERIC PFEIFFER

O NE ASPECT OF OLD age which has hitherto received insufficient consideration by researchers and by clinicians alike has been the sexual life of elderly persons. In fact, until recently, relatively little scientific information with regard to the range and scope of sexual behavior in the elderly has been available, either to the elderly themselves or to those who must care for and counsel them. But the picture has begun to change. With the publication of Kinsey's pioneering works (Kinsey, Pomeroy, and Martin, 1948, 1953) with the investigations of Masters and Johnson (1966) and, still more recently, with the Duke University publications on the natural history of sexual behavior in old age (Pfeiffer, Verwoerdt, and Wang 1968, 1969a, b) small but significant body of knowledge has now been identified. Nevertheless, information about sexual behavior in the aged still lags far behind similar information on adults or adolescents. Our society has to a considerable extent moved toward greater frankness in the study and discussion of many aspects of human sexuality. That is to say, the taboos concerning sex in adolescence and adulthood have largely been laid aside. Not so the taboo against sex in old age.

Reprinted by permission from *Behavior and Adaptation in Late Life*, E. Busse and E. Pfeiffer (Eds.), Boston: Little Brown and Company, 1969, 151-162.

THE TABOO AGAINST SEX IN OLD AGE

There is no doubt that a taboo against sex in old age exists and that it constitutes a serious impediment to systematic, indepth investigations into patterns of sexual behavior in old age. The taboo operates at several different, if clearly related, levels. First, it is evident among potential subjects and their relatives. A number of investigators have commented on the difficulty of recruiting aged subjects for studies which are clearly labeled sexual in nature (Kinsey, Pomeroy, and Martin, 1948, 1953; Masters and Johnson, 1966). Even when cooperation has been gained, the data which can be collected are generally of a very limited variety. At times the aged themselves may be glad to participate in such studies, but relatives who learn of their participation may become upset and insist that they withdraw from the study. A recent fictional account of a survey type of sex study also depicts the experience as clearly disturbing to some participants (Wallace, 1960).

Second, the taboo also operates among some physicians and behavorial scientists. Thus, referring physicians may express concern that such studies may prove upsetting to their patients, or they may contend that such matters are essentially private and should not be studied scientifically. As has been pointed out by Lief in several publications, physicians themselves may not be entirely comfortable with sexual matters since their training in general has but inadequately prepared them in this regard (Lief, 1965, 1968).

Finally, investigators themselves must learn to overcome a degree of initial hesitancy and embarrassment before they can comfortably inquire into the sexual lives of their elders. For instance, in the

Duke longitudinal study some of the young physician investigators found it difficult to inquire into the sexual lives, past or present, of aged women who had been single all of their lives. There were fourteen such women in the study panel; on only four of these were any sexual data obtained.

The Nature of the Taboo

What is the explanation of this taboo? One frequently stated opinion is that it is merely a hangover from a Victorian age (Rubin, 1965). But the tenacity with which it persists makes it seem likely that present-day processes are also active in maintaining it. Our society still holds that sexual activity should be engaged in primarily for procreative, only secondarily for recreative, purposes. In adolescence and adulthood, when the production of offspring is a possibility, sexual activity can be tolerated. But in old age the fiction that coital activity is being carried on for reproductive purposes can no longer be maintained.

It also seems likely that the taboo against sex in old age is, in part, an extension of the incest taboo. In our society children of all ages often experience a great deal of anxiety from observing or imagining their parents engaged in sexual activity. Since the elderly represent the parent generation, some of the discomfort may be accounted for on this basis.

Finally, the taboo against sex in old age may serve the interests of the regnant generation. By creating and fostering a stereotype of the elderly as an asexual group, the younger group perhaps seeks to eliminate the aged as competitors for sexual objects.

Actually, a series of fictions or cultural stereotypes exist with regard to sexual behavior in old age (Golde and Kogan, 1959; Rubin, 1965). The most important ones can be summarized briefly. Many people believe that sexual desire and sexual activity cease to exist with the onset of old age; or that sexual desire and sexual activity should cease to exist with the onset of old age; or that aged persons who say they are still sexually active are either morally perverse or engaged in wish-fulfilling deceptions and self-deceptions.

These stereotypes have only minimal relationship to the actual data and, as is true of stereotypes generally, make little allowance for individual variation. Only the phrase "onset of old age" is variably defined, from the menopause to retirement to extreme old age. Having considered the taboo against sex in old age and the several stereotypes which exist about the topic, the actual data can now be considered. Three series of studies will be reviewed and evaluated: the findings of Kinsey and his associates; those of Masters and Johnson; and the Duke longitudinal data.

KINSEY'S FINDINGS

Kinsey studied the sexual histories of 14,084 men (Kinsey, Pomeroy, and Martin, 1948). Included in this huge group were 106 men over age sixty, only eighteen of whom were over seventy. It is, therefore, not an exaggeration to say that the aged were underrepresented in Kinsey's sample. For this reason some of the statements which Kinsey makes must be viewed somewhat cautiously since they were, in a number of instances, based on extrapolations from data on younger age groups. Kinsey, nevertheless, reached a number of interesting conclusions which he felt were justified on the basis of his data. One of these was that men were sexually most active in late adolescence (ages 16 through 20) and that their activity then gradually declined and that the "rate at which males slow up in these last decades does not exceed the rate at which they have been slowing up and dropping out in the previous age group" (Kinsey, Pomeroy, Martin, 1948). This should be contrasted, however, with the fact that he then goes on to present on the succeeding page data on the rapid increase in the proportion of subjects who are impotent. His figures indicate that this rises from 20 percent at age sixty to 75 percent at age eighty. Kinsey also noted that married men, when compared with either single men or with men who had been previously married, had frequencies of sexual activity which were only slightly higher than those of their nonmarried counterparts.

Kinsey also studied some fifty-six women over age sixty (Kinsey, Pomeroy, and Martin, 1948). His conclusions regarding age-related changes in sexual behavior for the most part represent extrapolations from changes observed at younger ages. He noted a gradual decline in frequency of sexual intercourse between ages twenty and sixty but felt that this "must be the product of aging processes in the male" and that there is "little evidence of any aging in the sexual capacities of the female until late in her life" (Kinsey, Pomeroy, and Martin, 1948). Kinsey further observed that in contrast to the men, single and postmarital females had rates of sexual activity which ranked far below those of their married counterparts.

MASTERS AND JOHNSON REPORT

Masters and Johnson (Masters and Johnson, 1966) devote a considerably greater portion of their book to geriatric sexual responses than did Kinsey. Their data are divided into two categories: (1) findings with respect to sexual anatomy and physiology in old age, based on actual laboratory participation of a small group of aged subjects; and (2) findings with respect to sexual behavior in old age, based on interviews with a somewhat larger group of self-selected aged subjects. Masters and Johnson report that in their sample men past age sixty were slower to be aroused sexually, slower to develop erection, slower to effect intromission, and slower to achieve ejaculation. Accompanying physiological signs of sexual excitement, such as sexual flush and increased muscle tone, were also less pronounced than in younger subjects. The findings were similar for women. Degree of physiological response to sexual stimulation, as indicated by breast engorgement, nipple erection, sexual flush over the breasts, increased muscle tone, clitoral and labial engorgement, were diminished in women over age sixty. However, capacity to reach orgasm was not diminished, especially among those women who had had regular sexual stimulation.

Masters and Johnson interviewed 133 men above age sixty, fifty-two of whom were above age seventy. They present their conclusions somewhat dogmatically and often without sharing with the reader the actual data upon which these conclusions are based. They state that, "there is no question of the fact that the human male's sexual responsiveness wanes as he ages." Great emphasis is placed by them on the role of monotony in sexual activity in determining declining sexual activity. Why monotony should be more important in advanced age than earlier in life is not explained. Vincent has recently pointed out that monotony of sexual expression can be a significant problem in young marriages as well (Vincent, 1969). Masters and Johnson also conclude that men who have had a high sexual "output" during their younger years are likely to continue to be sexually active in old age. This is in congruence with the findings of Newman and Nichols who earlier reported a positive correlation between strong sexual feelings in youth and continued sexual interest in old age (Newman and Nichols, 1960).

Masters and Johnson also interviewed fifty-four women above age sixty, seventeen of whom were above seventy. They conclude on the basis of their sample that capacity for sexual intercourse with orgasmic response is not lacking in older women. Unfortunately, they do not address themselves to the actual incidence of continuing sexual interest or activity in these women. They agree with Kinsey that a sizable portion of the postmenopausal sex drive in women is related to the sexual habits established in earlier years.

Masters and Johnson also asked about masturbation in their sample of women. They conclude, again rather cavalierly, that, "masturbation represents no significant problem for the older-age-group of women." They further state that, "there is no reason why the milestone of the menopause should be expected to blunt the human female's sexual capacity, performance, or drive" and finally, that, "there is no time limit drawn by the advancing years to female sexuality." While these statements may be true from a physiological standpoint, they ignore the social and psychological realities involved. Regular or even occasional satisfaction of sexual needs through coital activity is no longer available for many aged women, and considerable conflict may attach to the practice of masturbation; for it is a fact that the majority of aged women will spend a considerable portion of their old age in widowhood, without a sexual partner. Thus time indirectly does set limits upon female as well as upon male sexuality.

THE DUKE LONGITUDINAL DATA

At the Duke University Center for the Study of Aging and Human Development,

a longitudinal, interdisciplinary study of older individuals has been carried out since 1954 and is still in progress. As part of the study which seeks to elicit somatic, psychological, and social changes associated with old age, data on past and present sexual behavior were also obtained. Subjects of the study were seen repeatedly at approximately three-year intervals. This technique made possible the observation of change occurring within individual subjects over time, not merely changes in groups of subjects, as is the case in cross-sectional studies. Information was obtained on the degree of enjoyment of sexual intercourse and intensity of sexual feelings, both at the present time and in younger years. Also sought was information on the present frequency of intercourse in those subjects who were still sexually active and on the reasons for and age of cessation of coital activity in those subjects who were no longer sexually active.

Initially 254 subjects, ranging in age from sixty to ninety-four years, and roughly equally divided between men and women, were studied. At subsequent examinations this number gradually dwindled as subjects died, became seriously disabled, and a few failed to continue in the study for a number of personal and situational reasons. Included in the study panel were thirty-one intact couples who provided the investigators with a unique opportunity to cross-validate the information provided by each of the two marriage partners. This was important methodologically because the reliability and validity of data on sexual behavior obtained by interview technique has at times been questioned.

The results of these studies have been presented in a number of related articles and papers (Pfeiffer, Verwoerdt, and Wang 1968, 1969a, b). Only a brief summary of them can be presented here. From the ongitudinal data the following major statements can be made. First, sexual interest and coital activity are by no means rare in persons beyond age sixty. Second, patterns of sexual interest and coital activity differ substantially for men and for women of the same age.

About 80 percent of the men whose health, intellectual status, and social functioning were not significantly impaired reported continuing sexual interest at the start of the study. Ten years later the proportion of those still sexually interested had not declined significantly. In contrast, in this same group of men 70 percent were still regularly sexually active at the start of the study but ten years later this proportion had dropped to 25 percent. Thus there was a growing discrepancy with advancing age between the number still sexually interested and those still sexually active.

In the sample of women whose health, intellectual status, and social functioning were good at the start of the study only about one-third reported continuing sexual interest. This proportion did not change significantly over the next ten years. Only about one-fifth of these same healthy women reported at the start of the study they were still having sexual intercourse regularly. Again this proportion did not decline over the next ten years. Obviously and somewhat surprisingly, then, far fewer women than men were still sexually interested or coitally active. How can this phenomenon be explained? The present author has suggested three tentative explanations. First, women may always have had lower levels of sexual interest than men. Kinsey reports a lower frequency of total sexual outlets for women than for men, at all ages (Kinsey, Pomeroy, Martin, and Gebhard, 1953). Our own data also lend some support to this notion; most men but only one third of the women in

our sample reported strong sexual feelings in their younger years (Pfeiffer, Verwoerdt, and Wang, 1969a). Whether these differences between the sexes exist as a result of a cultural or of a biological double standard, however, cannot be said at this time. Second, there is reason to believe that the clearly demarcated menopause in women, signaling the end of reproductive capacity, may indeed have a negative influence on sexual interest and activity in at least some women. A new longitudinal study at Duke University of persons between ages forty-five and seventy may shed some light on this supposition. Third, decline of sexual interest and activity in women may have occurred before their entry into the study (that is, before age 60). Our data indicate that the median age of cessation of intercourse occurred nearly a decade earlier in women than in men, ages 60 and 69, respectively (Pfeiffer, Verwoerdt, and Wang, 1968). Interestingly enough, the overwhelming majority of women attributed responsibility for the cessation of sexual intercourse in the marriage to their husbands; the men in general agreed, holding themselves responsible.

A number of other important findings also emerged from the study. Among these were the following.

1. As Kinsey had found for the younger ages, we found that in old age, too, married men did not differ markedly from non-married men in degree of reported sexual interest and activity. On the other hand, married women differed substantially from nonmarried women; only a very few of the latter reported any sexual activity, and only 20 percent reported any sexual interest.

2. While our cross-sectional data indicated a gradual *decline* in sexual interest and activity with increasing age, our longitudinal data revealed that some 20 to 25

percent of the men, but only a few percent of the women, actually showed patterns of *rising* sexual interest and activity with advancing age. Furthermore, rising patterns were more frequent among nonmarried than among married men.

3. Among the group of intact couples included in the study panel there was a very high level of agreement between husbands and wives with regard to reported frequency of sexual intercourse and reasons for stopping coital activity.

It must be admitted that the Duke longitudinal data on sexual behavior in old age are far from complete. Additional information is obviously needed to answer some of the following questions: What sexual conflicts and problems do the married and the nonmarried aged experience? What are their sexual fantasies, dreams, and concerns? How important is masturbation as a sexual outlet for those aged who no longer have a capable sexual partner available to them, and what conflicts does it arouse? To whom do the aged turn for help with their sexual or marital problems? Full and satisfying answers to these and other questions are not currently available, and more comprehensive studies are needed.

REFERENCES

Golde, P. and Kogan, N. A sentence completion procedure for assessing attitudes toward old people. *J. Geront. 14*:355-363, 1959.

Kinsey, A. C., Pomeroy, W. B., and Martin, C. R. *Sexual Behavior in the Human Male.* Philadelphia: Saunders, 1948.

Kinsey, A. C., Pomeroy, W. B., Martin, C. R. and Gebhard, P. H. *Sexual Behavior in the Human Female.* Philadelphia: Saunders, 1953.

Lief, H. I. Sex education of medical students and doctors. *Pacif. Med. Surg. 73*:52-55, 1965.

Lief, H. I. Sex and the medical educator. *J. Amer. Med. Wom. Ass. 23*:195-196, 1968.

Masters, W. H., and Johnson, V. E. *Human Sexual Response.* Boston: Little, Brown, 1966.

Newman, G., and Nichols, C. R. Sexual activities and attitudes in older persons, *J.A.M.A. 173*:33-35, 1960.

Pfeiffer, E., Verwoerdt, A., and Wang, H.S. Sexual behavior in aged men and women. Observations on 254 community volunteers. *Arch. Gen. Psychiat.* (Chicago) *19*:753-758, 1968.

Pfeiffer, E., Verwoerdt, A., and Wang, H.S. The natural history of sexual behavior in a biologically advantaged group of aged individuals. *J. Geront. 24*:193-198, 1969a.

Rubin, I. *Sexual Life After Sixty.* New York: Basic Books, 1965.

Verwoerdt, A., Pfeiffer, E., and Wang, H.S. Sexual behavior in senescence. I. Changes in sexual activity and interest of aging men and women. *J. Geriat. Psychiat.* In press.

Verwoerdt, A., Pfeiffer, E., and Wang, H.S. Sexual behavior in senescence. II. Patterns of sexual activity and interest. *Geriatrics 24*:137-154, 1969b.

Vincent, C. E. Sex and the young married. *Med. Aspects Hum. Sex. 3*:13-23, 1969.

Wallace, I. *The Chapman Report.* New York: Simon and Schuster, 1960.

MORALE, ADJUSTMENT, AND LIFE SATISFACTION

I N THEIR EFFORTS TO EXAMINE the social behavior of the aged, gerontologists in the 1930s and early 1950s made numerous attempts to delineate the needs of the elderly (Barron, 1954; Havighurst and Albrecht, 1953; Havighurst, 1952). One result of these efforts was to focus attention on the adjustment problems of older people. To this extent, many researchers examined the patterns and styles of adjustment characteristic of specific groups in society (Britton, 1953; Britton and Britton, 1951; Schmidt, 1951; Shanas, 1950). The success or failure to adjust, for example, was often related to such factors as income and social status. In general, however, the adjustment difficulties of the elderly drew attention regardless of occupational or social background (Burgess, 1950; Cavan *et al.*, 1949; Morgan, 1937).

As a result of these seminal investigations, gerontologists gained an appreciation for both the social *and* psychological aspects of adjustment. Personal adjustment and morale soon became associated with the perceptual and attitudinal character of the aged (Fried, 1949; Morgan, 1937; Kardiner, 1937; Landis, 1942). Accordingly, both attitudes and behavior assumed a complementary role in the adjustment process. This linkage was to prove particularly useful in examining such role transitions as retirement and widowhood (Hoyt, 1954; Tibbitts, 1954; Hauser and Shanas, 1952).

For the most part, however, the period was one of descriptive exploration in the discipline. The large quantities of data collected permitted researchers to not only explore the needs of older persons, but also to assess the ameliorative programs of state and federal agencies. In general, these efforts were seldom oriented around or by specific theoretical models.

Along with the lack of a theoretical base, research was often typified by cross-sectional methodologies (Barron, 1954; Morgan, 1937; Hauser and Shanas, 1952). As a result, the adjustment picture was frequently confused by attempts to correlate success or failure with such isolated factors as health, income, age, employment status, and the like. In addition, the prevailing view of adjustment and satisfaction assumed a declining character with time. To complicate the matter further, little concensus was apparent regarding the measurement of either variable (s). Few attempts were in evidence to specify the operations necessary for conceptual measurement.

On the other hand, the focus on the phenomenology of adjustment was expanded in the later 1950s and early 1960s. During this period of time, social as well as psychological measures were employed to assess the adjustment and satisfaction of the elderly (Anderson, 1958; August, 1956; Kuhlen, 1959; Streib, 1957). In addition, attempts were made to specify the character of the concepts (Trenton, 1963; Tobin and Neugarten, 1961; Streib, 1956), as well as to develop standardized measuring instruments (Neugarten and Havighurst, 1961). As a consequence, gerontologists were now able to compare and evaluate the results of their research.

Armed with improved measurement techniques and adopting the wisdom of longitudinal design, researchers set about incorporating their efforts into a series of theoretical models (see Section II). No longer limited to the correlation of relatively isolated variables, these formulations gave consideration to the psychological arena (Thompson, 1958) as well as the role transitions attendant upon old age (Emerson, 1959; Drinkwater, 1959). Most of these orientations account in part for the interplay of family and peer relations relative to the adjustment and satisfaction (i.e. morale) of the older person (Havighurst, 1960; Orbach and Shaw, 1957; Friedmann, 1958).

It is apparent that the work of this period added significantly to the gerontologist's arsenal of knowledge. The psychological dimensions of adjustment were now cast into explanatory models which permitted the testing of specific hypotheses regarding the aging process. Concepts were also broadened in their interpretation and operations carefully specified as to their measurement. In addition, the role relationships of the aged as well as the implications of role loss were combined with phenomenological data to predict the success or failure of subsequent adjustment. Such efforts went far beyond the mere specification of personality or "success types." Adjustment and satisfaction were regarded as functions of life style, perceptual accuracy, and socioemotional flexibility.

Several patterns characteristic of these earlier periods were to continue development in the late 1960s and early 1970s. One of these involved attempts to specify more carefully those factors related to good adjustment and life satisfaction (Adams, 1971). To the picture of adjustment, gerontologists have added such variables as ego strength (Cameron, 1967), housing quality (Lipman, 1969; Schooler, 1969), and family relationships (Kerckhoff, 1966). Similarly, there remains strong interest in the adjustment patterns of individuals and social groups (Goldsamt, 1967; Back and Gergen, 1966; Havens, 1968). For the most part, however, researchers have sought to incorporate both dimensions into specific theories or frameworks (Loeb, 1966; Neugarten, 1970). Among these, the *family life cycle* has proved one of the most useful.

Instrumental refinement has also continued to the present time. This development has followed on the heels of both methodological creativity and statistical sophistication. This has often meant the simultaneous use of several instruments, such as the likert scale and the semantic differential. Both measures suggest the assessment of social and psychological factors related to adjustment. In addition, behavioral observation has added an objective dimension to the measurement process. Together, these techniques have provided information which has led to the testing and reformulation of several contemporary theories.

Finally, contemporary efforts in theory development have not been oriented toward adjustment and morale *per se*. Instead, these formulations are sensitive to a range of aging phenomena. This more wholistic view of aging regards adjustment, morale, and satisfaction as by-products of both perceptual and social changes. In addition, there is new evidence from longitudinal studies to support a continuity view of aging behavior. This suggests that the continuation of a previously established pattern of behavior may be the most critical factor in the social and emotional well-being of the older adult. In essence, as long as the changes wrought by age and society do not overly disturb the "equilibrium of life," adjustment will prove relatively uneventful and morale and satisfaction should remain high.

The papers which follow illustrate the character of contemporary research relative to adjustment and satisfaction. To some extent, these selections continue the search for factors related to "successful aging." On the other hand, each author seeks to place his findings in theoretical perspective. In addition, considerable attention is given to conceptual and instrumental refinement.

The paper by Edwards and Klemmack represents an attempt to delineate which, if any, of the previously studied variables related to life satisfaction are the most efficient predictors of it. In addition, the authors strive to determine what combination of factors is most successful in explaining the variance in experienced satisfaction within a sample of older adults.

Data for the study were obtained through interviews with 507 middle-aged and older men and women residing in a Virginia 4 county area. Twenty-two independent variables were utilized in the study. Although many of the independent variables were found to be statistically related to life satisfaction, the results indicate that even minimal controls (e.g. socioeconomic status) frequently reduce the magnitude of most of the general relationships and often eliminate some that were initially statistically significant. In comparing the relative contributions of each variable in accounting for the variance in life satisfaction with age, the authors report socioeconomic status, perceived health status, and informal participation with nonkinsmen to be the best predictors of life satisfaction. Neither informal familial participation nor most of the social and personal background characteristics examined contribute significantly to the predicting of life satisfaction.

The paper by Cutler gives consideration to two additional factors in the life satisfaction-adjustment equation, the availability of personal transportation and residential location. The author hypothesizes that (1) life satisfaction should be higher among older persons for whom personal transportation is available than among those individuals having little access in this regard; and (2) a stronger relationship should obtain between personal transportation and life satisfaction among the aged who reside farther from local community facilities than among those whose residences are more proximate.

Data were obtained through interviews with 170 noninstitutionalized respondents aged sixty-five and older residing in a small community in central Ohio. The results indicate that the life satisfaction of the elderly *is* related to differentials in personal transportation availability. Older persons having such transportation access exhibit higher life satisfaction scores than those older persons now have transportation available for their use. In addition, "the consequences of transportation differentials for life satisfaction are somewhat greater for the aged whose residences are more distant from the centralized resources, facilities, and services of the community."

Spence examines the concept of futurity (i.e. the ability to characterize the immediate and distant future) relative to its implications for the adaptive patterns of the aged. His principal concern is whether those older persons who manifest a sense of futurity are also among the better adjusted. It is hypothesized that (1) those who are future-oriented will be more satisfied than those who are not, and (2) those who desire change will be less likely to be satisfied than those who do not desire change.

Spence's findings lend general support to both hypotheses. That is, planning is observed to be positively related to satisfaction, while desiring change is negatively related to satisfaction. Nevertheless, the author notes an interaction effect between the variablies planning and a desire for change. An inverse relationship is observed, for example, between making plans and age primarily among those people who do not desire change. In addition, an inverse relationship holds between desiring change and age principally for those who do not make plans. On the basis of these results, Spence suggests that, "in addition to futurity, a positive present orientation may also be contributing to the adaptive potential."

Still another dimension of the adjustment-morale picture is provided in the paper by Bultena. The author suggests that, for the most part, the major goals of individuals are not materially changed by their entry into old age. In this regard, the culturally-valued goals of an acceptable social status, economic success, good health, and independence continue to comprise important objectives for the older person. Nevertheless, the crises of later life may impose a number of obstacles to the realization of these goals. As a consequence of both the cultural goal seeking and decremental assumptions of old age, Bultena hypothesizes that, "the greater the discontinuity in life patterns between the pre- and postretirement periods, the greater will be the impact on the individual's ability to function successfully relative to the attainment of culturally-valued goals and thereby the greater the probability of his being demoralized."

The author's findings indicate morale to be positively related to socioeconomic status. That is, the proportion of respondents with low life satisfaction decreases with a corresponding increase in socioeconomic status. Decremental life changes are also observed to be associated with a low level of morale. In addition, Bultena notes that the impact of life changes on morale are mediated by the social structure. In this instance, the psychological costs of decremental changes appear to be disproportionately centered among those in the lower socioeconomic segments of the aged population.

The final paper in this section examines the implications of consistency theory with regard to the life satisfaction of older adults. The focus of this research concerns the consonance or dissonance between one's expectations relative to a role change (i.e. retirement) and his actual behavior following this transition. It is hypothesized that, "the transition from work to nonwork related roles should influence life satisfaction to the extent that postretirement expectations for behavior have been disconfirmed."

Data were obtained from pre- and postretirement interviews with 114 older males residing in an urban area of central Missouri. With the exception of the family area, the findings yield little support for the consistency hypothesis (i.e. expectational disconfirmation should be accompanied by negative changes in life satisfaction). Instead, evidence is presented which indicates the *type of disconfirmation* to be more central to the explanation of life satisfaction change than disconfirmation *per se*.

REFERENCES

Adams, D. L. Correlates of satisfaction among the elderly. *Gerontologist,* 1971, *11,* 64-68.

Anderson, J. E. Psychological aspects of the use of free time. In W. Donahue, W. W. Hunter, D. H. Coons, and H. K. Maurice (Eds.), *Free time: challenge to later maturity.* Ann Arbor: University of Michigan Press, 1958.

August, H. Psychological aspects of personal adjustment. In I. N. Gross (Ed.), *Potentialities of women in the middle years.* Lansing: Michigan State University Press, 1956.

Back, K. W., and Gergen, K. J. Personal orientation and morale of the aged. In I. H. Simpson and J. C. McKinney (Eds.) *Social aspects of aging.* Durham, North Carolina: Duke University Press, 1966.

Barron, M. L. A survey of a cross-section of the urban aged in the United States. In M. L. Barron (Ed.), *Old age in the modern world.* Edinburgh: E. & S. Livingstone, 1954.

Britton, J. H. The personal adjustment of retired school teachers. *Journal of Gerontology,* 1953, *8,* 333-338.

Britton, J. O., and Britton, J. H. Factors related to the adjustment of retired Y.M.C.A. secretaries. *Journal of Gerontology,* 1951, *6,* 34-38.

Burgess, E. W. Personal and social adjustment in old age. In M. Derber (Ed.), *The aged and society.* Champaign, Illinois: Industrial Relations Research Association, 1950.

Cameron, P. Ego strength and happiness of the aged. *Journal of Gerontology,* 1967, *22,* 199-202.

Cavan, R. S., Burgess, E. W., Havighurst, R. J., and Goldhamer, H. *Personal adjustment in old age.* Chicago: University of Chicago Press, 1949.

Drinkwater, R. W. Some role problems in middle life and their implications for subsequent adjustment. In *Proceedings of the fourth congress, international association of gerontology,* 1959, *3,* 452-459.

Emerson, A. R. The first year of retirement. *Occupational Psychology,* 1959, *33,* 197-208.

Fried, E. Attitudes of the older population groups toward activity and inactivity. *Journal of Gerontology,* 1949, *4,* 141-151.

Friedman, E. A. The work of leisure. In W. Donahue, W. W. Hunter, D. H. Coons, and H. K. Maurice (Eds.), *Free time: challenge to later maturity.* Ann Arbor: University of Michigan Press, 1958.

Goldsamt, M. R. Life satisfaction and the older disabled worker. *Journal of American Geriatric Society,* 1967, *15,* 394-399.

Havens, B. J. An investigation of activity patterns and adjustment in an aging population. *Gerontologist,* 1968, *8,* 201-206.

Havighurst, R. J. Social and psychological needs of the aging. *Annals of American Academy of Political and Social Science,* 1952, *279,* 11-17.

Havighurst, R. J. Life beyond family and work. In E. W. Burgess (Ed.), *Aging in western societies: a survey of social gerontology.* Chicago: University of Chicago Press, 1960.

Havighurst, R. J., and Albrecht, R. *Older people.* New York: Longmans, Green and Company, 1953.

Hauser, P. M., and Shanas, E. Trends in the aging population. In A. I. Langing (Ed.), *Cowdry's problem of ageing.* Baltimore: Williams & Wilkins Co., 1952.

Hoyt, G. C. The process and problems of retirement. *Journal of Business of the University of Chicago,* 1954, *27,* 164-168.

Kardiner, A. Psychological factors in old age. In A. Kardiner (Ed.), *Mental hygiene in old age.* New York: Family Welfare Association of America, 1937.

Kerckhoff, A. C. Family patterns and morale in retirement. In I. H. Simpson and J. C. McKinney (Eds.), *Social aspects of aging.* Durham, North Carolina: Duke University Press, 1966.

Kuhlen, R. G. Aging and life adjustment. In J. E. Birren (Ed.) *Handbook of aging and the individual.* Chicago: University of Chicago Press, 1959.

Landis, J. T. Social-psychological factors of aging. *Social Forces,* 1942, *20,* 468-470.

Lipman, A. Public housing and attitudinal adjustment in old age: a comparative study. *Journal of Geriatric Psychiatry,* 1969, *2,* 88-101.

Loeb, M. M., Pincus, A., and Mueller, B. J. A framework for viewing adjustment in aging. *Gerontologist,* 1966, *6,* 185-187.

Morgan, C. M. The attitudes and adjustments of recipients of old age assistance in upstate New York and metropolitan New York. *Archives of Psychology,* 1937, *214,* 1-131.

Neugarten, B. L. Adaptation and the life cycle. *Journal of Geriatric Psychiatry,* 1970, *4,* 71-87.

Neugarten, B. L., Havighurst, R. J., and Tobin, S. S. The measurement of life satisfaction. *Journal of Gerontology,* 1961, *16,* 134-143.

Orbach, H. L., and Shaw, D. M. Social participation and the role of the aging. *Geriatrics,* 1957, *12,* 241-246.

Schmidt, J. F. Patterns of poor adjustment in old age. *American Journal of Sociology,* 1951, *57,* 33-42.

Schooler, K. K. The relationship between social interaction and morale of the elderly as a function of environmental characteristics. *Gerontologist,* 1969, *9,* 25-29.

Shanas, E. The personal adjustment of recipients of old age assistance. *Journal of Gerontology,* 1950, *5,* 249-253.

Streib, G. F. Morale and the retired. *Social Problems,* 1956, *3,* 270-276.

Streib, G. F., and Thompson, W. E. Personal and social adjustment in retirement. In W. Donahue and C. Tibbitts (Eds.), *The new frontiers of aging.* Ann Arbor: University of Michigan Press, 1957.

Thompson, W. E., Pre-retirement anticipation and adjustment in retirement. *Journal of Social Issues,* 1958, *14,* 35-45.

Tibbitts, C. Retirement problems in American society. *American Journal of Sociology,* 1954, *59,* 301-308.

Tobin, S. S., and Neugarten, B. L. Life satisfaction and social interaction in the aging. *Journal of Gerontology,* 1961, *16,* 344-346.

Trenton, J. R. The concept of adjustment in old age. In R. H. Williams, C. Tibbitts, and W. Donahue (Eds.), *Processes of aging.* New York: Atherton Press, 1963.

Chapter 30

CORRELATES OF LIFE SATISFACTION: A RE-EXAMINATION

JOHN N. EDWARDS AND
DAVID L. KLEMMACK

INTENSIVE INVESTIGATION has been conducted for more than a decade concerning the biological, psychological, and sociological correlates of individual well-being, of which life satisfaction is one component. For example, a negative relationship has been noted in several studies between well-being and advancing age, poor health, and physical disability (Jeffers and Nichols, 1961; Kutner, Fanshel, Togo, and Langer, 1956; Lowenthal and Boler, 1965). Additional evidence has shown individual well-being to be related to a host of perceptual phenomena, including life space, relative deprivation, inadequacy, and aging itself (Hansen and Yoshioka, 1962; Phillips, 1961; Tobin and Neugarten, 1961).

Particular attention has been focused, though, on the sociological correlates of well-being and the more discrete dimension of life satisfaction. Among other relationships, numerous studies have consistently observed significant correlations between life satisfaction and socioeconomic status, marital status, size of community, and work status (Gurin, Veroff, and Feld, 1960; Hansen and Yoshioka, 1962; Kutner et al., 1956; Marshall and Eteng, 1970). Concomitant with this line of inquiry, there

Reprinted by permission from the *Journal of Gerontology*, 1973, *28*, 497-502.

has been a considerable focus on the role of social relations and activities in their influence on satisfaction, resulting in a continuing debate regarding the disengagement theory (Cumming and Henry, 1961; Tallmer and Kutner, 1970; Tobin and Neugarten, 1961; Youmans, 1969).

The Problem

What has been lacking in the abundant research to date, with one notable exception (Palmore and Luikart, 1972), has been an explicit attempt to determine which, if any, of the many variables related to life satisfaction are the most efficient predictors of it and what combination of factors is most successful in explaining the variance in experienced satisfaction. Cutler (1973), for instance, has recently demonstrated the desirability for such a determination after finding that involvement in voluntary associations makes no independent contribution to life satisfaction when the effects of health and socioeconomic status are held constant. Palmore and Luikart (1972) also point out that self-rated health, organizational activity, and internal control, that is, a belief in one's own efficacy, were most strongly related to satisfaction in their analysis of eighteen variables. Until such time as further explorations are made along this line, theory-building in gerontological studies will be seriously hampered. Without an empirical basis for ascertaining the variables to be included in a theory, theoretical efforts are not likely to be parsimonious and, even more seriously, are not likely to be found valid as they are subsequently tested.

To partially rectify the present situation, this inquiry is addressed to examining the effect of a broad range of variables on life satisfaction. Specifically, three questions are addressed (1) in general, what relationships exist in the present set of data between a variety of sociologically relevant factors and life satisfaction, (2) to what extent are these general relationships altered by the introduction of control variables, and (3) what is the relative contribution of the independent variables considered in explaining the variance in reported satisfaction? In considering these research questions, the independent variables taken into account pertain to socioeconomic status, personal and social background characteristics, formal social participation, informal involvement in familial relations, informal nonfamilial participation, and health status. Inasmuch as various aspects of these factors have been repeatedly employed in prior research, our basic concerns have to do with assessing the possibility that many observed relationships may be partialled out and with determining to what extent the different factors make an independent contribution in accounting for life satisfaction.

Data and Methods

The data presented here are derived from a larger study concerning the health, housing, and social participation of the middle-aged and elderly residing in a Virginia four-county area. The data were secured using a census enumeration district quota sample, resulting in a proportionate representation of males and females forty-five to sixty-four and those sixty-five and older. Reflecting the 4-county area population, the sample was predominantly white, Anglo-Saxon, and Protestant. Most of the subjects were long-term residents of the area, with 61 percent having lived for twenty years or more in their current neighborhood. Other than for a slight under-representation of persons classified as fall-

ing within the federal poverty guidelines, a comparison of these and other characteristics with the 1970 census parameters suggests the sample was representative of the region.

Life satisfaction, the dependent variable in this analysis, was measured by employing ten items from the Life Satisfaction Index modified by Adams (1969). The ten items include only those that Adams suggests are clearly interpretable as reflective of a specific subdimension of life satisfaction. The mean of the resulting indicator was 25.84 and the standard deviation 3.24. Based on our data, coefficient alpha was .90, suggesting the indicator was reliable (Nunnally, 1967).

Twenty-two independent variables included in the study were grouped into six major categories: socioeconomic status, personal and social background characteristics, formal social participation, informal interaction with kin, informal nonfamilial participation, and health status. The measures used for the variables in each of the categories were largely standardized ones. Socioeconomic status, for example, was comprised of the variables of education, income (total family income), and occupational prestige, the latter coded according to the Duncan scale (1961).

The category "personal and social background characteristics" encompassed age of respondent, sex of subject, marital status (married, never married, separated, divorced, or widowed), family size (number of related persons in the household), length of residence (number of years in the area), community size, and whether the head of the household was retired.

Formal participation was measured by (1) whether the respondent had voted in the 1964 and 1968 presidential elections and the 1970 congressional election, (2 the extent and intensity of participation in formal voluntary associations as indicated by the Chapin scale (1955), and (3) the intensity of involvement the subject had in church-related organizations.

Two indicators of kin participation were employed: (1) the frequency of contact with kinsmen outside the nuclear unit, and (2) the frequency of contact with offspring who no longer resided in the respondent's household.

Informal participation with nonkinsmen was indicated by the frequency with which the respondent interacted with neighbors; the number of times that friends, neighbors, and relatives were contacted by phone; the number of neighbors known; and the number of good friends claimed by the subject.

Health status, finally, was determined by three indicators. One such indicator concerned the perceived health of the respondent. Further indications of health status were obtained by eliciting information on the number of ailments the respondent had experienced within the last month prior to the interview and the number of ailments he or she had incurred within the previous year.

In addressing the research questions posed earlier, Pearson product-moment correlations were used to determine the general relationships between the independent variables and scores on the Life Satisfaction Index. Following this, the socioeconomic status variables were applied as controls and the partial correlations between the remaining independent variables and life satisfaction were derived. As a final procedure, standardized partial beta coefficients were computed using ordinary multiple regression with life satisfaction as the dependent variable. The beta coefficient provides a measure of the relative contri-

bution of each predictor in accounting for life satisfaction.

Findings

Looking first at the zero-order relationships between the independent variables and life satisfaction (Column 1, Table 30-I), it may be seen that most of the factors are related to satisfaction. Of the six major categories of factors, only one fails to significantly relate. Informal participation with kin, as noted in Column 1, is not statistically related to life satisfaction.

Inspecting the component variables of each of the categories of independent variables, several interesting relationships may be noted. Each of the indicators of socioeconomic status is positively associated with life satisfaction, family income having the highest correlation with it. Among the background characteristics, on the other hand, significant relationships exist between only three of the seven independent variables and the dependent variable. Those who are younger, currently married, and have larger families are more satisfied with life. In terms of formal social participation, belonging to and intensity of involvement in voluntary and church-related associations are directly related to reported satisfaction. In addition, most of the indicators of nonfamilial participation show a positive relationship with the dependent variable. High satisfaction is associated with a high frequency of visiting neighbors, phoning others, and knowing a large number of neighbors. Concerning the health status variables, perceiving oneself as being in good health is positively related to satisfaction with life, while the number of experienced ailments, either recent or immediately past ones, is unrelated.

Given these relationships, it is possible to explore the effect of control variables on

TABLE 30-I

RELATIONSHIP OF SELECTED VARIABLES WITH LIFE SATISFACTION

	Correlation with Life Satisfaction[a]	Partical Correlation with Life Satisfaction Controlling for Status[b]	Multiple Regression to Predict Life Satisfaction[c]
Socioeconomic status			
Education	.24*	—	.11
Income	.33*	—	.34*
Occupational status	.12	—	.12*
Background characteristics			
Age	—.14*	—.05	—.06
Sex	—.01	—.04	—.01
Marital status	.14*	.07	.10
Family size	.10*	.02	—.01
Time in area	—.07	—.01	—.05
Community size	—.02	—.08	—.12*
Retired (head of household)	—.06	—.06	—.08
Formal participation			
Voting	.05	—.08	—.14*
Voluntary association	.24*	.12*	.09
Church-related activities	.19*	.15*	.14*
Informal familial participation			
Visit relatives	.06	—	.02
Visit children	.02	—.02	—.03
Informal nonfamilial participation			
Visit neighbors	.16*	.18*	.14*
Phone others	.13*	.14*	.11*
Number of neighbors	.09*	.09*	.11*
Number of friends	.04	.04	—.01
Health			
Perceived health	.19*	.12*	.16*
Number of ailments last month	—.06	—.02	.04
Number of ailments last year	—.07	—.03	.01

[a]Zero-order Pearsonian correlation of each variable with life satisfaction.

[b]Partial correlation of each variable with life satisfaction controlling simultaneously for educational attainment, income, and occupational status.

[c]Partial beta coefficients (standardized) when predicting life satisfaction simultaneoulsy from all the remaining variables.

*Statistically significant at $p < .05$.

them. In particular our concern is whether the general relationships noted with respect to the background, formal participation, nonfamilial involvement, and health status variables remain related to reported satisfaction when control variables are intro-duced. Since socioeconomic status often ha[s] been identified as a critical factor in pre[-] vious research (Hansen and Yoshiok[a] 1962; Kutner *et al.,* 1956; Marshall an[d] Eteng, 1970; Thompson, Streib, and Kos[a] 1963), it was instituted as a control. Th[e] partial correlation between each variable and satisfaction with life, controlling for the three indicators of socioeconomic status, is presented in the second column of Table 30-I.

The results clearly show that some variables are related to life satisfaction independent of the effects of socioeconomic status while others are not. Controlling for socioeconomic status eliminated the statistically significant relationships between life satisfaction and age, marital status, and family size. All of the other variables found to be statistically significant in the first phase of the analysis remain so. In fact, the three indicators of nonfamilial informal involvement have somewhat higher relationships after controlling for socioeconomic status than before control, suggesting a slight suppression effect with this type of involvement.

The final question posed in the study concerns the relative effect of each variable in the prediction of life satisfaction. To this end, a multiple regression analysis was performed using life satisfaction as the dependent or criterion variable. The resulting regression coefficients were then standardized to facilitate comparisons of effects (Table 30-I, Column 3). Particularly since many of the variables contributed little or nothing to the prediction, the overall equation was fairly efficient, accounting for 24.35 percent of the variance in life satisfaction (multiple correlation = .49). Examination of the magnitude of individual coefficients points out that the primary determinant of life satisfaction is socioeconomic status, especially family income. The income coefficient is more than double that of any other in the equation. Perceived health also has a substantial positive relationship, which, in the context of this analysis, is independent of the effect of any and all of the remaining variables. In addi-

tion, the nonfamilial participation variables, particularly the combination of extent and intensity of neighboring, appear to have a substantial positive effect.

Discussion

In terms of the zero-order relationships reported here, substantial support for previous research is found. A variety of indicators bearing on socioeconomic status, personal and social background, formal participation, informal nonfamilial involvement, and health status are related to life satisfaction. Informal participation with kin, as has been indicated in some prior studies (Lemon *et. al.*, 1972), is not significantly related to perceived satisfaction.

Turning to the partial correlations, the findings indicate that some of the observed general relationships disappear when a control variable is introduced. Specifically, in controlling for socioeconomic status, all of the significant relationships are eliminated between the background characteristics and life satisfaction. Several other relationships, although they remain statistically significant, are substantially reduced in magnitude. Patently, this would suggest that the socioeconomic status variables are highly efficacious in accounting for and predicting life satisfaction.

This conclusion is reinforced by the multiple regression analysis presented above. In accounting for the variance in life satisfaction, the socioeconomic status variables are, as a category, the most efficient predictors among those considered. Family income, in particular, is the single most important variable in explaining reported satisfaction.

A predictive model of life satisfaction is also suggested, at least in skeletal form, by the regression analysis. Especially socioeconomic status, nonfamilial participation, and health status are pointed up as being the principal components of this model. Combined, they account for almost all of the explained variance in satisfaction. Although the causal ordering of the variables is open to question and remains a matter of speculation, it would appear that when a temporal sequence is considered, socioeconomic status should be treated as an independent variable, having both direct and indirect effects on satisfaction. Its indirect effects appear to be through informal participation and perceived health, which operate as intervening variables and are in turn directly related to experienced satisfaction. Regardless of the specific design of the model, however, the evidence emphatically suggests these three sets of factors are necessary components to be considered in any theory construction efforts dealing with life satisfaction.

Concerning current theory efforts, the data in part lend further support to the activity theory of aging, postulating that activity in general is important to the prediction of individual well-being. No support is found for role loss, as manifested in retirement, as being critical to the level of satisfaction one experiences. Formal activity, such as involvement in voluntary organizations, does not independently contribute to overall satisfaction. Furthermore, satisfaction is largely unaffected by the background characteristics that are usually hypothesized as specifying, either by increasing or decreasing, the general relationship between activity and life satisfaction.

Summary

The task of predicting and accounting for life satisfaction has been addressed in this research (a) by exploring the general relationships between twenty-two variables and life satisfaction, (b) by ascertaining the effects the introduction of control variables has on the general relationships, and (c) by determining the contribution made by each of the independent variables considered. On the basis of the findings, two major conclusions are noteworthy.

While many of the independent variables were found to be statistically related to life satisfaction at the zero-order level, thus paralleling the findings of a number of previous studies, the introduction of even minimal controls reduces the magnitude of most of the general relationships and eliminates some that were statistically significant. Holding socioeconomic status constant, the zero-order relationships between satisfaction and age, marital status, and family size are reduced to a nonsignificant level.

Comparing the relative contributions in accounting for the variance in life satisfaction, socioeconomic status, and family income in particular, was noted as the primary determinant. Additional variance was explained by perceived health status and participation in nonfamilial activities, especially those activities involving neighboring. Neither informal familial participation nor most of social and personal background characteristics contributed significantly to predicting life satisfaction. Participation in voluntary associations did not independently contribute to perceived satisfaction. In all, this suggests theory-building efforts should be directed to considering socioeconomic status, nonfamilial participation and health status as major components of future models designed to account for life satisfaction.

REFERENCES

Adams, D. L. Analysis of a life satisfaction index. *Journal of Gerontology*, 1969, *24*, 470-474.

Chapin, F. S. *Experimental designs in sociologi-

cal research. Harper, New York, 1955.

Cumming, E. M., and Henry, W. *Growing old.* Basic Books, New York, 1961.

Cutler, S. J. Voluntary association participation and life satisfaction: A cautionary research note. *Journal of Gerontology,* 1973, *28,* 96-100.

Duncan, O. D. A socioeconomic index for all occupations. In A. J. Reiss, Jr. (Ed.), *Occupations and social status.* Free Press, New York, 1961.

Gurin, G., Veroff, J., and Feld, S. *Americans view their mental health: A nationwide interview study.* Basic Books, New York, 1960.

Hansen, G., and Yoshioka, S. *Aging in the upper midwest: A profile of 6,300 senior citizens.* Community Studies, Kansas City, 1962.

Jeffers, F. C., and Nichols, C. R. The relationship of activities and attitudes to physical well-being in older people. *Journal of Gerontology,* 1961, *16,* 67-70.

Kutner, B., Fanshel, D., Togo, A., and Langer, T. S. *Five hundred over sixty.* Russell Sage Foundation, New York, 1956.

Lemon, B. W., Bengtson, V. L., and Peterson, J. A. An exploration of the activity theory of aging: Activity types and life satisfaction among in-movers to a retirement community. *Journal of Gerontology,* 1972, *27,* 511-523.

Lowenthal, M. F., and Boler, D. Voluntary vs. involuntary social withdrawal. *Journal of Gerontology,* 1965, *20,* 363-371.

Marshall, D., and Eteng, W. Retirement and migration in the north central states: A comparative analysis; Wisconsin, Florida, Arizona. Population Series #20, Dept. of Rural Sociology, Univ. of Wisconsin, 1970.

Nunnally, J. C. *Psychometric theory.* McGraw-Hill, New York, 1967.

Palmore, E., and Luikart, C. Health and social factors related to life satisfaction. *Journal of Health & Social Behavior,* 1972, *13,* 68-80.

Phillips, B. Role change, subjective age, and adjustment: A correlational analysis. *Journal of Gerontology,* 1961, *16,* 347-352.

Tallmer, M., and Kutner, B. Disengagement and morale. *Gerontologist,* 1970, *10,* 317-320.

Thompson, W., Streib, G. F., and Kosa, J. Effect of retirement on personal adjustment: A panel analysis. *Journal of Gerontology,* 1963, *18,* 165-169.

Tobin, S. S., and Neugarten, B. L., Life satisfaction and social interaction in the aging. *Journal of Gerontology,* 1961, *16,* 344-346.

Youmans, E. G. Some perspectives on disengagement theory. *Gerontologist,* 1969, *9,* 254-258.

Chapter 31

THE AVAILABILITY OF PERSONAL TRANSPORTATION, RESIDENTIAL LOCATION, AND LIFE SATISFACTION AMONG THE AGED

STEPHEN J. CUTLER

ALTHOUGH THE WIDESPREAD availability of the automobile has had profound implications for personal mobility, it is increasingly clear that the aged neither share equally in the advantages offered by personal transportation nor are they equally able to overcome the obstacles posed in its absence. Functional impairments, difficulties in income-maintenance, and the characteristics of transportation systems themselves have erected significant barriers to mobility for large segments of the elderly (Abt Associates, 1969; Cantilli and Shmelzer, 1971; US Senate, 1970; White House Conference on Aging, 1971). Placing further constraints on mobility is the situation in many smaller urban and rural communities where public and/or commercial (taxi) transportation are nonexistent (Cottrell, 1971; Twente, 1970). Yet, inasmuch as the description and documentation of these and related problems has only recently been undertaken and because the greatest share of attention is being given to the con-

Reprinted by permission from the *Journal of Gerontology,* 1972, *27,* 383-389.

centrated numbers of older persons living in larger urban areas, relatively little is known about the correlates of differentials in the availability of transportation (for a notable exception, see Carp, 1971a) or about the situation in this regard in other than the larger urban setting. The present research addresses itself to both questions by considering how differentials in the availability of personal transportation relate to the life satisfaction of the elderly and by considering this relationship, in conjunction with other critical variables, in the context of the smaller community.

Background and Hypotheses

The life satisfaction of the aged has been studied from a number of analytical perspectives (Adams, 1971; Riley and Foner, 1968). Among the most consistent findings are those which, contrary to the predictions of disengagement theory, show a positive relationship between life satisfaction and levels of social activity and interaction (Kutner, Fanshel, Togo, and Langner, 1956; Maddox, 1965, 1966; Palmore, 1968; Pihlblad and McNamara, 1965; Tobin and Neugarten, 1961). Yet, the extent to which activity and, consequently, life satisfaction are themselves dependent upon access differentials (which, broadly conceived, tend to enable or to facilitate the social engagement of the aged and which are defined, in part, by the availability of transportation) has, heretofore, received only limited empirical attention (Kaplan, 1970; Trela and Simmons, 1971). The general outline of the problem, however, is well stated by Clark (1971):

> Immobility . . . is life in an ever-shrinking world, forcing a slow attrition in many other areas of an individual's personal and social system and resulting in an impoverishment of all segments of life.

Similarly, but focusing more specifically on the absence of transportation, Carp (1971b) observes that:

> Lack of appropriate transportation constricts the life space of any person, limits his capacity for self-maintenance, restricts his activities and contacts with other people, and may contribute to his disengagement and alienation from society, and his experience of anomie.

On closer inspection, any presumed connection between the availability of transportation and the social and social-psychological functioning of the elderly is likely to be mediated by certain other factors. Relative access to the sites of social engagement, for example, is partially dependent on the availability of alternative means of transportation (Ashford and Holloway, 1972). In communities where public and/or commercial transportation facilities exist, those financially and physically able to use such services can maintain access to social activities in the absence of personal transportation. In those communities where public and commercial transportation do not exist, the availability of personal transportation becomes critical in determining the life space of the aged (Gerontological Society, 1969). Moreover, aspects of the ecological structure of the community must be taken into account (Lawton, 1970). When older persons live relatively close to the various locations of social engagement and interaction, then walking, in the absence of disabling functional impairments, can serve as a substitute, albeit less preferable (Carp, 1971c), to vehicular transportation. However, the greater the distance between residence and the locations of social activities, resources, and facilities, the lower the frequency of walking as a means of mobility (Carp, 1971c; 1972) and the more dependent is the older person on the availability of transportation for access

to these locations.

Thus, the availability of transportation can increase the capacity for mobility among the aged and thereby expand the range of social interaction, engagement, and activity; it can promote a sense of independence and reduce social isolation; it can lead older persons to feel that they have some control over their environment and reduce the import of what Lawton (1970) refers to as, "environmental docility." In short, transportation can maintain a differentiated, flexible, permeable, and multichanneled life-space (Gelwicks, 1971). Coupling these considerations with those outlined above (which deal with alternative means of transportation and ecological structure) leads to the two basic hypotheses of this study.

1. In the absence of public and commercial transportation, life satisfaction will be higher among older persons for whom personal transportation is available than among those for whom personal transportation is not available.

2. Where means of public and commercial transportation are not available and since dependence on transportation is assumed to be greater for those living more distant from the locations of social engagement, a stronger relationship between the availability of personal transportation and life satisfaction should be in evidence among the aged whose residences are farther from these locations than among those whose residences are more proximate.

Methods

The data for this study come from a larger survey of a randomly selected sample of 170 (representing an 85% response rate) noninstitutionalized respondents age sixty-five or older. Interviews, of fifty-minute duration on the average, were conducted over a four-week period in October and

November of 1970. The community of Oberlin, in which the survey was carried out, has a population of approximately 9,000 of which some 11 percent are in the sixty-five and older age category. The median age for these respondents is seventy-four, the median expected family income for 1970 was approximately $3,200, and the sample is composed of 121 females and 49 males and 137 whites and 33 nonwhites.

Two features of the community are of some importance for the analysis. First, dependence on personal transportation for mobility is high. There is no system of public transportation within the city, and while attempts at providing commercial transportation have been made, these attempts have been relatively short-lived and have been largely secondary activities adjunct to preexisting commerical establishments. With neither public nor commercial transportation available, vehicular mobility is for the most part a function of the availability of means of personal transportation. Second, the community displays a high degree of centralization in regard to its ecological structure in that most facilities are located within a one-quarter mile radius of the center of the city. Because a dispersed, neighborhood-based distribution of services, establishments, and facilities is not the case, differentials in access to these various locations are related, in part, to the distance of residence from the center of the city. Reflecting these aspects of the community, then, the primary independent variables are based on differentials in the availability of personal transportation and differentials in residential location in terms of distance from the center of the city.

Respondents unable to drive or who are able to drive but do not have means of personal transportation available to them for their own use are designated as being "without transportation" (48%) while those who are able to drive and have a car or other means of vehicular transportation available to them are designated as being "with transportation" (52%).

Distance of residence from the center of the city is determined by noting the location of a respondent's residence on a map on which a series of one-quarter mile concentric zones emanating from the center of the city are drawn. For present purposes, this variable is dichotomized into those older persons living up to one-half mile from the center of the city (65%) and those living more than one-half mile from the center of the city (35%).

Life satisfaction is measured through the use of fourteen items drawn from the A form of the Neugarten, Havighurst, and Tobin (1961) life satisfaction index. These items, tapping each of the five areas of life satisfaction, formed a summary index which is dichotomized at approximately the midpoint of the frequency distribution to yield groups of respondents having "low" (51%) and "high" (49%) life satisfaction scores.

As all data are presented in dichotomous form, the χ^2 test of statistical significance with Yates' correction for continuity is used throughout the analysis. However, Fisher's exact test is employed to determine the significance level for any table having a total $N \leq 30$ or having an expected cell frequency ≤ 5. Finally, since attention will be directed not only to absolute percentage differences and to levels of statistical significance but also to the relative strength of the relationships between the availability of personal transportation and life satisfaction among several control categories, adjusted coefficients of contingency are presented to facilitate these comparisons.

Results

The first hypothesis proposes that the availability of personal transportation will facilitate the social interaction and engagement of older persons by allowing for the maintenance or expansion of social and social-psychological life-space. A higher proportion of the aged having means of personal transportation available to them, therefore, should have high life-satisfaction scores than those without transportation. The data presented in Table 31-I do provide support for this hypothesis: 58 percent of the aged with transportation available to them are high on the life-satisfaction index whereas only 37 percent of those without transportation have high life satisfaction scores ($p < .02$). Thus, the capacity for mobility, as indicated here by the availability of personal transportation, would appear to be associated with higher life satisfaction. Restrictions on mobility, on the other hand, as indicated by the absence of personal transportation in the context of a community which does not provide alternative modes of transportation, are associated with lower levels of life satisfaction.

TABLE 31-I

RELATIONSHIP BETWEEN AVAILABILITY OF PERSONAL TRANSPORTATION AND LIFE SATISFACTION

Life Satisfaction	Without Transportation	With Transportation
Low	63%	42%
High	37	58
(N)	(75)	(89)
C_{adj}		.291

$$\chi^2 = 6.429 \quad p < .02$$

The second hypothesis, however, specifies that the importance of transportation will vary as a function of the distance of residence from the locations of social en-

gagement. Because dependence on transportation should be greater among older persons whose residences are more distant from these centralized locations in this community, the relationship between the availability of transportation and life satisfaction should be stronger among this group than it is among those older persons whose residences are more proximate. The data given in Table 31-II are in accord with this hypothesis also. For older persons living more than one-half mile from the center of the city, 73 percent of those with transportation and only 22 percent of those without transportation are high on the life satisfaction index ($p < .01$). Having personal transportation available appears to be of somewhat lesser importance, in terms of life satisfaction, for older persons living within one-half mile of the center of the city. While there is some slight tendency among persons living closer and having transportation to have higher satisfaction scores than those without transportation, the greater dependence on transportation among the aged who reside more than one-half mile from the center of the city is reflected in the difference between the magnitudes of the contingency coefficients (.612 for those living beyond $\frac{1}{2}$ mile and .085 for those living up to $\frac{1}{2}$ mile). Thus, the absence of transportation appears to pose less of a problem for the aged living closer to the center of the city insofar as it is manifested in life satisfaction and may indicate that walking is a more viable alternative in maintaining access under these circumstances.

There are several additional considerations which necessitate a more detailed examination of these findings. Previous research has pointed to a positive relationship between life satisfaction and both socioeconomic and health status (Adams,

TABLE 31-II

RELATIONSHIP BETWEEN AVAILABILITY OF PERSONAL TRANSPORTATION AND
LIFE SATISFACTION, CONTROLLING FOR DISTANCE OF RESIDENCE FROM
CENTER OF CITY

Life Satisfaction	½ Mile or Closer		More than ½ Mile	
	Without Transp.	*With Transp.*	*Without Transp.*	*With Transp.*
Low	58%	52%	78%	27%
High	42	48	22	73
(N)	(57)	(52)	(18)	(37)
C_{adj}		.085		.612
		ns		$\chi^2 = 10.701$ $p < .01$

1971; Riley and Foner, 1968). In the present sample, socioeconomic status, as measured by a dichotomized Hollingshead two-factor index of social position for the head of the household, and subjective assessment of health are similarly related to life satisfaction ($p < .001$ in both instances). It is also to be noted that socioeconomic status and subjective assessment of health are associated with the availability of personal transportation ($p < .01$ in both instances) with the higher status or the healthier respondents more likely to have personal transportation available to them than those of lower socioeconomic status or those in poorer health (Carp, 1972). The cumulative importance of these relationships, especially in regard to the data concerning those living at greater distances from the center of the city, is that the higher life satisfaction of the aged who have transportation available to them compared with those not having transportation might be a function of their being of higher socioeconomic status or in better health. To determine whether this is the case, Tables 31-III and 31-IV present the second-order relationships between residential location, availability of transportation, and life satisfaction controlling for socioeconomic and health status, respectively.

The data in Table 31-III again show little relationship between the availability of personal transportation and life satisfaction for the aged living within one-half mile of the center of the city regardless of socioeconomic level. Among the respondents of low socioeconomic status living beyond one-half mile from the center of the city, a rather marked relationship between having personal transportation and life satisfaction is in evidence: 91 percent of those without transportation have low scores on the life-satisfaction index while only 36 percent of those with transportation are low on the index ($p < .025$). Among the respondents of high socioeconomic status living beyond one-half mile from the center of the city, 50 percent of those without transportation are low on the life-satisfaction index while only 24 percent of those with transportation have low scores. Although the absence of a statistically significant relationship in the latter instance indicates that the availability of transportation is more critical for the life satisfaction of those of lower socioeconomic status, comparison of the contingency coefficients and the percentage differences between those living closer to and those living farther from the center of the city suggests that transportation is generally more important for the elderly living at the greater distances.

TABLE 31-III

RELATIONSHIP BETWEEN AVAILABILITY OF PERSONAL TRANSPORTATION AND LIFE SATISFACTION, CONTROLLING FOR DISTANCE OF RESIDENCE FROM CENTER OF CITY AND SOCIOECONOMIC STATUS

| | *High Socioeconomic Status* | | | | *Low Socioeconomic Status* | | | |
| | *½ Mile or Closer* | | *More than ½ Mile* | | *½ Mile or Closer* | | *More than ½ Mile* | |
Life Satisfaction	*Without Transp.*	*With Transp.*	*Without Transp.*	*With Transp.*	*Without Transp.*	*With Transp.*	*Without Transp.*	*With Transp.*
Low	35%	31%	50%	24%	72%	78%	91%	36%
High	65	59	50	76	28	22	9	64
(N)	(20)	(29)	(6)	(25)	(36)	(23)	(11)	(11)
C_{adj}	.059		.313		.095		.697	
	ns		ns		ns		$p<.025$	

TABLE 31-IV

RELATIONSHIP BETWEEN AVAILABILITY OF PERSONAL TRANSPORTATION AND LIFE SATISFACTION, CONTROLLING FOR DISTANCE OF RESIDENCE FROM CENTER OF CITY AND SUBJECTIVE HEALTH ASSESSMENT

| | *Better Health* | | | | *Poorer Health* | | | |
| | *½ Mile or Closer* | | *More than ½ Mile* | | *½ Mile or Closer* | | *More than ½ Mile* | |
Life Satisfaction	*Without Transp.*	*With Transp.*	*Without Transp.*	*With Transp.*	*Without Transp.*	*With Transp.*	*Without Transp.*	*With Transp.*
Low	50%	40%	67%	26%	68%	75%	89%	33%
High	50	60	33	74	32	25	11	67
(N)	(32)	(35)	(9)	(31)	(25)	(16)	(9)	(6)
C_{adj}	.059		.313		.106		.707	
	ns		ns		ns		$p<.05$	

Consistent results are seen for the data given in Table 31-IV. Taking into account the magnitude of the percentage differences, the absence of statistical significance, and the moderately low coefficients of contingency, it can be concluded that transportation differentials bear little relationship to life satisfaction among the older persons living closer to the center of the city whether they consider themselves to be in good or in poor health. Among those living more than one-half mile from the center of the city, however, differentials in the availability of personal transportation are once again of some importance. Among the aged in poorer health, 89 percent of those without transportation have low life-satisfaction scores while only 33 percent of those with transportation available to them are low on the life-satisfaction index ($p < .05$). For these living more than one-half mile from the center of the city and judging themselves to be in better health, 67 percent of those without transportation and only 26 percent of those with transportation have low life-satisfaction scores. In short, transportation differentials are of greater importance for the life satisfaction of the aged living at greater distances from the centralized facilities of the community, although such differentials are especially important for the aged who live at the greater distances and who are in poorer health.

Conclusion

Of the several modes of access to the resources and facilities of a community and to social interaction, walking, private automobiles, public and commercial transportation, financial, functional, and psychological characteristics of the aged interact to generate considerable variation in the extent of their utilization (Carp, 1971c). Where these alternatives are further circumscribed, as they are in this community

by the absence of intracity buses and taxis, dependence on the remaining means of mobility is heightened and differentials in their availability and utilization become particularly critical in delineating the nature and expanse of the life-space of older persons. What this research supports, then, is the notion that mobility restrictions, as they constrict life-space and narrow the social world of the aged, are associated with low levels of life satisfaction. Moreover, the analysis reaffirms the importance of considering how variable aspects of the environment relate to the morale or adjustment of the aged (Lawton, Kleban, and Singer, 1971; Schooler, 1970). In general terms, transportation differentials have a greater impact on life satisfaction when an older person's location in the ecological structure of the community tends to preclude the use of certain mobility options (i.e. walking) and when the means of overcoming environmental obstacles (i.e. distance) are not readily at hand.

Summary

In the context of a community which has neither public nor commercial transportation facilities, the life satisfaction of the aged is related to differentials in the availability of means of personal transportation. Older persons having personal transportation available to them have higher life-satisfaction scores than those older persons not having transportation available for their use. However, the consequences of transportation differentials for life satisfaction are somewhat greater for the aged whose residences are more distant from the centralized resources, facilities, and services of the community. Low levels of life satisfaction are especially characteristic of older persons who do not have personal transportation available and who live more than one-half mile from the center of the city.

For those living closer to the center of the city, life satisfaction is unrelated to transportation differentials. Finally, the highest proportions of older persons with low life-satisfaction scores are found among those who do not have personal transportation available to them, who live at the greater distances, and who are of lower socioeconomic status or in poorer health.

REFERENCES

Abt Associates. *Travel barriers: Transportation needs of the handicapped.* Springfield, Va.: National Technical Information Service, 1969.

Adams, D. L. Correlates of satisfaction among the elderly. *Gerontologist,* 1971, *11,* 64-68.

Ashford, N., and Holloway, F. M. Transportation patterns of older people in six urban centers. *Gerontologist,* 1972, *12,* 43-47.

Cantilli, E. J. and Shmelzer, J. L. (Eds.), *Transportation and aging: Selected issues.* Washington: U. S. Government Printing Office, 1971.

Carp, F. M. Retired people as automobile passengers. *Gerontologist,* 1972, *12,* 66-72.

Carp, F. M. On becoming an ex-driver: Prospect and retrospect. *Gerontologist,* 1971, *11,* 101-103. (a)

Carp, F. M. The mobility of retired people. In E. Cantilli and J. Shmelzer (Eds.), *Transportation and aging: Selected issues.* Washington: U. S. Government Printing Office, 1971. (b)

Carp, F. M. Walking as a means of transportation for retired people. *Gerontologist,* 1971, *11,* 104-111. (c)

Clark, M. Patterns of aging among the elderly poor in the inner city. *Gerontologist,* 1971, *11,* 58-66.

Cottrell, F. *Transportation of older people in a rural community.* Oxford, Ohio: Scripps Foundation, 1971.

Gelwicks, L. E. The older person's relation with the environment: The influence of transportation. In E. Cantilli and J. Shmelzer (Eds.), *Transportation and aging: Selected issues.* Washington: U. S. Government Printing Office, 1971.

Gerontological Society. Report of a Special Committee. Research and development goals in social gerontology. *Gerontologist,* 1966, *9,* No. 4, Pt. II, 37-54.

Kaplan, J. *Transportation of the aging in Richland County and Ohio.* Columbus: Dept. of Mental Hygiene, 1970.

Kutner, B., Fanshel, D., Togo, A. M., and Langner, T. S. *Five hundred over sixty: A community survey on aging.* New York: Russell Sage Foundation, 1956.

Lawton, M. P., Kleban, M. H., and Singer, M. The aged Jewish person and the slum environment. *Journal of Gerontology,* 1971, *26,* 231-239.

Lawton, M. P. Ecology and aging. In L. A. Pastalan and D. H. Carson (Eds.), *Spatial behavior of older people.* Ann Arbor: University of Michigan-Wayne State University, Institute of Gerontology, 1970.

Maddox, G. L. Persistence of life style among the elderly. *Proceedings of the 7th International Congress of Gerontology,* Vienna: Viennese Medical Academy, 1966.

Maddox, G. L. Fact and artifact: Evidence bearing on disengagement theory. *Human Development,* 1965, *8,* 117-130.

Neugarten, B. L., Havighurst, R. J., and Tobin, S. S. The measurement of life satisfaction. *Journal of Gerontology,* 1961, *16,* 134-143.

Palmore, E. B. The effects of aging on activities and attitudes. *Gerontologist,* 1968, *8,* 259-263.

Pihlblad, C. T., and McNamara, R. L. Social adjustment of elderly people in three small towns. In A. M. Rose and W. A. Peterson (Eds.), *Older people and their social world.* Philadelphia: F. A. Davis, 1965.

Riley, M. W., and Foner, A. *Aging and society: An inventory of research findings.* New York: Russell Sage Foundation, 1968.

Schooler, K. K. Effect of environment on morale. *Gerontologist,* 1970, *10,* 194-197.

Tobin, S. S., and Neugarten, B. L. Life satisfaction and social interaction in the aging. *Journal of Gerontology,* 1961, *16,* 344-346.

Trela, J. E., and Simmons, L. W. Health and other factors affecting membership and attrition in a senior center. *Journal of Gerontology,* 1971, *26,* 46-51.

Twente, E. E. *Never too old: The aged in community life.* San Francisco: Jossey-Bass, 1970.

U. S. Senate. *Older American and transportation: A crisis in mobility,* Washington: U. S. Government Printing Office, 1970.

White House Conference on Aging. *Transportation: Background and issues.* Washington: U. S. Government Printing Office, 1971.

Chapter 32

THE ROLE OF FUTURI-TY IN AGING ADAPT-ATION

Donald L. Spence

In this paper the concept of futurity will be examined for its implications in the adaptive patterns of older *Ss*. Miller and Lieberman (1965) found, in a sample of institutionalized older women, that, "an inability to characterize the immediate and distant future" was one of two concepts related to "negative" adaptation. In their particular study the adaptation was to an extensive change in the *S's* sociophysical environment. Although both healthy and mentally impaired aged were involved, adequacy of psychological functioning as indicated by the Murry TAT, Mental Status Questionnaire, and staff ratings was not significantly related to negative outcome. Only depressive affect, as indicated by a lack of futurity and a negative evaluation of past life, significantly differentiated between those who failed and those who succeeded in their adaptation to the change. Adaptation was indicated by the absence of mortality, physical illness, or psychological deterioration.

On the other hand, Kastenbaum (1963) found, in comparing younger with older *Ss*, a loss for the aged in personal futurity, "both in density of future events and degree of extension into the future." By distinguishing between cognitive and personal

Reprinted by permission from the *Gerontologist*, 1968, *8*, 180-183.

futurity, it was shown that older people do not lose the ability to use time as a cognitive tool for "organizing and interpreting experience," but they do lose the ability to perceive themselves in some personal future situation.

If futurity has adaptive consequences in circumstances involving change, and there is a decline in personal futurity with age, then what are the implications of futurity for aging-adaptation generally? Is futurity an aspect of the adjustment situation of older persons? Or, in situations of relative stability, is there a lack of relationship between futurity and adjustment?

In this paper, the question explored is whether those older persons who manifest a sense of futurity are also the better adjusted.

Method

The sample is composed of 226 community residents, drawn from among the elderly of the City of San Francisco. These *Ss* represent those still available from a larger original sample of 600 persons (Lowenthal, Berkman, Brissette, Buehler, Pierce, Robinson, and Trier, 1967). All *Ss* were sixty years of age or over at the time of their first interview in 1959 or early 1960. A second and third interview were conducted at one-and two-year intervals, respectively. The data upon which the present study is based was collected during the third interview.

Futurity: Among the interview materials was the question, "How much do you plan ahead the things you will be doing next week or the week after?" Sixty-two percent of the *Ss* responded in such a way as to indicate that they do plan ahead. It was felt, however, that an additional difference existed between those persons who were planning because they desired change and those whose plans related more simply to the organization of their future activities. Fifty-two percent of the *Ss* indicated by their responses that they desired some change in their present circumstances, while 48 percent desired "no change." Therefore, the *Ss* were separated into four groups:

(1) *Unsettled planners,* those who made plans and desired change (n = 74, 32.7%).

(2) *Composed planners,* those who made plans but did not desire change (n = 66, 29.2%).

(3) *The disgruntled,* those who did not make plans but desired change (n = 44, 19.5%).

(4) *The complacent,* those who did not make plans or desire change (n = 42, 18.6%).

The unsettled and composed planners are future-oriented; the disgruntled and the complacent are not future-oriented.

ADJUSTMENT: The measure of adjustment used in this paper is a morale score based on a series of seven questions primarily concerned with the *Ss'* mood-state. The development of this measure involved subjecting these seven and a number of similar items to a Tryon cluster analysis (Tryon, 1959). Scores from this particular cluster when dichotomized become a measure of high and low satisfaction (Clark and Anderson, 1967).

HYPOTHESES: First, it is hypothesized that those who are future-oriented are more likely to be satisfied than those who are not.

(1) The composed planners are more likely to be satisfied than the complacent.

(2) The unsettled are more likely to be satisfied than the disgruntled. Second, it is hypothesized that those who desire change are less likely to be satisfied than those who do not desire change.

(1) The unsettled are less likely to be satisfied than the composed planners.

(2) The disgruntled are less likely to be satisfied than the complacent.

Results

In Table 32-I, it can be seen that all four of the corollaries are supported. According to the statistical analysis of these data (Sutcliffe, 1957), the two principal relationships are statistically significant and independent. That is, planning is positively related to satisfaction, desiring change is negatively related to satisfaction, and

TABLE 32-I

PERCENTAGE OF SATISFIED *Ss* AMONG FOUR ORIENTATION TYPES

	Unsettled	Composed	Disgruntled	Complacent
High satisfaction	44.6	59.1	22.7	40.5
Low satisfaction	55.4	40.9	77.3	59.5
N's	(74)	(66)	(44)	(42)

Statistical relationships (multiple classification design involving analysis of frequency data in a manner similar to analysis of variance)

	χ^2	d.f.	P
Satisfaction (high) by planning (makes plans)*	8.73	1	<0.01
Satisfaction (high) by desiring change (does not desire change)	5.40	1	<0.05
Planning by desiring change	0.06	1	NS
Satisfaction by planning by desiring change	0.05	1	NS

*Words in parentheses indicate the direction of the relationship.

TABLE 32-II

PERCENTAGE OF SATISFIED Ss AMONG FOUR ORIENTATION TYPES
CONTROLLING FOR SOCIOECONOMIC STATUS

	% Satisfied			
	Unsettled	*Composed*	*Disgruntled*	*Complacent*
High SES	50.0	63.5	27.3	50.0
Low SES	28.6	42.9	18.2	23.1

Statistical relationships (omitting those already shown in Table 32-I)	χ^2	d.f.	P
Satisfaction (high) by SES (high)	11.26	1	<0.001
Planning (makes plans) by SES (high)	6.92	1	<0.01
Desiring changes (does not desire change) by SES (high)	3.13	1	<0.10
Satisfaction by planning by SES	0.13	1	NS
Satisfaction by desiring change by SES	0.00	1	NS
Planning by desiring change by SES	0.53	1	NS
Satisfaction by planning by desiring change by SES	0.00	1	NS

there is no interaction effect between the three variables.

It is possible, however, that some fourth variable is interacting with the dependent and independent variables. Socioeconomic status, for example, may make it more probable that people would plan while at the same time provide satisfaction. With high socioeconomic status it is also less likely that people would desire change.

Actually, three control variables were introduced into the analysis: socioeconomic status, sex, and age. The indicators of socioeconomic status were the results of combining income, rent paid, and neighborhood rating. Median splits on each of the indicators were combined and split again forming two categories (Lowenthal *et al.*, 1967). As to age categories, the original sample was drawn to include equal

TABLE 32-III

PERCENTAGE OF SATISFIED Ss AMONG FOUR ORIENTATION TYPES
CONTROLLING FOR SEX

	% Satisfied			
	Unsettled	*Composed*	*Disgruntled*	*Complacent*
Males	56.3	66.7	33.3	44.8
Females	35.7	52.8	13.0	30.8

Statistical relationships (omitting those already shown in Table 32-I)	χ^2	d.f.	P
Satisfaction (high) by sex (males)	5.77	1	<0.02
Planning (makes plans) by sex (males)	4.12	1	<0.05
Desiring change by sex	2.19	1	NS
Satisfaction by planning by sex	0.00	1	NS
Satisfaction by desiring change by sex	0.58	1	NS
Planning by desiring change by sex	1.97	1	NS
Satisfaction by planning by desiring change by sex	0.00	1	NS

TABLE 32-IV

PERCENTAGE OF SATISFIED Ss AMONG FOUR ORIENTATION TYPES
CONTROLLING FOR AGE

| | % Satisfied | | | |
	Unsettled	*Composed*	*Disgruntled*	*Complacent*
75 and over	31.2	46.7	26.7	42.3
65 – 74	42.8	45.8	13.3	37.5
60 – 64	53.3	77.8	28.6	37.5

Statistical relationships (omitting those already shown in Table 32-I)

	χ^2	d.f.	P
Satisfaction (high) by age (younger group)	6.93	2	<0.05
Planning (makes plans) by age (younger group)	16.19	2	<0.001
Desiring change by age	3.22	2	NS
Satisfaction by planning by age	2.50	2	NS
Satisfaction by desiring change by age	0.92	2	NS
Planning (does not make plans) by desiring change (does not desire change) by age (oldest group)	4.90	2	<0.10
Satisfaction by planning by desiring change by age	1.22	2	NS

numbers of persons in the age groupings sixty to sixty-four, sixty-five to seventy-four, and seventy-five and over. It is this baseline age which has been used in this analysis.

Table 32-II shows the same relationships as in Table 32-I for each of a high and low socioeconomic grouping. Although planning and satisfaction are both positively related to socioeconomic status, and desiring change is negatively related, there is no interaction of variables in either of the three-variable relationships or in the overall four-variable relationship. In other words, the relationship of socioeconomi status to satisfaction is independent of th relationships between the other variables The strength and direction of the origina relationships are unaffected by the intro duction of socioeconomic status as a con trol variable.

The introduction of sex as a contro variable is presented in Table 32-III. Agai the strength and direction of the origina relationships are unaffected. There are n significant interactions involving the vari able of sex. Men are more likely to pla

TABLE 32-V

PERCENTAGE OF Ss WHO MAKE PLANS AMONG THREE AGE GROUPINGS
CONTROLLING FOR DESIRING CHANGE

| | % Making Plans | | |
	60 — 64	*65 — 74*	*75+*
Desires change	68.2	65.1	36.6
Does not desire change	77.1	75.0	51.6

Statistical relationships

	χ^2	d.f.	P
Planning by age for those desiring change	2.22	2	NS
Planning (does not plan) by age(oldest group) for those not desiring change	16.55	2	<0.001

TABLE 32-VI

PERCENTAGE OF Ss WHO MAKE PLANS AMONG THREE AGE GROUPINGS
CONTROLLING FOR PLANNING

	% Desiring Change		
	60 — 64	*65 — 74*	*75+*
Makes plans	52.6	53.8	51.6
Does not make plans	63.6	65.2	36.6

Statistical relationships	χ^2	d.f.	*P*
Desiring change by age for those who plan	0.04	2	NS
Desiring change (does not desire change) by age (oldest group) for those who do not plan	6.60	2	<0.05

than women, and men are more likely to be satisfied. However, the consequence of planning is to increase the probability of satisfaction equally for men and women, roughly 22 percent.

Finally, age is introduced as a control variable (Table 32-IV). The relationships involving age are not straightforward. Age interacts significantly with the variables planning and a desire for change. The nature of this interaction involves two aspects. First, the inverse relationship between making plans and age holds primarily for those people who do not desire change (Table 32-V). Second, the inverse

relationship between desiring change and age holds primarily for those who do not make plans (Table 32-VI). This implies, that, as people age, it is those who desire change who continue to plan. Since desiring change is negatively associated with satisfaction, what happens to the relationship between planning and satisfaction as one ages?

An answer to the above question can be found in Table 32-VII. Although there was not a significant interaction between age, planning and satisfaction in the overall analysis, a trend suggesting a reduction of relationship with age is clearly estab-

TABLE 32-VII

PERCENTAGE OF SATISFIED Ss AMONG THOSE WHO DO AND DO NOT
PLAN CONTROLLING FOR AGE

	% Satisfied	
	Makes Plans	*Does not Make Plans*
75 and over	38.7	36.6
65 — 74	44.2	21.7
60 — 64	64.9	31.8

Statistical relationships	χ^2	d.f.	*P*
Satisfaction by planning for those 75+	0.06	1	NS
Satisfaction (high) by planning (makes plans) for those 65 — 74	8.21	1	<0.005
Satisfaction (high) by planning (makes plans) for those 60 — 64	17.22	1	<0.001

lished. Calculating separate χ^2 statistics for each age group shows planning and satisfaction strongly related for the younger *Ss* with the relationship all but disappearing for those seventy-five and over.

By looking back at Table 32-IV it can be seen that the above decline in the relationship between planning and satisfaction is independent of the increase in the relationship between planning and desiring change. For those *Ss* seventy-five and over the consequences of planning for satisfaction is consistent regardless of one's desire or lack of desire for change. The percentage difference between the unsettled and the disgruntled is 4.5, between the composed and the complacent, 4.4.

Discussion

Since the above data are cross-sectional and not longitudinal, it is difficult to draw conclusions of a general nature. The only control variable which affected the strength and direction of the original relationships was age. There were clearly fewer future-oriented *Ss* in the oldest group. Composed planners were most likely satisfied at all ages. However, the general decline in satisfaction with age is contradicted by an increase in satisfaction among the complacent. This seems consistent with Kastenbaum's explanation that, "some elderly people consider that they have lived out their life plan" (Kastenbaum, 1963). There is, therefore, a self-imposed restriction of their personal futurity. This does not contradict Miller and Lieberman's (1965) idea of the functional consequences of futurity, as the community residents of the present sample have not been forced to alter their circumstances. Given changing circumstances, would these same complacent *Ss* shift again to a future orientation? This question remains unanswered as does the question of the type of future orientation to which they would shift. Since being un-

settled decreases one's chances of satisfaction, it questions the general functional consequences of futurity and suggests that, in addition to futurity, a positive present orientation may also be contributing to the adaptive potential. This, it seems, questions Kastenbaum's alternative explanation that the decline in futurity with age is "accidental;" that is, "that specific conditions have occurred in the particular individual's total life situation which have brought about the observed restriction" (Kastenbaum, 1963).

Composed planning at any age implies, at least, an acceptance of present circumstances, as does complacency. Being unsettled does not imply such an acceptance. Since being unsettled is less dysfunctional at a younger age when it is more realistic to assume that one can alter circumstances, it is suggested that among the very old satisfaction results from accepting one's circumstances or, more likely, having circumstances one can accept.

REFERENCES

Clark, M., and Anderson, B. G.: *Culture and aging: an anthropological study of older Americans*, Charles C Thomas, Springfield, Ill., 1967.

Kastenbaum, R.: Cognitive and personal futurity in later life. *J. Individ. Psychol., 19:* 216-222, 1963.

Lowenthal, M. F., Berkman, P. L., Brissette, G.G., Buehler, J. A., Pierce, R. C., Robinson, B. C., and Trier, M. L.: *Aging and Mental Disorder in San Francisco.* Jossey-Bass, Inc., San Francisco, 1967.

Miller, D., and Lieberman, M. A.: The relationship of affect state and adaptive capacity to reaction to stress. *J. Geront., 20:*492-497, 1965.

Sutcliffe, J. P.: A general method of analysis of frequency data for multiple classification design. *Psychol. Bull.,* 54:134-137, 1957.

Tryon, R. C.: Domain sampling formulation of cluster and factor analysis. *Psychometrika, 24:*113-135, 1959.

Chapter 33

LIFE CONTINUITY AND MORALE IN OLD AGE

Gordon L. Bultena

Research has provided frequent documentation that some forms of personal pathology, such as anomia are disproportionately concentrated in the lower socioeconomic segments of American society. This is consistent with the theoretical position advanced by Merton (1957) and Meier and Bell (1959) that such pathologies tend to be precipitated out of a structural situation in which there is a disjunction for the individual between cultural goals and the institutionalized means for their attainment.

The analysis presented here is directed to applying this theoretical model to an explanation of demoralization as an age-related phenomena. That advancing age often is accompanied by diminished morale has been a frequent finding of research on aged populations. Role theory suggests that this relationship may reflect the fact that status and role changes in old age tend progressively to be decremental in character.

Specifically, individuals in reaching old age increasingly are caught up in role changes (more often involuntary than voluntary) which attenuate their capacity to attain cultural goals. The blockage of these goals in turn precipitates diverse problems of personal disorganization, of

Reprinted by permission from the *Gerontologist*, 1969, *9*, 251-253.

which demoralization, involutional melancholia, and suicide are but a few manifestations.

This theoretical approach assumes that the major goals of individuals are not materially altered by their entry into old age and that the culturally-valued goals which attract younger persons (such as acceptable social status, economic success, good health, energetic living, and independence) continue to comprise important objectives for the older age groups. While Rose (1965) has discerned the emergence of an aged subculture in American society, it is clear that this subculture is not yet of sufficient social visibility to provide a specialized set of normative patterns for the aged which serve as alternatives to those promulgated in the greater society.

Retirement from work comprises a critical role change in the life of the elderly male; a transition that stands in sharp contrast to the occupational changes experienced earlier in the life cycle which for most tend progressively to strengthen personal access to cultural goals. Retirement typically brings decrements in the individual's position, namely, diminished social status, a decline in income, loss of instrumental functions, decreased role clarity, and often a constriction in life space. In this respect it increases the likelihood of the individual's experiencing a sense of hopelessness and despair and of being alarmed over his need to retreat from familiar life ambitions.

Other role changes common to the aging process similarly serve to weaken access to prized goals. The biological process of aging results in diminished energy levels, often translated into a conception of oneself as old, tired, and decrepid, the import of which is great in a society which prizes youthfulness, zest, and activity. Similarly, advancing age brings an increased prominence of widowhood, dependence on others, a withering away of age-mates and group supports, chronic disease, and incapacitating illness.

In line with this argument, it may be hypothesized that the greater the discontinuity in life patterns between the pre- and postretirement periods, the greater will be the impact on the individual's ability to function successfully relative to the attainment of culturally-valued goals and thereby the greater the probability of his being demoralized. This approach is consistent with Rosow's (1963) contention that the key to good adjustment lies in a continuity in life patterns between middle and old age. However, while continuity in life patterns is hypothesized here as important to personal adjustment in old age, the impact of life changes on morale is further seen as mediated by the individual's position in the social structure. The amenities afforded by a higher economic position cushion the psychological costs entailed in many of the role transitions which commonly accompany the aging process.

Specifically, three hypotheses are tested with our data. First, consistent with previous findings with regard to the correlates of personal pathology, it is hypothesized that low morale is more prominent among retired males in the lower socioeconomic groups than among those in the higher status positions.

Second, that low morale is greatest among those who have undergone the most pronounced decremental changes in life patterns between the preretirement period and their contemporary situation.

Third, that the consequences for morale of these life changes are mediated by the individual's position in the social structure, with the most deleterious effect being evidenced in the lower segments of the class structure.

Materials and Methods

SAMPLE: The data are from interview in 1967 with 284 retired men in three communities in Wisconsin. The respondent were obtained through two procedures First, an area-probability sample coupled with a screening interview to ascertain retirement status provided respondents in a metropolitan community (170,000 population). Second, a random sample of retired males in two rural trade centers was drawn from complete census enumerations in these communities. The respondents ranged in age from sixty-three to ninety-nine, with the median age being seventy-four. All were fully retired, with two-thirds having been retired for at least five years.

MEASUREMENT OF VARIABLES: Life satisfaction was measured by a modified form of the Life Satisfaction Scale. The derivation and validation of the original scale has been described elsewhere (Neugarten, Havighurst, and Tobin, 1961). The modified scale contained thirteen agree-disagree items designed to tap the respondent's general satisfaction with his current life situation (Wood and Wylie, 1966). The scores on this scale ranged from zero to twenty six, and for purposes of the analysis were categorized into three groups, "high morale" (22-26), "medium morale" (13-21) and "low morale" (0-12).

Socioeconomic status was measured by a composite score derived from three variables: occupation, education, and preretirement income. The scores ranged from zero (indicating low status) to twenty-one (high status) with a median score of eight These were categorized into four groups

Continuity-discontinuity patterns were ascertained for three variables: general life situation, health, and organizational participation. The respondents were asked for each of these variables to contrast their present situation with that prevailing in the period just prior to their retirement.

TABLE 33-I

PERCENTAGE DISTRIBUTION ON LIFE SATISFACTION BY SOCIOECONOMIC STATUS

			Life-Satisfaction Score			
Socioeconomic Status Score			High (%)	Medium (%)	Low (%)	
Low	(0 — 4)	(N = 67)	33	40	27	100
	(5 — 8)	(N = 83)	34	54	12	100
	(9 — 13)	(N = 68)	54	37	9	100
High	(14 or more)	(N = 42)	40	55	5	100

$$\chi^2 = 20.99, 6df, p < 0.005$$

TABLE 33-II

PERCENTAGE DISTRIBUTION ON LIFE SATISFACTION, BY NATURE OF CHANGE IN LIFE PATTERNS

		Life-Satisfaction Score			
Change in Life Pattern		High (%)	Medium (%)	Low (%)	
Perceived life change (general)					
None	(N = 28)	57	39	4	100
Very little	(N = 76)	50	40	10	100
Some	(N = 99)	39	52	9	100
A great deal	(N = 76)	24	50	26	100

$$\chi^2 = 24.02, 6df, p < 0.001$$

Perceived change in organizational participation					
More active	(N = 20)	60	40	0	100
Same as before	(N = 147)	45	43	12	100
Less active	(N = 71)	31	55	14	100
Much less active	(N = 41)	27	46	27	100

$$\chi^2 = 16.12, 6df, p < 0.05$$

Perceived change in health					
Much better or better	(N = 28)	46	50	4	100
Same	(N = 158)	49	42	9	100
Worse	(N = 75)	25	55	20	100
Much worse	(N = 19)	6	47	47	100

$$\chi^2 = 37.86, 6df, p < 0.001$$

χ^2 was employed to test the statistical significance of differences. The .05 level of significance was used.

Results

The data reported in Table 33-I provide support for the hypothesis that socioeconomic status is associated with life satisfaction. The proportion of respondents with low life-satisfaction scores increases progressively from 5 percent in the upper status categories to 27 percent for those at the lower socioeconomic levels (Table 33-I).

The relationship of continuity-discontinuity patterns of life satisfaction is reported in Table 33-II. It is found that the more decremental the change between the preretirement period and the current situation, the greater the probability of the individual's having low morale. Whereas only 4 percent of those reporting no change in their general life situation obtained low life-satisfaction scores, one fourth of those reporting "a great deal" of change had low scores. A diminished level of involvement in organizational activities similarly is found to be associated with low morale, with one fourth of those who reported themselves as, "much less active now" obtaining a low life-satisfaction score. No one who was more active, and only one tenth of those whose activity level had not changed since retirement, ranked low in life satisfaction (Table 33-II).

Similarly, nearly one-half of those who indicated that their health had deteriorated greatly since retirement had a low life-satisfaction score, compared to only 4 percent of those whose health had improved

and 9 percent of those reporting no chang in their health status (Table 33-II).

The data reported in Table 33-III pro vide a test of the hypothesis that the im pact of role discrepancies on morale i more severe at the lower than at the uppe status levels. This hypothesis generally i confirmed in the analysis. While over on third of those with low status who pe ceived a substantial change in their live since retirement ranked low in life satis faction, only 12 percent of a comparabl group of high status respondents had lo scores. Similarly, the proportion of re spondents whose level of organizationa participation had slipped in retirement an who also ranked low in life satisfaction i approximately three times as great at th lower than at the upper status levels (Tabl 33-III).

The difference in morale between up

TABLE 33-III
PERCENTAGE DISTRIBUTION ON LIFE SATISFACTION OF THOSE EXPERIENCING A DECREMENTAL LIFE CHANGE SINCE RETIREMENT, BY SOCIOECONOMIC STATUS

Nature of Decremental Change		Life-Satisfaction Score			
		High	Medium	Low	
Life has changed a great deal since retirement		*Proportion*			
High status	(N = 26)	34	54	12	100
Low status	(N = 44)	16	48	36	100
		$\chi^2 = 6.33$, $2df$, $p < 0.05$			
Less active in organizational activities					
High status	(N = 38)	42	50	8	100
Low status	(N = 64)	23	52	25	100
		$\chi^2 = 6.49$, $2df$, $p < 0.05$			
Health has become worse or much worse					
High status	(N = 25)	28	60	12	100
Low status	(N = 64)	17	52	31	100
		$\chi^2 = 3.85$, $2df$, $p < 0.20$			

Note. — The distribution on socioeconomic status was dichotomized for purposes of this analysis, with low status representing a score of 0 to 8 and high status a score of 9 to 21.

er and lower status persons experiencing decremental change in health is not found to be statistically significant. However, the pattern is the same as the other two perceived life changes, with a deterioration in health most often being accompanied by low morale among those of lower socioeconomic status (Table 33-III).

Summary

The relationship of life continuity-discontinuity patterns to morale was tested for a sample of retired men in Wisconsin. As hypothesized, it was found that morale was related positively to socioeconomic status and that decremental life changes were associated with a low level of morale. It was revealed further that the impact of life changes on morale was mediated by the social structure, with the psychological costs of decremental changes being disproportionately centered among those in the lower socioeconomic segments of the aged population.

REFERENCES

Meier, D., and Bell, W. Anomia and the achievement of life goals. *American Sociological Review*, 159, *24*, 189-202.

Merton, R. Social structure and anomie. *Social theory and social structure*. Glencoe, Ill.: Free Press, 1957.

Neugarten, B. L., Havighurst, R. J., and Tobin, S. The measurement of life satisfaction. *Journal of Gerontology*, 1961, *16*, 134-143.

Rose, A. The subculture of the aging: A framework for research in social gerontology. In A. Rose and W. Peterson (Eds.), *Older people and their social world*. Philadelphia: F. A. Davis, 1965.

Rosow, I. Adjustment of the normal aged: Concept and measurement. In R. Williams, C. Tibbitts, and W. Donahue (Eds.) *Processes of aging*, vol. 2. New York: Atherton Press, 1963.

Wood, V., and Wylie, M. An analysis of a short self-report measure of life satisfaction: Correlation with rater judgments. Paper presented at the 19th annual meeting of Gerontological Society, New York, 1966.

Chapter 34

COGNITIVE DISSONANCE AND THE LIFE SATISFACTION OF OLDER ADULTS

BILL D. BELL

MUCH OF THE LITERATURE in social gerontology focuses attention upon the increasing numbers of older people in the population while at the same time emphasizing the declining proportion of these persons in the active labor force (Brotman, 1968a, b; Donahue, Orbach, and Pollak, 1960; Sheldon, 1958). In accordance with this developing perspective, many phenomena associated with occupational retirement have come under close scrutiny. The writings of Busse and Kreps (1963), Carp (1972), Friedmann and Havighurst (1954), Goodstein (1962), Lipman (1961), Rosow (1967), Streib and Schneider (1971), and Thompson and Streib (1957), for example, illustrate the growing concern for the effects of retirement on the social adjustment and morale of older persons.

While much of the early correlational research has been displaced as a result of Merton's (1957) stress on data-based theoretical procedures, many of the traditional orientations in gerontology continue to overlap one another (Bell, 1973). In addition, contradictory predictions relative to the same independent variables frequently

Reprinted by permission from the *Journal of Gerontology*, 1974, 29, 564-571.

are observed with the simultaneous application of more than one perspective (e.g. social class supposedly exhibits a positive relationship to life satisfaction in the case of consistency theory and a negative relationship in terms of the crisis perspective). As a consequence, it is difficult to discern in the literature a comprehensive test of any given theory relative to the question at hand. For this reason, the research to follow selects a single orientation (consistency theory) and examines only the assumptions and predictions of this perspective with regard to retirement and life satisfaction. Of immediate concern is the relationship of confirmed or disconfirmed expectations for behavior relative to one's phenomenal expression of satisfaction.

Theoretical Perspective

The consistency orientation is, to some extent, a variant of role theory. This is particularly true to the extent that the concept expectation is employed in this formulation. More generally, however, the perspective derives out of cognitive consistency theories which postulate a relationship between cognitions and behavior. Cognitive elements (or simply, cognitions) refer to understandings, opinions, beliefs, expectations, or feelings one has relative to himself or his environment (Festinger, 1957). Consistency theorists argue, in general, that the complement of cognitive elements constitute a cognitive system (Heider, 1946). It is further suggested that this system tends toward a state of simplicity and harmony establishing balance or consistency among the various elements (Allen, 1968). In this regard, it is postulated that inconsistent cognitions arouse an unpleasant psychological state which leads to behaviors designed to reestablish consistency. The latter relationship is held to be psychologically satisfying in nature.

Research on the effects of consistency and man's desire for a predictable environment received considerable impetus from Aronson's (1968), Aronson and Carlsmith's (1962), and Bramel's (1968) extensions of Festinger's (1957) theory of cognitive dissonance. According to this theory, if an individual expects a certain event to occur and it does not, he will experience dissonance because his cognition that he expects the events to occur is inconsistent with his knowledge that the event did not occur. As dissonance is presumably an unpleasant psychological situation, disconfirmation should result in negative affect. On the other hand, if disconfirmations do occur, dissonance should lead to a cognitive restructuring on the part of the person in an effort to maximize consonant elements (Abelson, Aronson, McGuire, Newcomb, Rosenberg, and Tannenbaum (1968).

In the gerontological literature, the consistency framework is reflected in the writings of those stressing the significance of attitudes in relation to given events. Writers, such as Carp (1972), Dubin (1956) Gordon (1960), Rosow (1963), Shanas (1958), Thompson (1958), and Weiss and Kahn (1959), for example, frequently reference the importance of attitudes in discussions of postretirement behavior. For Streib and Schneider (1971), in particular, preretirement attitudes are seen as the most important predictor of a satisfactory adjustment to retirement.

It should be pointed out, however, that few writers have provided a clear statement regarding their use of the attitude variable. To appreciate this point, one need only view the concept from the present perspective. In this regard, an attitude toward a given event is held to reflect one's expectations for behavior relative to that event. Not only is it generally unclear in the aging literature as to what expectations are being tapped (e.g. expectations toward one's behavior? toward the behavior of others? toward both?), it is also difficult to specify the influence of these expectations relative to one's actual behavior. In addition, the measurement process in such studies is frequently hampered by conceptual difficulties, cross-sectional designs, and measurement delays.

For the purposes of the present research, therefore, it will be helpful to view an attitude as composed chiefly of individual expectations. In this sense, the focus of attention is upon those expectations held uniquely by a single subject person in reference to his own behavior. Such a conceptualization permits a meaningful examination of the relationship between preretirement attitudes and postretirement satisfaction within the framework of consistency theory.

The Sample

The present data derive from a series of two interviews with a group of male respondents residing in an urban area of central Missouri. The initial interview was made in the Spring of 1973 prior to the retirement of the individuals in question. Respondents near retirement age were selected from lists supplied by (1) local labor organizations, (2) area churches (including the Salvation Army), (3) the local office on aging, (4) an older Americans transportation service, (5) the Social Security Administration, (6) a recreational agency for older persons, and (7) numerous interested individuals in the study community. Information was obtained as to the employment status, residence, health, and marital status of each person. Accordingly, the sample consisted of 145 employed, white males living within the city limits of the community in question. Each individual's spouse was living and resided with the respondent. In addition, each subject was in relatively good health from the standpoint of physical mobility and owned or had access to appropriate means of transportation. All interviews were conducted in the homes of the respondents.

The following spring (1974), a second or postretirement interview was conducted with the same subjects. As fifteen respondents had not relinquished active employment, six had moved to another community, five chose not to be reinterviewed, two had lost a spouse during the year, and three had died, the final sample consisted of 114 retired males meeting all study criteria. The mean length of time since retirement was 5.6 months.

The individuals in question ranged in age from fifty-three to seventy-two years (the mean age was 68.2 years). Occupationally, the sample was composed of farmers, service workers, and laborers (29.7%); clerical, sales, operatives, and craftsmen (31.5%); and professional, technical, and managerial workers (38.8%). From the standpoint of national comparison, data cited by Brotman (1968a) and Carp (1972) suggest the present distribution to be overly representative of upper occupational levels. This suggestion is borne out by two related indicators, education and income. The mean educational level of the sample, for instance, was 11.9 years, a figure slightly above the national average for all age groups (McKee, 1969). In addition, the median postretirement income for the sample was $450 per month. This figure is more than $100 greater than that suggested by Streib and Schneider (1971).

Major Variables

EXPECTATIONS: From the standpoint of consistency theory, an expectation was viewed as a cognitive element or dimension referencing anticipated relationships between the holder and aspects of his environment. In the present research, particular attention was focused on the respondent's individual expectations for behavior subsequent to retirement. To this extent, expectations were assessed through phenomenal reports. The unit of measurement was one of *time*. Specifically, the number of hours per month the preretiree expected to spend in each of three role areas (family, voluntary associations, and community) was obtained.

From an operational standpoint, family and kinship behavior involved all interaction between the respondent and those persons (with the exception of his spouse) related to him through blood or marital ties. This included visits, telephone calls, letters, or any other means of communication between the respondent and his kin. Voluntary association behavior, on the other hand, encompassed the individual's involvement in such formal organizational structures as civic clubs, professional societies, fraternal organizations, and the church. Included here were activities both directly and indirectly related to organizational goals. Finally, community behavior consisted of interaction with close friends and neighbors (defined as such by the respondent) as well as involvement in nonformal civic and political activities (e.g. canvassing for civic causes, political campaigning and voting, participation in community events, etc.).

By comparing the preretirement expectations of time with postretirement reports of behavior, a judgment was possible relative to the confirmational nature of expectations in the areas of family, voluntary associations, and community. The relationships were expressed by the formula $T_2 - T_1 = -$, 0, or $+$. In this instance, T_1 denoted the amount of time the respondent expected to spend in a given area subsequent to retirement; T_2 represented the actual amount of time currently spent in each of the role areas. The minus and plus designations depicted a situation of disconfirmed expectations; a zero denoted expectational confirmation.

DISSONANCE: In a conceptual sense, dissonance was held to be a dissatisfying psychological state engendered by inconsistent cognitive elements (Abelson *et al.*, 1968). In the present instance, dissonance was viewed as a consequence of expectational disconfirmation. This suggestion was based on the assumption that if an individual expects a certain event to occur and it does not, he will experience dissonance, since his cognition that he expects the event to occur is inconsistent with his knowledge that the event did not occur. Disconfirmation, then, whether of a positive or negative character, gives rise to negative affect; hence, diminished satisfaction.

Although dissonance was not operationalized in the present study, its presence was assumed in instances where individual expectations were not confirmed. In terms of the expectational-behavioral formula, $T_2 - T_1 = -$, 0, or $+$, the minus and plus conditions were considered characterized by dissonance. The zero situation, on the other hand, was one of confirmation and thus not characterized by dissonant elements. As a consequence, the greatest negative affect and hence the most dramatic satisfaction changes were expected in the minus and plus conditions.

LIFE SATISFACTION: Life satisfaction was regarded as the phenomenal experience of pleasure, with self and others, relative to past or present social circumstances. In essence, satisfaction represented a statement of personal morale with respect to time and place. In the present study, life satisfaction was assessed by means of a single item.

Pre- and post-retirement satisfaction were measured by means of the following question: "On the whole, how satisfied would you say you are with your way of life today?" In responding, the subject ranked himself along a five-point scale ranging from one (not satisfied at all) to five (very satisfied). Although the scale has face validity, many of the items suggested by Neugarten, Havighurst, and Tobin (1961) were positively correlated with the measure. Specifically, ratings of present happiness, absence of concern over health, and feelings of usefulness, correlated significantly, at the .001 level, with ratings of satisfaction (r's $= +.35; +.68;$ and $+.33$, respectively). In the analysis to follow, scale values were utilized as measures of the pre- and post-retirement satisfaction of each respondent.

RETIREMENT: Retirement was considered a period of time characterized by the absence of occupationally-oriented behaviors. From an operational standpoint, individuals were classified as retired on the basis of two criteria. In the first instance, the person was no longer engaged in those activities that were once held to constitute his occupation or profession. To this extent, his present means of financial support were derived from pensions, investments, or other compensatory sources. Second, the individual subjectively defined himself as retired through an affirmative response to the question, "Do you consider yourself retired?" Those respondents who failed to meet both criteria were excluded from the sample.

Research Hypothesis

In the present study, the transition from work to nonwork related roles should influence life satisfaction to the extent that postretirement expectations for behavior have been disconfirmed. In other words,

TABLE 34-I
THE RELATIONSHIP BETWEEN EXPECTATIONAL DISCONFIRMATION AND
CHANGE IN LIFE SATISFACTION

Area of Role Behavior	r	N	%	Significance Level
The family	—.25	114	100.0	.001
Voluntary associations	+.06	114	100.0	.211
The community	—.12	114	100.0	.069

the greater the expectational disconfirmation, the more negative the change expected in life satisfaction.

The Findings

The relationship of life satisfaction change to change in expectational-behavioral family orientations can be seen in Table 34-I. In this instance, the correlation of expectational disconfirmation (both of a positive and negative nature) with subsequent changes in life satisfaction is significant and in the predicted direction ($r = -.25$; $p<.001$). That is, the greater the expectational disconfirmation relative to family behavior, the more negative the change evidenced in life satisfaction. This finding remained consistent for the various categories of age, income, health, status, and retirement duration.

Somewhat different results obtain in the case of associational orientations. As is evident from Table 34-I, the correlation of expectational disconfirmation with subsequent changes in life satisfaction is weak and nonsignificant ($r = +.06$; $p<.211$).

With regard to the community area, on the other hand, the correlation of expectational disconfirmation with subsequent changes in life satisfaction is in the predicted direction ($r = -.12$; $p<.069$). Although nonsignificant in this instance, the correlation does suggest a tendency for expectational disconfirmation in the community sector to be associated with negative changes in life satisfaction. Such a tendency is consistent with the present hypothesis.

A logical alternative to the consistency hypothesis, however, would suggest a consideration of the specific type of expectational disconfirmation relative to its effect on life satisfaction. That is, it would seem reasonable that behavior which exceeds one's expectations in a given area (i.e. positive disconfirmation) should evoke little anxiety for the individual concerned. On the other hand, disappointments (i.e. negative disconfirmations) should be characterized by considerable negative affect. Under these circumstances, it would not be the degree of disconfirmation which influences life satisfaction as much as the direction of that disconfirmation. In essence, then, positive disconfirmation should be associated with increases in life satisfaction, whereas negative disconfirmation should bring about decreases in this variable.

Table 34-II illustrates the relationship between the type of expectational disconfirmation and changes in life satisfaction. In the area of family behavior, it can be seen that a significant relationship obtains between these variables ($r = -.23$; $p<.002$). On the other hand, this association is opposite to the direction predicted. That is, the correlation is such as to suggest that for the present respondents, the more positive the disconfirmation (i.e. the more time invested in the family beyond that expected with retirement), the more negative the

TABLE 34-II

THE RELATIONSHIP BETWEEN THE TYPE OF EXPECTATIONAL
DISCONFIRMATION AND CHANGE IN LIFE SATISFACTION

Area of Role Behavior	r	N	%	Significance Level
The family	—.23	114	100.0	.002
Voluntary associations	+.01	114	100.0	.464
The community	—.06	114	100.0	.221

change in life satisfaction. As before, this finding remained relatively consistent for the various categories of age, income, health, status, and retirement duration.

In the voluntary association area, the relationship between the type of expectational disconfirmation and change in life satisfaction is decidedly weak and nonsignificant ($r = +.01$; $p<.464$). Controls for age, health, and retirement duration yielded complex findings. A negative relation obtained, for example, in the poor health category ($r = -.21$; $p<.016$). This association was even stronger when age and health were considered together ($r = -.39$; $p< .027$). On the other hand, nonsignificant correlations were observed in the case of healthy ($r = +.03$; $p<.366$) and older respondents ($r = +.08$; $p<.234$). In addition, a positive association held in the case of relatively recent and healthy area residents ($r = +.23$; $p<.036$). In general, however, these findings are not supportive of the present hypothesis.

With respect to the community area, the relationship between the type of expectational disconfirmation and change in life satisfaction is nonsignificant ($r = -.06$; $p<.221$). It seems evident that the type of expectational disconfirmation experienced in the present instance plays little role in the matter of life satisfaction change subsequent to retirement. The present hypothesis, therefore, is not substantiated on the basis of these findings.

Discussion

From the perspective on the present data, a negative relationship obtained in the family area between expectational disconfirmation and change in life satisfaction. On the other hand, subsequent analysis revealed the explanation for this finding to lie in the type of disconfirmation as opposed to disconfirmation *per se*. That is, the more positive the disconfirmation relative to family behavior, the more negative the change evidenced in life satisfaction. Several factors might account for this finding. In the first place, family interaction is qualitatively different from that characterizing the work setting (Lipman, 1961). To this extent, one's behavior relative to his coworkers probably involves rewards unobtainable within the family context. Then, too, increased interaction in this setting may serve only to magnify hostilities previously latent in the face of infrequent (preretirement) contacts. In addition, the diminished personal status accompanying occupational retirement (Reiss, 1961) places the person in a dependent as opposed to an independent relationship relative to family members. Coupled with the prospect of declining interactional opportunities outside the family (Srole, 1956), forced interaction in such a setting might be expected to result in lowered satisfaction. In the present instance, this was especially true of younger ($r = -.27$; $p<.001$), recently retired individuals ($r = -.48$; $p<$

.001) in poor health $(r = -.59; p<.001)$.

In the case of voluntary associations, no relationship was observed between disconfirmation and change in satisfaction. In this instance, the type of disconfirmation also bore little or no relationship to the issue of satisfaction change. Several factors appear operative here. First, there was a tendency for the younger, lower status persons to experience satisfaction diminution with associational participation. The reverse was true for high status respondents. In this regard, it is well to recall that the reasons for associational participation differ among individuals and often within and across status categories (McKee, 1969). In addition, the character of voluntary associations differ significantly among status groupings (Rose, 1960). It may be assumed, then, that the value to the individual of such settings varies accordingly. For many people interaction represents a valued aspect of life and experience. For others, the organization functions primarily to fill a vacancy in time. In the latter instance, the organization may constitute the only available source of meaningful social activity.

A factor of equal importance, however, is the response of association co-members to the newly-retired participant. For many organizations, such as labor unions, fraternal orders, etc. continued or increased participation is frequently seen as an effort to "hang on" to membership (Friedmann and Havighurst, 1954). In instances where one's contribution to the life of the organization is reduced by low income, poor health, and other factors, he seldom receives the feedback necessary to sustain a positive self-image and hence a high level of satisfaction. In addition, settings of this type place a negative emphasis upon unemployment. As a result, the individual may find himself in a situation where he has few interactional alternatives, is more in-

volved than he desires to be, and receive noncomplimentary feedback from organiza tional participants.

In the community area, a negative bu nonsignificant relationship obtained be tween expectational disconfirmation an change in life satisfaction. Once again however, the type of disconfirmation bor little relationship to the issue of satisfac tion change. In way of explanation, i should be pointed out that community in teraction was primarily with friends and neighbors; 61.2 percent of the respondents for example, interacted only with friend and neighbors prior to retirement. Follow ing retirement, 66.1 percent of all subject confined their community behavior to thes persons. Given these circumstances, it i possible to conceive of the community sec tor as a hybrid of the previous two. Th person's position in relation to his friend and neighbors, for instance, is akin to tha of his family members. Similarly, many in formal facets of community interactior parallel those of associational settings Hence, to the extent that one's status witl friends and neighbors reflects the loss o occupational roles, a negative correlatior similar to that evidenced in the family would be expected. On the other hand since informal community activities ar often associated with valued formal organi zational settings (Carp, 1967), a positive correlation would obtain relative to satis faction change. Consequently, this dua community focus might account for th rather weak correlation observed at pres ent.

Perhaps the most obvious limitation o this research is found in the consistency framework itself. This formulation is some what deterministic in its suggestion tha dissonance always arises when relevant cog nitions are brought into conflict. In th present instance, conflict was supplied b expectational disconfirmation. Nevertheless, with the exception of the family area, research findings did not substantiate the predictions of this orientation. Instead, some evidence has been produced which indicates the type of disconfirmation to be a more critical explanatory factor than disconfirmation *per se*.

It is well to recall that most of the research on consistency theory has been conducted in a laboratory setting (Abelson *et al.*, 1968). In addition, the college sophomore has proven the most readily obtained subject. These observations raise a series of questions when placed along side the present results. Is dissonance, for example, a phenomenon *only* of the young? That is, is dissonance characteristic of one generation and not another? The answer to this question may prove less enlightening than that of a second, namely, do the implications of dissonance and consistency apply outside the laboratory? Although not measured directly, dissonance does not appear to satisfactorily explain the present outcomes. Indeed, even when the type of dissonance is explored separately, only in the area of family behavior does it seem appropriate.

Another weakness of the present orientation is its failure to consider the time element. As has been remarked, the second series of interviews were conducted an average of 5.6 months after the retirement of these respondents. A third series of interviews might have yielded still different findings. Unfortunately, the consistency framework provides no indication as to either the mode or amount of time involved in dissonance resolution. Not considered, for example, is the fact that different individuals can tolerate different degrees of ambiguity (dissonance?). Nor is it recognized that individuals live with numerous inconsistencies throughout the major portion of their lives (Aronson,

1968). Then, too, one must consider the possibility that many of the individuals in the present study fail to see their behavior as disconfirming of their expectations and, consequently, not productive of dissonance.

In a similar fashion, it should be borne in mind that the phenomenon of retirement is not new to Western culture. To be sure, Carp (1972), Streib and Schneider (1971), and others regard it as an institution in its own right. As such, it is possible to consider the question of socialization, particularly anticipatory socialization (Merton, 1957), to a new position in the social structure. If this process is indeed operative, it would seem reasonable to suggest that individuals facing retirement might scale down their expectations for postretirement behavior prior to retirement. This would, of course, result in little or no dissonance with respect to the actual termination of employment. In essence, then, dissonance may be an irrelevant issue for the greater proportion of retiring males.

Summary

The present paper examined the implications of consistency theory with regard to the life satisfaction of older adults. Pre- and post-retirement interviews with 114 older males in an urban area of central Missouri were subjected to investigation. With the exception of the family area, pre- and post-retirement analysis yielded little support for the consistency hypothesis (i.e. expectational disconfirmation will be accompanied by negative changes in life satisfaction). Instead, some evidence was displayed which indicates the *type of disconfirmation* to be more central to the explanation of life satisfaction change than disconfirmation *per se*. In the family, for instance, the more positive the disconfirmation indicated, the more negative the change evidenced in life satisfaction. For voluntary association and community sectors, on the other hand, disconfirmation (both positive and negative) as well as the specific type of disconfirmation bore little relationship to the issue of satisfaction change. The findings do, however, suggest differential "rewards" to characterize the role areas in question.

REFERENCES

Abelson, R. P., Aronson, E., McGuire, W. J., Newcomb, T. M., Rosenberg, M. J., and Tannenbaum, P. H. *Theories of cognitive consistency: A sourcebook,* Rand McNally, Chicago, 1968.

Allen, V. Uncertainty of outcome and postdecision dissonance reduction. In R. P. Abelson, E. Aronson, W. J. McGuire, T. M. Newcomb, M. J. Rosenberg, and P. H. Tannenbaum (Eds.), *Theories of cognitive consistency: A sourcebook,* Rand McNally, Chicago, 1968.

Aronson, E. Dissonance theory: progress and problems. In R. P. Abelson, E. Aronson, W. J. McGuire, T. M. Newcomb, M. J. Rosenberg, P. H. Tannenbaum (Eds.), *Sourcebook on cognitive consistency.* Rand-McNally, New York, 1968.

Aronson, E., and Carlsmith, J. M. Performance expectancy as a determinant of actual performance. *Journal of Abnormal Social Psychology,* 1962, *65,* 178-182.

Bell, B. D. *Life satisfaction among the occupationally retired: A tri-theoretical inquiry.* Doctoral dissertation, Univ. of Missouri—Columbia, 1973.

Bramel, D. Dissonance, expectation, and the self. In R. P. Abelson, E. Aronson, W. J. McGuire, T. M. Newcomb, M. J. Rosenberg, and P. H. Tannenbaum (Eds.), *Sourcebook on cognitive consistency.* Rand-McNally, New York, 1968.

Brotman, H. Who are the aged: a demographic view. In *Occasional papers in gerontology.* Univ. of Michigan-Wayne State Univ., Nov., 1968.

Brotman, H. A profile of the older American. Address read before the *Conference on Consumer Problems of Older People.* Administration on Aging, No. 208, New York, 1968.

Busse, E. W., and Kreps, J. M. Criteria for retirement: A reexamination. *Gerontologist* 1963, *4,* 115-120.

Carp, F. M. The impact of environment on old people. *Gerontologist,* 1967, *7,* 106-108.

Carp, F. M. *Retirement.* Behavioral Publications, New York, 1972.

Donahue, W., Orbach, H. L., and Pollak, O. Retirement: The emerging social pattern. In C. Tibbitts (Ed.), *Handbook of social gerontology.* Univ. of Chicago Press, Chicago, 1960.

Dubin, R. Industrial workers' worlds. In E. Larrabee and R. Meyerson (Eds.), *Mass leisure.* Free Press, Glencoe, IL., 1956.

Festinger, L. *A theory of cognitive dissonance.* Stanford Univ. Press, Stanford, 1957.

Friedmann, E. A., and Havighurst, R. J. *The meaning of work and retirement.* Univ. of Chicago Press, Chicago, 1954.

Goodstein, L. D. Personal adjustment factors and retirement. *Geriatrics,* 1962, *17,* 41-45.

Gordon, M. Changing patterns of retirement. *Journal of Gerontology,* 1960, *15,* 300-304.

Heider, F. Attitudes and cognitive organization. *Journal of Psychology,* 1946, *21,* 107-112.

Lipman, A. Role conceptions and morale of couples in retirement. *Journal of Gerontology,* 1961, *16,* 267-271.

Merton, R. K. *Social theory and social structure.* Free Press, Glencoe, IL., 1957.

McKee, J. B. *Introduction to sociology.* Holt, Rinehart, and Winston, New York, 1969.

Neugarten, B. L., Havighurst, R. J., and Tobin, S. S. The measurement of life satisfaction. *Journal of Gerontology,* 1961, *16,* 134-143.

Reiss, A. J. *Occupations and social status.* Free Press of Glencoe, New York, 1961.

Rose, A. M. The impact of aging on voluntary associations. In C. Tibbitts (Ed.), *Handbook of social gerontology.* Univ. of Chicago Press, Chicago, 1960.

Rosow, I. Adjustment of the normal aging: concept and measurement. In R. H. Tibbitts and W. Donahue (Eds.), *Processes of aging,* Vol. II. Atherton Press, New York, 1963.

Rosow, I. *Social integration of the aged.* Free

Press, New York, 1967.

Shanas, E. Facts versus stereotypes: The Cornell study of occupational retirement. *Journal of Social Issues*, 1958, 2, 61-63.

Sheldon, H. *The older population of the United States.* New York, John Wiley & Sons, New York, 1958.

Srole, I. Social integration and certain corollaries. *American Sociological Review*, 1956, 21, 709-716.

Streib, G. F., and Schneider, C. J. *Retirement in American society: Impact and process.* Cornell Univ. Press, Ithaca, 1971.

Thompson, W. E. Preretirement anticipation and adjustment in retirement. *Journal of Social Issues*, 1958, 2, 35-63.

Thompson, W. E., and Streib, G. F. Personal and social adjustments in retirement. In W. Donahue and C. Tibbitts (Eds.), *The new frontiers of aging.* Univ. of Michigan Press, Ann Arbor, 1957.

Weiss, R., and Kahn, R. On the definition of work among American men. Univ. of Michigan, Institute for Social Research, Ann Arbor, 1959. (mimeo.)

Section VIII

THE MINORITY ELDERLY

PERHAPS NO AREA IN gerontology received less attention during the 1930s and early 1950s than the minority elderly. During this period, gerontologists were involved in sketching the outlines of the discipline and in delineating several specific issues (e.g. morale, retirement, and the adjustment of older persons). In harmony with this approach, demographic studies were in abundance (Kiser, 1950; Thompson, 1933; Valaoras, 1950). Accordingly, the problems of the elderly were catalogued; patterns of adjustment described; and ameliorative programs of aid evaluated. In general, the focus of attention was the elderly *per se.* With few exceptions (Hacker, 1951), "the aged" were regarded as a relatively homogeneous group manifesting a series of common needs.

Toward the end of this period, however, a new focus began to emerge. The issues of common need and concern were to form the basis for an aging subculture (Barron, 1953). To an extent, the aged in the latter decades of life were felt to demonstrate a growing sense of identity with one another. To most gerontologists, this group consciousness was regarded as functional for the older person. Such feelings and associations made adjustment to life situations considerably easier and provided the social and emotional support necessary to cope with a rapidly changing environment.

These early perspectives, however, were essentially descriptive in nature. Few theories were available to orient research efforts or to place specific findings in context. In addition, most studies were generally limited to cross-sectional surveys of large populations of older persons. As a consequence, little could be said of the problems or potentialities unique to a given minority.

The minority status of the aged served as a focal point for debate among gerontologists in the late 1950s and early 1960s. During this time, the subcultural aspects of the aged were delineated (Rose, 1965) as were those features indicative of their minority standing (Streib, 1965). In general, while features of collective awareness were acknowledged to characterize older adults, these dimensions were often limited by such factors as social class membership and residential locale. For the most part, the group consciousness and subcultural identification of the aged could better be explained by localized conditions than by an over-arching perspective fixed within chronological limits.

Although demographic concern continued (Sheldon, 1958), attention began

315

to focus upon specific segments of the aged population. In this regard, both rural and urban studies appeared relative to such groups as the urban poor (Bogue, 1963; Niebank and Pope, 1965), Jews (Wershow, 1964), and blacks (Harrington, 1963). As a result of these and other efforts, research interest in gerontology shifted toward the minority aged as groups in their own right. On the other hand, however, these settings remained somewhat of a curiosity to researchers. While theories of aging multiplied during this period, little attempt was made to apply and/or test these formulations relative to the minority sector. In addition, longitudinal methodologies were rarely employed with these individuals. Consequently, the minority perspective on age was cast aside in favor of other issues.

The late 1960s and early 1970s were to witness an expansion in demographic research (Brotman, 1968; Goldscheider, 1966; Zelinsky, 1966). The issue of an aging subculture laid to rest, gerontologists turned their attention in earnest to the minority aged (Blau and Berezin, 1968). Chief among those groups receiving consideration were blacks of both rural and urban character (Jackson, 1967; 1971; Kent, 1971; Smith, 1967; Solomon, 1970). On the basis of these studies, older blacks as a group lost their homogeneous image as researchers demonstrated significant variations within this minority. Along with blacks, Mexican-Americans (Carp, 1968; Leonard, 1967; Moore, 1971), Jews (Lawton *et al.,* 1971), and Americans of East Asian ancestry (Kalish and Yuen, 1971) became subjects of research interest. Women also, especially widows, came under close scrutiny (Berardo, 1968; Youmans, 1967). In addition to a problem focus, the patterns of adjustment characteristic of such groupings became part of the contemporary research picture (Kent, 1971; Maddox, 1969).

The most significant change in perspective, however, came in the early 1970s as gerontologists sought to test the theories and insights of previous research in the minority arena. Aided by developments in methodological design and statistical application, researchers explored the affect of a number of variables associated with the minority experience. In this regard, kinship ties were found to be more significant in minority settings with respect to the adjustment and morale of the aged. In addition, the "community" proved a more important source of social identity for the aged minority member. While these efforts succeeded in revealing several weaknesses in theory construction relative to the aged, the final contributions of these contexts have yet to be fully realized.

The writings which follow illustrate the contemporary approach to the minority aged. In most instances, the papers emphasize the advantages to be gained by research in these settings. Also highlighted are a series of recent findings relative to several minority groups. To a considerable extent, these authors view the term "minority" as applicable to other than traditional or "visual" categories of persons within the general population.

The paper by Moore addresses itself to an area of aging research only recently recognized as vital to social gerontologists, the minority aging. Specifically, the author attempts to demonstrate that the various characteristics of minority groupings make them ideal "natural laboratories" for the delineation of significant aspects of the aging process as well as the testing of a number of propositions and hypotheses from currently popular theories.

Minority groups with their own special histories, their experience with cultural discrimination, their institutionalization of numerous "coping structures," and their need to adjust to rapid social change, not only affords the gerontologist a rare look at the generation gap experience, but also "permits the researcher to specify a set of traditional values regarding age itself as a principal value difference between old and young." In addition, Moore argues that the focus on the minority aged and how they cope with various forms of prejudice and discrimination can help clarify what is meant by "minority status" when applied to the older person. Finally, the closeness of many minority groups in terms of residential location (e.g. ghettos, reservations or barrios) permits an exploration of the extent to which potential community supports do in fact help the aging process.

Jackson's purpose is to examine the current research regarding aged Negroes in an effort to determine the degree of correspondence between these findings and a number of cultural stereotypes. Besides focusing on aged Negroes in general, the author attempts to examine the influence of urban and rural differences on the picture. Her data scan the period from 1960 to 1968.

For the most part, the Negro aged are seen to depart from such stereotypes as those which hold that their marital statuses are significantly different from those of the white aged. Both groups fail to differ significantly in this regard. With respect to the stereotype that Negro life expectancies are typically less than whites, the author cites research which suggests that Negroes may live longer at later age periods. As to whether the Negro aged place more importance upon their families, are more religious, in poorer health, or less active than their white counterparts, controls for socioeconomic status tend to reduce any stereotypical difference to nonsignificance. Under these circumstances, "aged Negroes are no more religious than white aged; and their organizational participation . . . may even be somewhat higher. Their health is probably better than or no worse than that of whites." The principal difference among the Negro aged as well as among their white contemporaries are seen to center in the rural-urban dimension.

The paper by Crouch is an exploration of the nation's second largest minority, the Mexican-Americans. The author is particularly interested in two, related questions: (1) how older Mexican-Americans view old age, and (2) how they perceive three primary institutions from which informal or formal programs of aid emanate, the family, the church, and the government.

Data for the study were obtained through in-home interviews with 291 older Mexican-Americans residing in a Standard Metropolitan Statistical Area in West Texas. The findings indicate old age to be negatively viewed by this minority group. In addition, old age is usually considered to begin at or below sixty years. These views on age, however, are shown to be closely related to the respondent's socioeconomic status. The data on the perception of support institutions suggests that these older persons generally recognize a deemphasis on the extended family. In addition, " (the respondents) feel that the church has a social action as well as a sacred function and believe that the Anglo government could be a potent agency for support." The author feels that the Mexican-American aged are not substantially different from other Anglo aged populations.

The last two papers in this section focus upon two groups not often thought of as minorities, the elderly poor of the inner city and widows. The size of these groupings as well as their rather high degree of internal similarities among participants mark them as objects of study as well as curiosity.

For Clark, the inner-city aged constitute a unique group in modern society. For the most part, these individuals have been forced into the core areas of the city due to financial and other circumstances. On the other hand, this group of people often lack many of the family and other supports often characterizing ethno-minority groups. As a consequence, the life of the inner-city aged may become especially impoverished and marked by both personal isolation and social invisibility.

While the evidence amassed by the author suggests the plight of the inner city aged to be quite bleak (i.e. incidents of malnutrition are higher in this group, shelter is poor and at a minimum, medical services are often inaccessible, and mobility is hampered both physically and socially), when seen from another perspective the picture brightens considerably. Viewed from the standpoint of a process, the city represents a potential for promoting human survival as well as human misery. Clark feels that the key to the puzzle lies in the aged's phenomenal perception of their social and physical situation.

The paper by Lopata suggests that widows can be considered a minority group for a number of reasons. First and foremost in the criteria for minority status is that of differential treatment by a dominant group. The author delineates the situations in which this differential treatment occurs as well as the manner by which it is employed. Secondly, she notes that the external "signs" of sex, poverty, and "oneness" tend to serve as clues of stimuli for majority reactions. These external features of minority status are as distinctive as color or mode of dress. As a consequence, the reactions of the dominant culture tend not to be limited to a single generational cohort, but are reflected in the actions and behavior of all age groups. One evidence of the effect of these differential reactions has been the withdrawal of the once-active widow from the ongoing social life about her.

REFERENCES

Barron, M. L. Minority group characteristics of the aged in American society. *Journal of Gerontology*, 1953, *8*, 477-482.

Berardo, F. Widowhood status in the United States: perspectives on a neglected aspects of the family life cycle. *Family Coordinator*, 1968, *17*, 191-203.

Blau, D., and Berezin, M. A. Some ethnic and cultural considerations in aging. *Journal of Geriatric Psychiatry*, 1968, *2*, 3-5.

Bogue, D. J. *Skid-row in American cities*. Community and Family Study Center, University of Chicago, 1963.

Brotman, H. B. *Who are the aged: a demographic view*. Ann Arbor: University of Michigan-Wayne State University Institute of Gerontology, 1968.

Carp, F. *Factors in utilization of services by Mexican American elderly*. Palo Alto, California: American Institute for Research, 1968.

Goldsheider, C. Differential residential mobility of the older population. *Journal of Gerontology*, 1966, *21*, 103-108.

Hacker, H. M. Women as a minority group. *Social Forces*, 1951, *30*, 60-69.

Harrington, M. *The other America*. New York: Macmillan, 1963.

Jackson, J. J. Social gerontology and the Negro: a review. *Gerontologist*, 1967, *7*, 168-178.

Jackson, J. J. The blacklands of gerontology. *Aging and Human Development*, 1971, *2*, 156-171.

Kalish, R. A., and Yuen, S. Americans of east Asian ancestry: aging and the aged. *Gerontologist*, 1971, *11*, 36-47.

Kent, D. P. The elderly in minority groups: variant patterns of aging. *Gerontologist*, 1971, *11*, 26-29.

Kent, D. P. The Negro aged. *Gerontologist*, 1971, *11*, 48-51.

Kiser, C. V. The demographic background of our aging population. In *The social and biological challenge of our aging population: proceedings of the Eastern States Health Conference*. New York: Columbia University Press, 1950.

Lawton, M. P., Kleban, M. H., and Singer, M. The aged Jewish people and the slum environment. *Journal of Gerontology*, 1971, *26*, 231-239.

Leonard, O. E. The older Spanish-speaking people of the southwest. In E. G. Youmans (Ed.), *Older rural Americans*. Lexington, Kentucky: University of Kentucky Press, 1967.

Maddox, G. L. Growing old: getting beyond the sterotypes. In R. R. Boyd and C. G. Oakes Eds.), *Foundations of practical gerontology*. Columbia, South Carolina: University of South Carolina Press, 1969.

Moore, J. W. Mexican-Americans. *Gerontologist*, 1971, *11*, 30-35.

Niebank, P. L., and Pope, J. B. *The elderly in older urban areas*. Philadelphia: Institute for Environmental Studies, University of Pennsylvania, 1965.

Rose, A. M. The subculture of the aging: a framework for research in social gerontology. In A. M. Rose and W. A. Peterson (Eds.), *Older people and their social world*. Philadelphia: F. A. Davis, 1965.

Sheldon, H. D. *The older population of the United States*. New York: John Wiley & Sons, 1958.

Smith, S. H. The older rural Negro. In E. G. Youmans (Ed.), *Older rural Americans*. Lexington, Kentucky: University of Kentucky Press, 1967.

Solomon, B. Ethnicity, mental health and the older black aged. In B. Solomon (Ed.), *Ethnicity, mental health and aging*. Los Angeles: University of Southern California Gerontology Center, 1970.

Streib, G. F. Are the aged a minority group? In A. W. Gouldner (Ed.), *Applied sociology*. New York: The Free Press of Glencoe, 1965.

Thompson, W. S., and Whelpton, P. K. *Population trends in the United States*. New York: McGraw-Hill Book Co., 1933.

Valaoras, V. G. Patterns of aging of human populations. In *The social and biological challenge of our aging population: proceedings of the Eastern States Health Conference*. New York: Columbia University Press, 1950.

Wershow, H. J. The older Jews of Albany park—some aspects of a subculture of the aged and its interaction with a gerontological research project. *Gerontologist*, 1964, *4*, 198-202.

Youmans, E. G. Family disengagement among older urban and rural women. *Journal of Gerontology*, 1967, *22*, 209-211.

Zelinsky, W. Toward a geography of the aged. *Geographical Review*, 1966, *56*, 445-447.

Chapter **35**

SITUATIONAL FACT-ORS AFFECTING MINORITY AGING

JOAN W. MOORE

IT IS PART OF THE scientific credo that research should be motivated by the promise of knowledge that will contribute to the general understanding of phenomena. This credo is sometimes hard to follow in the study of aging. By and large the plight of the aging subjects is pathetic and the urgent desire to come up with an answer to some of their problems often prompts us to narrow research, often wildly over generalized.

If this is true for aging in general, it is even more so for minority aging: as other papers in this section clearly show, this segment of the American population has an exponential share of the nation's problems. Nonetheless, a case can be made that whatever research we do on minority aging, no matter how narrow or problem-oriented, can begin to contribute substantially to the understanding of aging in general if we can agree on some research priorities.

The argument in this paper is simple. Whether we talk about individuals, group behavior, or the aged as a collectivity, most of our generalizations are based on the study of a limited sample, primarily middle-majority Anglos. We do not really know how much such sample limitations con-

strain these generalizations, for example, generalizations about "disengagement," about the "generation gap," and about the aged as a "minority group." The life experiences and present situations of the minority aged can present such general theoretical issues in a fresh and often clearer light.

Let us look for a moment at a few things that go into the making of an American minority and see what can be learned from them about aging. This examination of necessity omits much of relevance to any particular minority or to the understanding of minorities *per se*. It is focused on what is inherent in the minority situation that is important to the study of aging rather than to minority status. All five of the characteristics to be mentioned have relevance for the aging of all Americans. With the minorities these characteristics are clearer.

First, each minority has a *special history,* a collective experience that has placed its members in their present position in the American social system. That special history differs from one minority to another, but in all cases it entails subordination. The particular process was different: conquest, prolonged conflict, and expropriation in the case of American Indians and Mexicans; slavery and its aftermath for the blacks; migration into special economic slots for Puerto Ricans, Mexicans, and Asians, a transplanted European culture of racism in the case of all groups. Since the "generation gap" is in no small part a resultant of the reinterpretation of collective history, the position of the minorities in having a *special* history makes the study of this controversial issue a bit easier, as we shall enlarge upon below.

Second, in every case this special history has been accompanied by *discrimination,*

Reprinted by permission from the *Gerontologist,* 1971, *11,* 88-93.

and the development of strong and predominantly negative *stereotypes* about the minority. Although the content of the particular stereotype and the nature of the discrimination has varied from one group to another, in every case members of the minority populations have been viewed by the larger society as special and as requiring special treatment in all institutional areas. This characteristic has relevance for all Americans, in that we are increasingly concerned about the *age* category as a basis for minority status. The combination of two categorical bases for discrimination, minority status *and* old age, offers special interest for the gerontologist, as detailed below.

Third, in every case some *variant subculture* has been developed in the minority. In some cases, like many American Indian tribes, the subculture is strong and distinctive. In some cases, like the Jews and the blacks, the subculture has been much closer to that of the dominant culture. The subculture includes value sets of significance to aging, e.g. values about the importance of work or physical prowess to personal identity. It also may include specific definitions of the timing of statuses and norms relating to behavior in particular age statuses. In addition, these subcultures differ one from another. The combination of these features promises further insight into the generation gap, as discussed below.

Fourth, in almost all cases (whether in reservation, ghetto, or barrio) substructures have developed, and often been institutionalized, that could very loosely be termed *"coping structures."* The Negro church, the Mexican-American family structure, the Jewish voluntary association, the Chinese benevolent society, all of these have supported the minority individual in his difficulties in coping with economic uncertainty and a hostile and exclusionary larger society. "Coping" here is used to refer to many things, ranging from help with bare survival needs (as with the extension of the family network), to avenues for meaningful social participation, internal prestige and power (as with the Negro church), to a diffuse but still important opportunity for a sense of belonging to *some* collectivity (provided by all residential concentrations of minorities). These ingroup supports, with their variability, offer considerable promise of fruitful study in the general process of aging.

Finally, all of these things have been *changing rapidly* and with increasing obviousness.

All of these features of the general minority situation have special relevance for the aged. All of them are exaggerations, amplifications, researchable deviations of what is happening for all Americans. The entire society is changing, although changes for minority persons are more easily seen and more accessible to study. One of the most critical issues in social gerontology is the problem of role continuity and discontinuity, how either one develops, how continuity or discontinuity in various roles are handled by people of widely varying social characteristics and background. The minority person offers the "natural laboratory" for at least the gross delineation of significant aspects of the aging process. Of course, the proper scientific controls are lacking: attempts to place the minorities on a precise continuum, where minority A and B share all but, say, dark skin, have met with perennial frustration. But all such attempts have led to a clarification of the processes involved, and this is greatly to be desired, given the present state of development of social gerontology.

Let us now turn to some specific illustrations of issues in social gerontology that might fruitfully be approached through the study of minority groups. One of the most conspicuous in terms of popular interest is the question of the importance of the "generation gap" to the aging individual. As an obvious consequence of rapid social change, the value differences between old and young in society have given rise to a variety of speculations about their effects. Most such speculations are concerned with integration of the society at large; very few have attempted to search out the implications of a severe generation gap for particular age groups. For gerontologists, it would seem that defining the generation gap and its significance for aging would be of prime importance. It is obviously quite different to grow old in a society in which your children and grandchildren agree with you totally about your life work compared with a society in which, at the very least, one may feel the need to "keep up" with the times, and at the worst, one feels alienated from the new values apparently espoused by the young. Research is, in fact, being conducted on such matters (Bengston, 1969), but in the larger system, such research must of necessity be extremely broad.

Studying minorities would permit specification of *particular* values in the hypothesized generation gap, and particular kinds of continuities and discontinuities that might be related to "successful" aging.

For example, the special history of many minorities is now being redefined. This redefinition entails action by the young based on their reevaluation of the collective past. This particular form of the "generation gap" has been hypothesized by one psychiatrist (Elam, 1970) as having some specific consequences for the successful accomplishment of age-specific psychological tasks, that is, ego integrity among the black aged. He argues that the black revolution provides more positive input for the old black

than does the "normal aging" person's reflection on a past lifetime, since the past for many blacks has been one of frustration and failure. The young people's reinterpretation of collective problems helps the old black give a positive meaning to his failures. At least it removes the stigma of failure as a consequence of personal inadequacy. In this respect, the reinterpretation of the collective special history helps the black, old person make positive sense out of his unique experiences and helps him to ego integrity rather than despair. By contrast, a social worker has put forth some specific counter-hypotheses about the relevance of this reinterpretation of black history for the attainment of ego integrity, arguing that the young people's rejection of the past as the "only possible way" tends to produce despair in the old black (Solomon, 1970). Both arguments emphasize a specific change in values which is specifically relevant to a universal problem in aging, namely the frame of reference used by the old person in evaluating his life experiences.

There are alternatives for the blacks. For example, the old black may reaffirm that his own particular life *had* significance, that "Uncle Tomism" was the only possible, and an honorable, way. This may involve a rejection of the young person's reinterpretation, a particular form of the generation gap. Or, following Elam, he may take greater pride in the collective future, certainly a form of generational solidarity. Finally, following Solomon, he may be confused, resentful, or bewildered by the reinterpretations taking place around him.

Thus the existence of a special collective history, which provides the context within which the aging minority individual must interpret the meaning of his particular life, can permit the researcher to specify a significant dimension of the "generation gap." This task is more difficult in the larger society because of the greater diffuseness of the relationship between the aging individual's particular history and the collective experience on the one hand and the reevaluation of that collective experience by the young on the other hand.

Because minority populations have developed subcultures, they permit another kind of specification of what might be meant by "generation gap" and its consequences for the elderly. American Indian tribes represent the best case. The traditional role of the elderly varies widely from tribe to tribe: in the northwest coast tribes, the young men assume the work and political responsibilities of the tribe, while in southern Arizona and California, it is the older man. No matter what the norms, any changes (and recent changes have been drastic) means a change in the role of the aged (Kelly, 1969). These changes, of course, are tightly interwoven with changes in the social structure of the tribal society, and in particular with the kinship structure. But it still seems valid to isolate them analytically. Thus studying the generation gap among minority groups permits the researcher to specify a set of traditional values regarding age itself as a principal value difference between old and young. By contrast, "the role of the aged" is far less clear-cut in the society as a whole, and the changes are far less specifiable as a consequence.

Another example of the kind of issue that can be elevated from the plane of normative rhetoric is the blurred question of whether the aged in American society are themselves a minority group. This much overworked metaphor can be given some specificity in a population with a lifetime of discrimination. Active discrimination and pervasive stereotypes are the normal environment of most minority persons from early childhood. If, in fact, old age carries some of these social and psychological handicaps, does the life experience of discrimination and prejudice on the basis of minority characteristics prepare one for this new kind of discrimination? Is the elderly minority person more able to cope with yet another negative categorization? Or does the lifetime of discrimination wear him down so that he is especially vulnerable to this new form of discrimination?

In this formulation any such questions are, of course, fatuous. But their very fatuity casts light on one of the problems in the transformation of rhetoric to research. Discrimination which pervades the life experience of the minority person has been studied from many perspectives, ranging from the economic to the psychological. Individual and collective ways of "coping" are now in the process of being more intensively analyzed. In particular, the importance of reference groups is now being emphasized. The focus on minority aged and how they cope with this new form of prejudice and discrimination can help us clarify what is meant by "minority status" when applied to the old person. We can explore the relative significance of family members, age peers and juniors, members of the same ethnic group and members of other ethnic groups, potential employers (who are still salient for many minority aged), potential landlords, and the whole host of individuals with whom the minority person, poor or middle-class, must deal. We can explore the shifts in significance of these various groups with aging. We can explore the importance of class status. We can explore the variations in the content of stereotype, how they vary from, say, landlord to younger member of the same minority group, and how the old minority person responds to these issues. Most important, we can see if the discrimination entailed in being "put on the shelf" is similar to that entailed in the active rejection characterizing younger *and* older minority persons.

The existence of ghetto, reservation, or *barrio* institutions suggests another opportunity for gerontologists interested in age in general. By and large, Anglo old people in metropolitan areas do not live in tightly knit communities, unless there are some very special circumstances (Rosow, 1967). By contrast, poor minority old people may live in socially integrated communities. The strength of bonds in the minority kinship group and in the minority ghettos varies widely, from, say a high point in some Indian reservations to, perhaps, a low point in some of the more conflictful metropolitan ghettos. Potential community supports for the aging person have generally eroded in the society at large. The study of minority aged persons permits an exploration of the extent to which such community supports do in fact help the aging process.

In addition, potential kinship and community supports among the minorities are undergoing drastic change, providing yet another opportunity for generalizable research. For example, many observers have suggested that the old black woman is in some respects "better off" than the old white woman because the combination of poverty and a prolonged period of childbearing have tended to permit her to retain a meaningful functional role. A grandmother is often involved in active mothering both of her own children born late in life and of her children's children. This is true for other minorities as well and tends to be part of the norms attached to that status. Further, the role of the old person in a poor family may be significant because he may make a substantial contribution to the whole family's economic welfare. The small sums provided by Social Security or other pension or welfare plans may be a substantial portion of the household income. In addition, many elderly poor continue to work at unskilled and service jobs until very late in life, also providing income resources for all. The prevailing minority situation of poverty, in short, may have one minor side benefit for the aging individual in that a survival-oriented family system provides a potential contribution to his continued sense of personal worth.

This "benefit," however, is probably bought at the expense of increased fatigue and anxiety. Very few families will reject a higher standard of living in order to maintain the old person's functional role. Ironically, any improvement in the family's economic status may erode what little contribution the existing system might have made to the successful aging of the old poor minority person, (Elam, 1970; Moore, 1971; Solomon, 1970).

Another opportunity for study presents itself here, however. In some minority communities, new roles are being sought for old people. For example, community control of schools on one Indian reservation has meant that the old are finding a revived role as the repository of tribal tradition: something of the same is potentially present in all ethnic studies programs. Thus change in some minority communities may be regarded as releasing the old people for new roles: self-conscious programs of cultural exploration have developed that may provide an opportunity for research on the invention of functional roles for the elderly.

Kinship supports are one aspect of ingroup supports for the aging individual: many of the same generalizations can be applied to other ghetto institutional supports. As indicated, ghetto supports vary from place to place and minority to minority. They may range from total support to nothing much more than the comfort that comes from being with people who look like oneself and talk like oneself after a lifetime of prejudice and discrimination on "the outside." Under present conditions such ghetto supports are precarious at best. They also shrivel along with collective progress just as the emotional supports in the family may erode away with individual progress. For example, the Mexican areas of formerly lively settlements in middle-western cities have shrunk to a few restaurants and a few old people, while the economically mobile second and third generations follow the classic patterns of movement to "better" areas of the town. In addition such ghettos are frequently located in those parts of town most susceptible to redevelopment either by means of urban-renewal projects or private development and expansion efforts. Barrio or ghetto supports may thus be particularly susceptible to destruction. They are rarely replaced in whatever alternative housing may be provided for those relocated.

Adjustments of minority old people that depend on the minority community may be precarious. People at the bottom of any social hierarchy can rarely impose the conditions of their life: their adjustments are thus easily disrupted. Nowhere is this more probable than with the minority old person.

The same factors that militate against a minority person's well-being at earlier ages continue to operate without abatement: in many respects, things are worse. Though an able-bodied young man may suffer from job insecurity, an old man with a lifetime of job insecurity will also face a future without retirement benefits. For a very high proportion of minority elderly, this grim statement represents reality. Past collective problems are, if anything, increased with age. As the society as a whole becomes more bureaucratized, the badly educated person of any group becomes relatively worse off: minority elderly lag far behind the dominant group in such resources as education, linguistic fluency and so on, that might help them overcome problems as they arise (Moore, forthcoming). It is also plain that the gap between Anglo and minority elderly will increase in future decades.

The discussion of in-group support, kin and communal, and their changes and their variations provides obvious opportunities not only for research on existing situations but also for the development of programs. Such programs might build on the strengths of past situations, while avoiding the precariousness of minority adaptations in the past. If there is any validity to the hypothesis that collective and individual progress will erode kin and communal supports for the aged, it seems ridiculous for practitioners not to attempt some kind of ameliorative effort. In turn, such efforts may provide fruitful research opportunities. The "natural laboratory" provided by local variations in community strength need not be left untouched.

The discussion in this paper has illustrated ways in which five special characteristic situations of American minorities could help illuminate general issues in the study of aging. These general issues relate to three levels of analysis: the functioning of aging individuals, the functioning of aging individuals in groups, and the functioning of the aged as distinctive collectivities. Minorities require that we enlarge our generalizations and deepen our conceptual framework.

REFERENCES

Bengston, V. Generational differences: Correlates and consequences, Unpublished ms., 1969.

Elam, L. C. Critical factors for mental health in aging black populations. Paper delivered at workshop on Ethnicity, Mental Health, and Aging, Los Angeles, Calif., April, 1970.

Kelly, W., and Levy, J. Indians. Paper delivered at NICHD Conference on Ethnic Differences in Retirement, Tucson, April 1969.

Moore, J. Retirement and the Mexican American Aged, *Proceedings of the NICHD Con-*ference on Ethnic Differences in Retirement, 1971.

Rosow, I. *Social integration of the aged.* New York: Free Press, 1967.

Solomon, B. Ethnicity, mental health and the older black aged. In *Ethnicity, mental health and aging.* Los Angeles: University of Southern California, Gerontology Center, 1970.

Chapter 36

AGED NEGROES: THEIR CULTURAL DEPARTURES FROM STATISTICAL STEREOTYPES AND RURAL-URBAN DIFFERENCES

Jacquelyne J. Jackson

Cultural Departures from Statistical Stereotypes

NEEDLESS TO SAY, the operational definitions of "cultural departures" and "statistical stereotypes" used, as well as judgments made about the "adequacy" of programs, planning, and evaluation for meeting the needs of Negro elderly, were directly affected by my interpretations of the current status of knowledge about and programs and planning for aged Negroes.

As has been noted elsewhere (Jackson, 1967; 1968), very little is known about aged Negroes. Yet, if one essential criterion in determining, e.g. the adequacy of programs, planning, and evaluation for meeting the needs of the elderly is that crystallized by Eisdorfer (1968) in another context as that of "basic information on the aging process and the impact of aging upon the individual and his community," it would follow that most such programs, planning, and evaluation for most aged, regardless of race and ethnicity, are, no doubt, yet inadequate.

Reprinted by permission from the *Gerontologist*, 1970, *10*, 140-145.

(An incidental, in the sense of falling without the realm of this paper, point is that of the "touchy" issue of racial segregation or of racial desegregation for programs in which aged persons would be expected to interact face-to-face. Should there be racial desegregation in "X" program? If so, why so, when so, where so, and how so? Although this may be more pronounced in the South, it is probably an "itchy" issue in the North as well. It is certainly an issue much influenced by various stereotypes regarding the Negro and other aged groups.)

Since so little is known about aged Negroes, no exhaustive nor precise delineation of cultural departures by aged Negroes from statistical stereotypes can now be proffered. However, a general discussion of some of their cultural departures may be especially useful for program, planning, evaluation, and personnel for the elderly.

Three general areas which may be focused upon are (a) statistical stereotypes derived largely from data collected by the U.S. Bureau of Census and variously interpreted by that agency and others; (b) statistical stereotypes obtained from empirical findings in social gerontological and other related studies; and (c) what may be termed the "laymen's 'statistical stereotypes.' "

One example of a cultural departure by aged nonwhites (i.e. 60 + years of age, 92% of whom were Negroes in the 1960 census) from a statistical stereotype of nonwhites generally is that nonwhites did *not* differ significantly by marital status from aged whites in 1960.

Since, this fact may startle some, χ^2 results are provided in Table 36-I. Overall, the largest proportional difference by marital status between these nonwhites and whites was that more nonwhites than whites were widowed. The second largest such lifference for males was that more non-whites were in the category of "spouse absent" than were whites; for females, more whites were "single" than were nonwhites.

The trend toward an increasing significant difference between the marital statuses of nonwhites and whites for younger age groups, however, suggests that as the younger nonwhite population becomes older, the marital statuses of aged nonwhites (or at least of aged Negroes) will vary from the 1960 pattern. If so, significant racial differences by marital status may appear among a future older population. Especially may more older Negro males be spouse-less, increasing, perhaps, the need for even more institutionalized and other secondary supportive and protective services.

In 1965, Negro aged (i.e. 65+ years of age) were 6.1 percent of the total Negro population, a smaller proportion than that of all aged in the total population of the United States, because they tend to die earlier than whites. But, contrary to the usual statistical stereotype, it appears that whites do *not* have *lower* mortality rates or life expectancies in every age group.

and 1961 (specifically 1900–1902, 1909–1911, 1919–1921, 1929–1931, 1939–1941, 1949–1951, and 1959–1961). They concluded that, "By age seventy-five, however, the life expectancy differential had reversed itself with whites having life expectancy of 8.7 years and nonwhites one of 9.5 years. This crossing seemed to have occurred at about the age of sixty-eight."

They contended that this phenomenon of racial reversal of life expectancy is probably not related to such factors as sex, cause of death, point in time, mortality measure, nor data error. Rather, the causal model, "which appears most consistent with the data is one which does not rely on a biological explanation alone but which depends upon the interaction of biological and social variables." Calloway's emphasis on socioenvironmental variables to explain this reversal (Jackson, 1967) tends to support this conclusion.

However, Brotman suggested that data are too sparse and reporting too faulty to be able to even demonstrate such a pattern of racial reversal of mortality rates or life expectancies. He believes that, just as there

TABLE 36-I

χ^2 RESULTS FOR WHITE-NONWHITE MARITAL STATUSES BY SEX, 1960[a]

Marital Status	White-Nonwhite Males			White-Nonwhite Females		
	χ^2	df	p	χ^2	df	p
Single	0.6261	5	<.98	1.2477	5	<.90
Spouse present	1.1455	5	<.90	0.3863	5	<.99
Spouse absent	2.4179	5	<.70	0.4038	5	<.99
Divorced	0.0324	5	<.99	0.0098	5	<.99
Widowed	4.3987	5	<.30	2.2725	5	<.80

[a]Source of raw data: U. S. Bureau of the Census. *U. S. Census of Population: 1960*. Detailed Characteristics, U. S. Bureau of Census, 1963, Table 176.

Thornton and Nam (1968) examined mortality rates for whites and nonwhites in seven age groups (commencing with 25–34 years, and proceeding, by i = 10, to 85+ years) roughly between the years 1900

is no significant differences by marital statuses between older whites and nonwhites, there is also *no* significant difference in their mortality rates or life expectancies. This, too, may be an issue in need of resolution. It is also highly probable that if older Negroes obtain significantly better preventive and other health care under Medicare, and if Medicaid is also extended significantly to the younger Negro population, this racial reversal, if it does exist, may well be erased.

Racial reversal or not, it is now the case that (a) most Negroes die earlier, (b) perceive of themselves as being "old" earlier, and (c) are, in fact, *old* earlier than are whites.

As an aggregate, aged Negroes depart from census-type statistical stereotypes of all aged in several other ways. For example, their incomes and education levels are lower than the averages; their housing is more substandard. Other noncensus data show that they are also less likely to be aware of available sources than the aged generally. But, there are also some aged Negroes who depart culturally and statistically from the average aged, Negro or white, for their incomes and educational levels are higher, their housing better, and they have effective manipulative skills for utilizing available and creating new resources than the aged generally.

Briefly, empirical findings in social gerontology and related fields contain certain statistical stereotypes from which aged Negroes especially tend to depart. Such literature too often depicts, e.g. aged Negroes as having extremely weak family structures and assistance patterns, extremely high religious activity and interest, poor or extremely poor health; and almost no organizational participation.

For most aged Negroes with families, the family is the primary source of assistance (to the extent of its ability) and of primary group relationships. When socioeconomic status is controlled, aged Negroes are no more religious than white aged; and their organizational participation, again

with SES constant, may even be somewhat higher. Their health is probably better than or no worse than that of whites.

The "laymen's 'statistical stereotypes'" vary, but the author feels that, within the Negro community, the aged have been thought of in much more favorable terms than the stereotypes which are assigned to the aged by white Americans. While white Americans may have been busy emphasizing youth, Negro Americans have been busier emphasizing survival, and the social roles assigned to Negro aged were delineated and significant. But, one of the funny things happening along the road to integration, pluralism, or separatism is that of decreasing significance attached to Negro aged by Negroes. This apparent phenomenon is probably a concomitant of the decreasing economic importance of Negro aged for their families.

What is more important are two general conclusions about aged Negroes and their cultural departures from statistical stereotypes: (a) obviously, more valid and reliable statistical stereotypes about Negro aged are needed; and (b) morally, we, as social gerontological researchers and practitioners, ought ever be on guard to prevent the unfavorable "laymen's 'statistical stereotypes'" about aged Negroes from becoming what Merton (1957) termed "self-fulfilling prophecies."

Rural-Urban Differences

The rural-urban differences among Negro aged (i.e. 65 years of age and over) have received little attention in the literature. But, of course, there are certain differences which yet need to be ferreted out for further consideration in rural and urban programs, planning, and evaluation for these aged.

The focus on such differences within this paper, unfortunately, is highly limited

It is primarily restricted to selected demographic data from the 1960 Census and selected findings about urban and rural aged Negroes in two Georgia counties, as described by Jackson and Ball (1966).

Most of the demographic data were only available for nonwhites rather than for Negroes specifically. Since, however, Negroes were 93.6 percent of all nonwhites, sixty-five plus years of age, in 1960 (91.8 and 95.1%, respectively for Negro males and females), the term "Negroes" and "nonwhites" may be used synonymously.

As can be readily seen in Table 36-II, nonwhite aged in urban, rural nonfarm, and rural farm areas showed little variation by the factors delineated therein. More were married in the rural farm than in the remaining two areas. More males in the rural farm and more females in the urban areas were in the labor force than were their counterparts. Striking perhaps to some may be the fact that considerably less than 1 percent of these aged persons were in group quarters of any kind (including institutions) in 1960.

While this table is useful in providing a broad overview of basic social characteristics of its depicted population, its data are obviously much too scanty to assist substantially in planning and evaluating programs for Negro aged. The type of data described by Jackson and Ball (1966) provide a useful, but partial complement to such data.

Using noninstitutionalized Negroes, sixty-five plus years of age, in one rural (N = 70) and one urban (N = 62) Georgia county, they investigated certain rural-urban differences. Their findings should be regarded as tentative, in that the urban sample was somewhat skewed by marital status.

A brief description of the samples: the mean age of the rural and urban respond-ents, most of whom were Georgia natives, was seventy-four and seventy-two years, respectively. Approximately 38 and 31 percent of the rural and urban males, and 70 and 40 percent of the rural and urban females were widowed. Most respondents had less than a sixth-grade education, and their major lifetime occupations were either as farmers or laborers. The majority were no longer in the labor force, and, for most, their monthly incomes averaged less than $100. These two samples differed significantly (χ^2, $p > 0.05$) by age, sex, marital, employment, and educational status, major lifetime occupation, monthly income, and religious affiliation.

χ^2 results also showed that the rural and urban samples varied significantly ($p > 0.05$) by:

(1) *income sources* (essentially more rural than urban aged were dependent upon welfare funds only);

(2) *health factors* (greater frequency of utilization of health services by the urban groups; urban males reported the least number of health problems; more rural than urban aged would first "turn to" their families in case of illness, while more urban than rural aged would first "turn to" a hospital; more urban than rural aged placed the greatest responsibility upon a governmental agency for providing them with medical care, while more rural than urban subjects placed a greater responsibility for such care upon their families);

(3) *material possessions* (home ownership was higher among the rural than among the urban aged; some rural respondents had no running water and indoor toilets);

(4) *family and household factors* (rural families were larger; a greater proportion of urban parents received assistance from their children; the rural and urban parents varied in type of assistance desired from

TABLE 36-II
SELECTED DEMOGRAPHIC CHARACTERISTICS FOR NONWHITES 65+ YEARS
OF AGE, BY URBAN, RURAL NONFARM, AND RURAL FARM AREAS, 1960[a]

Characteristic	*Urban*	*Rural Nonfarm*	*Rural Farm*
% Nonwhites, 65+ years of age, in total nonwhite population	5.7	7.4	6.2
Median age, Negroes only	70.8 yrs.	71.5 yrs.	70.8 yrs.
Q	4.2 yrs.	4.6 yrs.	4.2 yrs.
Median school years, nonwhite			
Males: 65 — 69 yrs.	5.3	3.6	3.8
70 — 74 yrs.	5.0	3.4	3.7
75+ years	4.4	3.0	3.3
Females: 65 — 69 yrs.	6.1	4.5	4.7
70 — 74 yrs.	5.7	4.3	4.5
75+ years	5.0	4.7	3.8
Marital status			
% Nonwhite males:			
Single	7.4	5.4	3.8
Married	64.4	69.3	74.5
Widowed	25.0	23.5	20.6
Divorced	3.2	1.8	1.1
% Nonwhite females:			
Single	4.7	3.6	3.4
Married	29.4	36.8	45.0
Widowed	63.4	58.5	50.8
Divorced	2.5	1.1	0.8
Average family size in same household:			
Husband-wife, head 65 — 74	3.06	3.51	4.09
head 75+	2.84	3.10	3.61
Other male head, 65+	3.30	3.74	4.24
Female head, 65+	3.20	3.57	4.05
% in Labor Force:			
Males: 65 — 69 yrs.	39.8	34.5	61.6
70 — 74 yrs.	26.1	23.0	47.9
75 — 79 yrs.	18.8	15.0	34.7
80 — 84 yrs.	12.3	9.4	19.4
85+ yrs.	8.6	5.5	12.4
Females: 65 — 69 yrs.	22.0	13.7	13.5
70 — 74 yrs.	13.0	7.9	7.8
75 — 79 yrs.	7.9	4.9	5.3
80 — 84 yrs.	4.4	2.8	3.8
85+ yrs.	3.8	1.6	1.8
Median individual income (1959)			
Male: 65 — 74 yrs.	$1,433	$782	$773
75+ yrs.	$ 859	$601	$620
Female: 65 — 74 yrs.	$ 688	$550	$545
75+ yrs.	$ 617	$534	$531
% In group quarters	.04	.04	.002

[a]Source of raw data: U. S. Bureau of the Census. *U. S. Census of Population:* 1960. Detailed Characteristics, U. S. Bureau of Census, 1963.

hildren) ;

(5) *friendship and social contact* (more ural than urban females, and more urban han rural males preferred homogeneous ge-group associations; males reported a arger friendship group than did females; nore urban than rural males and more ural than urban females felt that their ocial contact was greater than it was ten ears ago) ;

(6) *church participation* (church attendance was more frequent for rural than rban females, and for urban than rural nales, more of the rural subjects participated in at least one church-sponsored rganization than did the urban subjects) ;

(7) *desirability of a home for the aged* vhereas almost all of the nonwelfare re-'pients in the samples favored a home for ne aged, for others, not for themselves, gnificantly more of the rural than urban elfare recipients favored such a home, ;ain, for others, but not primarily for nemselves) ; and

(8) *attitude toward death* (measured ery crudely, with a negative attitude be-ig defined as a fear of death, the urban spondents were more positively oriented ward death than were the rural subjects).

These, then, are some suggested vari-les which may be useful in differentiating tween specific rural and urban Negro ;ed subjects in the "Deep South." In all obability, most of these tentative com-rative findings could be replicated in rther studies of other Southern, Negro-ed rural and urban groups. Certainly, course, many other variables need to be mpared and tested, if we are to uncover e relevant rural-urban differences among ese aged.

Summary

The major purposes of this paper were ose of suggesting some areas where aged Negroes tend to become "cultural depar-turers" from statistical stereotypes and of also suggesting certain variables which may be useful in distinguishing between rural and urban aged Negroes.

Essentially, both tasks were only partial-ly successful, due to the scarcity of avail-able data about aged Negroes, and, no doubt, to the value judgments imposed upon those data.

Given those limitations, however, Negro aged tend to depart from such statistical stereotypes as those which hold that their marital statuses are significantly different from those of white aged; that their life expectancies are typically less than those of whites (they may be longer at the later age periods) ; that they differ significantly from whites by importance placed upon their families, or that they are more religi-ous, in poorer health, or less active in formal organizations than whites.

Some variables which may be useful in distinguishing between rural and urban Negro aged in southern areas, at least, in-clude those of income sources, material possessions, health, family, and household factors, friendship and social contact, church attendance and participation in church-related organizations, and attitudes toward the desirability of homes for the aged and toward death.

REFERENCES

Brotman, H. Private conversations with the author, Oct. 30-31, 1968.

Eisdorfer, C. Patterns of federal funding for research in aging. *Gerontologist,* 1968, *8,* 3-6.

Jackson, J. J. Social gerontology and the Ne-gro: A review. *Gerontologist,* 1967, *7,* 168-178.

Jackson, J. J. Negro aged and social gerontol-ogy: A critical evaluation. *Journal of Social & Behavioral Sciences,* 1968, *13,* 42-47.

Jackson, J., and Ball, M. A comparison of rural and urban Georgia aged Negroes. *Journal of* the *Association of Social Science Teachers,* 1966, *12,* 30-37.

Merton, R. K. *Social theory and social structure.* Glencoe, Ill.: Free Press, 1957.

Thornton, R. J., and Nam, C. B. The lower mortality rates of nonwhites at the older ages: An enigma in demographic analysis. In *Research reports in social science.* Tallahasee: Florida State University, Institute for Social Research, Vol. II, No. 1, 1968.

U. S. Bureau of Census. *Detailed characteristics United States summary, 1960. Final Report PC (1)-1 D.* Washington: U. S. Government Printing Office, 1963.

Chapter 37

AGE AND INSTITUTIONAL SUPPORT: PERCEPTIONS OF OLDER MEXICAN-AMERICANS

BEN M. CROUCH

SINCE WORLD WAR II that segment of American society called elderly or aging has received an increasing amount of attention from government officials, scientists, and welfare institutions. The basic objectives of this attention have involved understanding the process of aging and its consequences and ameliorating the frequently disadvantageous position of older persons through various types of programs. This paper reports findings on (1) how older Mexican-Americans view old age and (2) how they perceive three primary institutions from which informal or formal programs of aid emanate: the family, the church, and the government.

The attempt to understand the process of aging and to provide programs for the older segment of society means that officials must deal with a population that is as heterogeneous as society in general. In the face of this heterogeneity, important questions arise concerning differences in the aging process among divergent older populations. Similarly, social, cultural, ethnic, and regional differences among older groups raise questions about the means of providing programs as well as the substance

of the programs themselves.

What is needed is information on aging and ameliorative programs in terms of various subpopulations of older Americans. Older Mexican-Americans represent a significant subpopulation in that they are part of the nation's second largest minority. With few exceptions (Carp, 1968; Leonard, 1967), however, there has been little systematic research dealing directly with this older group. Currently almost all of the information available must be gleaned from census reports and from incidental treatments in community studies of Mexican-Americans.

Methodology and Sample Description

The present study was carried out in a Standard Metropolitan Statistical Area in West Texas. Data were gathered through interviews in the homes of respondents. As all those interviewed used Spanish as their first language, and most as their only language, the interviews were carried out by a trained Mexican-American coed whose ethnicity and fluency in both English and Spanish helped to circumvent problems of rapport and language.

For purposes of this study older Mexican-American was defined as anyone of this ethnic background fifty years of age or older. Because there existed no central list of such persons from which a sample could be drawn, it was necessary to seek names and addresses from various agencies and churches. Potential interviewees were also obtained by asking for names over a local Spanish-speaking radio station. These sources yielded over 300 names of which 291 were actually contacted. By extrapolating from 1960 census data, it was estimated that a sample of this size constituted about 40 percent of the total population of

Reprinted by permission from the *Journal of Gerontology*, 1972, 27, 524-529.

older Mexican-Americans in the city at the time of the survey. Clearly, the sample was not random and excluded rural residents, largely because they proved very difficult to locate. In spite of these limitations, however, no apparent systematic biases were observed in the resulting sample. For purposes of analysis, respondents were grouped into four age categories: fifty to fifty-nine, sixty to sixty-four, sixty-five to sixty-nine, seventy and over.

The characteristics of the older Mexican-Americans in the sample reflect the social position of this minority as a whole. The median number of years of formal education completed by the 129 males and 163 females in the sample was less than one year; only one respondent had finished high school. Work experiences were largely semi- or unskilled. Over one half of the females had never worked and those that had were employed predominately as private household workers. Fifty-five percent of the males had worked as laborers with another 25 percent employed as craftsmen or operatives. Only 23 percent were making $200 or more per month; almost all of these were under sixty and employed full time. The modal income category for the remainder of the sample was $50 to 70 per month. This income most frequently came from part-time work, support from children, and social security.

Results and Discussion

Perception of Old Age

As a whole, this sample of older Mexican-Americans perceives old age and the process of aging to be undesirable. Fifty-five percent indicated they felt this way while only 13 percent stated that old age was good. Many who said that it was good reflected the determinism which has traditionally been characteristic of this culture, e.g. "God willed it, so it must be good."

The respect and prestige traditionally accorded an older person in the Mexican-American culture could conceivably cause such a person to view aging in a positive light. It appears, however, that the negative effects of advancing years in terms of health and employment within an urban setting offset any benefits of these traditional cultural values.

In general the age at which the majority of this sample perceives old age to begin is at or below sixty. Nearly two thirds of the sample responded in this fashion. Forty-five percent perceived the beginning of old age to be between fifty and fifty-five. Apparently those older Mexican-Americans are not greatly influenced by the legal overtones of the age of sixty-five in American society; only 8 percent indicated this age.

This proclivity to perceive old age as starting at or below the age of sixty is probably related to socioeconomic status. Prior research has revealed that persons with a low socioeconomic background usually view old age as beginning sooner chronologically than persons of higher socioeconomic status. Leake (1962) reported that upper class executives saw themselves maturing slowly, while working-class men felt that old age began in their fifties. As previously noted, this sample occupied the lowest social position in terms of education and occupation. Because of this low social position, there is a heavy reliance upon physical labor. As a result, most of the older Mexican-Americans in this sample apparently perceived themselves as having passed their prime before the mid-century mark.

In a comparison of Anglo men and women with respect to the point old age begins, Leake (1962) observed that on the average women felt they become old at a later chronological age than men. This difference was not observed in the present sample. In fact, there was a tendency for women to report an earlier onset of old age than men. That female perceptions of old age did not differ greatly from those reported by males is probably due to the family patterns of lower-class Mexican-Americans. While the males usually spent their prime engaged in manual labor, having and rearing large families with little or no pre- and post-partum care took their toll on the females. Fifty-eight percent of all the respondents in this sample had seven or more living children while only 3 percent had no children at all. Given family demands and the fact that, unlike other racial or ethnic groups, Mexican-American females do not significantly outlive males (Ellis, 1962), it is not surprising that Mexican-American women do not see old age beginning later than their men.

Although old age is usually conceived in terms of years, perhaps more revealing are subjective perceptions of when old age begins. In answer to an open-ended question, about 45 percent indicated the beginning of old age in both chronological and subjective terms or in subjective terms alone. These subjective responses were placed in one of the following four categories for analysis: when one's health breaks down; when one needs help to live; when one feels old and useless; when one can no longer work. The last two responses were the most frequent with each accounting for about 30 percent of the subjective responses. It was interesting to note that younger respondents were somewhat more likely than older respondents to mention inability to work; at the same time, the frequency of the other three subjective responses, particularly uselessness, tended to increase with age.

Perceptions of Institutional Support

In providing support and aid to older Americans, three institutions are of paramount importance: the family, the church, and the government.

The Family: Penalosa (1967) noted that much of the current writing on the nature of the Mexican-American population generally represents an "anachronistic misconception." The values of this minority are no longer dictated by traditional folk culture. This contention by Penalosa is reflected in the findings concerning perceptions of the family held by older Mexican-Americans. Traditionally, it has been the duty of the family to care for and support the older members. Reciprocally, the older person has expected this prescribed support. The subjects in this sample, however, depart from this traditional pattern in that the majority did not manifest expectations of support from the family. Sixty-one percent indicated that the family does not have an obligation to support the older persons, whereas only 38 percent stated that the family does have such an obligation. This finding is particularly noteworthy in the light of responses to the following questions: Of the resources responsible for helping to care for older Mexican-Americans, that is, the family, the church or the government, which one has had the greatest obligation? Forty-nine percent indicated that the family has had the greatest obligation, 5 percent indicated the government, and less than 1 percent indicated the church; the balance of the sample did not give a specific response, usually stating that they did not know. Thus, approximately one half of the sample testified that in the past the family has been the primary supporting institution, while only 38 percent stated that the family still has any obligation.

Carp (1968, see also Clark, 1959), in her study of older Mexican-Americans, reports that children prefer to care and provide for elderly parents; failure to do this, in fact, constitutes deviance. Present findings suggest that while children may still desire to support their parents (children were not interviewed) most elderly parents felt that they are not so obligated. In this regard then, these older Mexican-Americans do not strongly hold to traditional extended family patterns. The explanation for this departure from traditional patterns most probably lies in the effect of urban life.

It was expected that the older persons in the sample would tend to perceive the family as having a greater obligation to older family members than would younger persons in the sample. This expectation was based on research findings reported by Francesca (1958) that even within an urban setting the older age groups would tend to hold to the traditional norms more. It was found, however, that regardless of the age category, most respondents felt that the family owed no obligation to its older members. Apparently, the departure from traditional patterns of familial expectations is not age-specific. When feelings about the family's obligation were examined in terms of the respondent's sex, the same pattern emerged. Two-thirds of both males and females felt that the family had no obligation to its older members.

The Church: Data on the perception of the church were collected via two open-ended questions: What is the church doing for older Mexican-Americans? And what should the church be doing for older Mexican-Americans? In answer to the first question regarding the current activity of the church, 81 percent felt that the church was doing little or nothing or did not know of any activity specifically on behalf of older Mexican-Americans. More important for understanding perceptions of the church, however, are the responses to the second question, which involves expectations. To

analyze differences in perceptions of what the church should be doing, a simple index of satisfaction with the church was utilized. Statements to the effect that the church should do nothing or continue to function as it has in the past were taken as evidence of satisfaction. Statements which manifested a desire for the church to do more in some or in all areas of aid to older Mexican-Americans were taken to reflect dissatisfaction.

According to Burma (1954), older Mexican-Americans tend to be more devout and involved with the church. From this it might be expected that older respondents would be more often satisfied with the church than younger respondents. This tendency did in fact exist. However, more striking was the fact that even in the oldest group, 52 percent was dissatisfied; approximately two thirds of each of the younger age groups shared this negative perception of the church.

The Government: A third source of aid in old age is the government and its programs. Familiarity with local, state, and federal programs was quite limited, although such programs were available. Respondents were asked in an open-ended question if they knew of any financial aid programs for old persons. While several programs were named, the majority of each age group mentioned only Social Security. One quarter to one third of the respondents in each age group identified both Social Security and Old Age Assistance, and a much smaller percentage of each group responded by naming three different programs.

Respondents were then asked to identify programs in a somewhat different context. Specifically, they were asked what government programs they knew of that were or could be beneficial to them. Here responses were limited to Social Security and Medicare with only 2 percent of the sample mentioning both programs. The pattern of responses had a tendency to be age-specific. While over one half of the respondents under sixty years of age named Social Security, no more than 17 percent of any older group did so. Conversely, whereas only 34 percent of those under sixty named Medicare, approximately two thirds of each older group did so. This pattern probably results first from the fact that most respondents in the upper age ranges worked at jobs not covered by social security, and second, from the fact that persons sixty-five years old (or close to it) have perhaps been more familiarized with Medicare. It is interesting to note further that as age increases so does the proportion of subjects indicating that they do not know of government programs which would be useful to them. When responses to this question were examined in terms of sex, it was found that males were slightly more likely to know of the Medicare program than females. Similarly, nearly twice as many females (28 to 15%) claimed to know of any programs of use to them. This finding suggests that females may be somewhat less cosmopolitan than males, probably because the female's world has been traditionally limited to the home.

TABLE 37-I

WHAT SHOULD THE GOVERNMENT PROVIDE

Everything	45%	(100)
Medical and physical aid	10%	(21)
Food and clothing	3%	(6)
Nothing	11%	(24)
Don't know	31%	(68)

Perhaps more important than familiarity with specific programs are old Mexican-American's expectations of an Anglo government. Asked what they felt the government should provide, a large percentage of each age group felt that the government should provide aid in all areas of need (Table 37-I). Vague responses that the government should offer "everything," "anything" or just "help" signify that this older population tends to feel that the Anglo government is powerful enough to provide support in every area. A sizable percentage in each age group also answered that they did not know what the government should do. Here is evidence that although older Mexican-Americans are aware of their problems and that they want government aid, they frequently are unable to articulate problems as a target of government programs.

Conclusions

It seems reasonable to expect that the existence of a specific cultural tradition largely maintained by the predominant use of Spanish as a first language would contribute to major differences between older Mexican-Americans and other older Americans. However, results reported here suggest that the divergence is minimal, at least in terms of perceptions of old age and selected institutions of support. The key to understanding respondents' feelings that old age begins rather early lies not in their ethnicity but in their socioeconomic status. That is, feelings about old age are colored by the point at which one reaches and passes his prime; for persons who rely on manual work as most lower-class persons have traditionally done, one's prime is passed relatively early. This sample had a decidedly negative evaluation of the status of old age.

The data on the perception of support institutions suggests that these older Mexican-Americans generally recognize a de-emphasis of the extended family, feel that the church has a social action as well as a sacred function and believe that the Anglo government could be a potent agency for support. Contrary to traditional Mexican culture, most respondents in the sample felt that the family does *not* have a support obligation to aged members. It is to the more formal institutions that these older people tend to look. The church, traditionally an important institution in the Mexican-American community, tends to be viewed as somewhat remiss in helping older residents; a majority of each age group was dissatisfied with the performance of the church in helping older Mexican-Americans. The Anglo government, while distant and impersonal, is nevertheless seen as a very important source of aid. A large percentage of each age group felt that the government should provide everything. These observations suggest that older Mexican-Americans are not strongly locked into a traditional culture. Indeed, in terms of perceptions and expectations of three support agencies, respondents appear to be quite Anglicized.

Summary

This paper reports findings of a survey of older Mexican-Americans. The objective was to obtain data on how older members of this minority perceived old age itself and how they felt about the family, the church, and the Anglo government as sources of support in old age. Old age was viewed negatively and usually as beginning at or below sixty years. It was reported that re-spondents had less of an expectation of aid from the family than the church or the government. It was concluded that older Mexican-Americans appear not to be substantially different from other older Americans; rather, they appear to be quite Anglicized in their perceptions of old age and institutional support.

REFERENCES

Burma, J. *Spanish speaking groups in the United States.* Durham: Duke University Press, 1954.

Carp, F. *Factors in utilization of services by Mexican American elderly.* Palo Alto, Calif: American Institute for Research, 1968.

Clark, M. *Health in the Mexican-American culture.* Berkeley: University of California Press, 1959.

Ellis, J. M. Spanish-surname mortality differentials in San Antonio, Texas, *Journal of Health & Human Behavior,* 1962, *3,* 119-120.

Francesca, Sister (OLVM). Variations of selected cultural patterns among three generations of Mexicans in San Antonio, Texas. *American Catholic Sociological Review,* 1958, *19,* 25-34.

Leake, C. D. Social status and aging. *Geriatrics,* 1962, *17,* 785.

Leonard, O. E. The older rural Spanish-speaking people of the Southwest, In E. G. Youmans (Ed.), *Older rural Americans.* Lexington: University of Kentucky Press, 1967.

Penalosa, F. The changing Mexican American in Southern California. *Sociology & Social Research,* 1967, *51,* 404-417.

Chapter 38

PATTERNS OF AGING AMONG THE ELDERLY POOR OF THE INNER CITY

MARGARET CLARK

A S WE KNOW, cities in America are housing more and more ethnic minority
populations, and more and more aged people as well. These trends are clearly the result of a deterioration of the quality of life
in downtown areas. The aged poor, like
the ethnic poor, have been unable to "join
the flight of younger and affluent families
to suburbia to avoid the noise, smog, dirt,
social tension and poor housing of the central city" (Birren, 1970). Both groups are
held in part by the inexpensive housing;
when the slum neighborhoods in which
they live are razed, they move on to other
tenements, other skid row hotels, other
furnished rooms.

This paper will discuss this group of
aged people, the poor of the inner city,
both in terms of what we already know
about them and in terms of the kinds of
additional information that would be useful, either in planning for their needs or
in understanding more about aging and
adaptation to its circumstances.

The aged poor of the inner city have
seldom been studied as a discrete group.
Most large sample studies of the elderly
have concentrated on institutional popula-

Reprinted by permission from the *Gerontologist*,
1971, *11*, 58-66.

tions where numbers of older people are
readily available. The author uses the term
"institution" here in its broader sense to
include senior centers, "adult communities" or retirement villages, and "golden
age clubs," as well as hospitals and old age
homes. Nor have there been small-sample
studies done, of the kind usually conducted
by urban anthropologists, because the elderly poor in cities are usually white and
Euroamerican in ethnicity, they have
missed such scholarly attention which has
rather been focused on minorities and
other exotic groups. Numerous survey
studies, however, have spotted the inner-
city aged and identified them as a unique
group in our aging population (Clark and
Anderson 1967; Lowenthal and Berkman,
1967; New York State Department of Mental Hygiene, Mental Research Unit, 1961;
Srole, Langner, Michael, Opler, and Rennie, 1962; and others). Suddenly, we have
become aware that "geriatric ghettos" have
sprung up within the last two decades in
the downtown areas of our principal cities.

This phenomenon is relatively new in
America. Many factors (historical, economic, and political) can account for this
age-specific concentration of people. It is
consistent with the general social pattern
of the polarization of many low-status
groups in our society and their segregation
from the mainstream of American life.

Many members of this group are largely
"invisible" (Harrington, 1963) and are
missed in the standard polls and surveys.
We seldom see them on the main arterials
of the city; rather, we find them huddled in
the city's interstices, in the small side streets
and less frequented byways. Their apartments and rooms are in the basements or in
the rear of buildings, or in walk-up hotels.
They can be found shopping in small
neighborhood stores rather than in the

large emporiums or supermarkets. They are also invisible because our current culture, with its primary concerns of productivity and profits, has trained us to dismiss such people from our range of perception. Even in studies specifically designed to locate these people and identify their problems, the very techniques of research themselves may be chosen to preserve an emotional distance from the subjects.

We need to know more about this group, other than what can be culled here and there from demographic or survey data. We need to know about their patterns of survival in the inner city. How has their poverty affected the process of aging among them? Is this process substantially different from other, more fortunate groups of aged people? We have some indication that the downwardly-mobile, who have slipped into poverty during their later years, fare worse psychologically than those who have endured this condition all their lives (Brill, Weinstein, and Garratt, 1969). However, in contrast, we can also pinpoint a hardy breed of older people who, although not indigenous to the downtown areas, have learned its rules of survival very well.

Above all, we need to know the *experience* of growing old in a geriatric ghetto in terms of the perceptions of those who must live it. We shall never fully understand the experience until we can see it through their eyes and comprehend it on their terms. Accordingly, there is a great need for more phenomenological studies of this group, research that allows subjects to think and act and speak for themselves.

The City as a Process

To understand the urban aged and their experiences, attention must be given to the city as a social institution that has evolved from the earliest times of human history (Mumford, 1961; Strauss, 1968). Certain districts have always been set aside in cities for special categories of people (traders, foreigners, the military, seats of government, etc.), but rarely have we seen concentrations of old people into certain districts as evidenced today.

Why do we find large concentrations of old people living here? Are they people who have always lived in these districts but who were left behind in the Great Rush to the suburbs after the Second World War? Have they been drawn here out of economic necessity or personal choice? Many of us might believe that the last place we would want to grow old in is in the heart of a large American city in these times. Inflated prices make a mockery of the fixed pension; the law of the inner city can be heartless and unconcerned with the welfare of the feeble and helpless; and in an atmosphere that almost crackles with violence, potential or actual, what chances does an older person have to escape robbery or bodily harm? (He is often, is fact, the ideal victim.) Under these circumstances, we ought to be witnessing a concerted effort on the part of the inner-city aged to escape from this trap, but we do not. As it is true of ghetto life everywhere, there is possibly some comfort for the aged urban poor in "being with one's own" and sharing with others a mistrust and fear of others outside the enclave. For most, however, there is nowhere else to go, so they must make the best of it, rationalizing away the real disadvantages and real injustice of their misery. Despite these painful realities (and the need to deny them), we can discern, through reports from the people themselves, that inner-city living is in some ways functional to their survival.

For about five years (1959-1964), an interdisciplinary research group at Langley Porter Neuropsychiatric Institute in San

Francisco studied a large group of aged subjects in various conditions of mental and physical health. Many of these people were from substantial neighborhoods in outlying areas of the city, but an appreciable number comprised a group that could qualify as inner-city, poor aged. From findings on this group the author has selected a number of problem areas around which to organize the following discussion. Of particular value are a series of intensive interviews with selected subjects. From their own testimony, we can see how inner-city life is functional and dysfunctional in the following major areas of concern:

NUTRITION: The procurement of food, whether nutritious or not, is very important to these informants. References to cafeterias and restaurants are frequent. The corner groceryman takes on an imposing stature in their eyes, for he is both food-supplier and banker, extending credit and cashing the monthly OAS or Social Security checks. An enforced move from one room to another in a different district can be perceived as a catastrophe if the cafeteria that offers cut-rate breakfasts is now six rather than two blocks away from home base. The frequency of these references can be misleading, however. Most of the meals are prepared in one's own quarters, often over an electric hot-plate or gas-ring. Some men even make arrangements with older women in their building to come in and fix meals at a certain rate (four meals a week for a dollar, for example). But even as rare as restaurant visits might be, the references still recur.

In a recent monograph on nutrition and aging (Howell and Loeb, 1969), it was noted:

> A variable that has been considered to be positively related to dietary intake and nutrition in the elderly is social interaction. Although little systematic data have been collected, the evidence does seem to support the general hypothesis.

Within this group, a high level of malnutrition has been related to social isolation, while one study, at least, suggests that eating with others tends to upgrade the nutritional quality of the diet (Schwartz, Henley, and Zeitz, 1964). The many references to public eating places might, therefore, be more related to the need for social interaction (or mental stimulus) than to the needs of nutrition *per se*. Further study is needed to explore this relationship between eating and sociability. Even the most cursory reflection will suggest that the relationship is not a simple one. Eating alone in a public place can be experienced as a lonelier event than eating at home alone. Idly viewing city life from the windows of a cheap cafeteria might serve only to emphasize how little a role in society one has left. Doubtless, eating out is a complex experience for the aged poor of the inner city, but what little information we have would suggest a positive adaptive relationship between eating and some conviviality.

Educational programs for better nutrition among the urban poor have not been successful for several reasons. Once again, the targets for such programs are hard to reach, and even where some contact is made, it is unlikely that the programs have substantively changed eating habits. These are particularly resistant among those who have immigrated into the inner city during their maturity from rural or foreign cultures. The former pattern of a substandard diet is not easily replaced, let alone *augmented* with more nutritional foods. As a group, the elderly are the least likely to respond to such suggested changes, even where such changes could easily fit into their meager budgets.

SHELTER: Very few of the central city elderly own their own homes. The older citizen is a renter: 70 percent of households in New York City with heads sixty-five and older rent (Canton, Rosenthal, and Mayer, *n.d.*), while four fifths of the San Francisco sample discussed here (Clark and Anderson, 1967) were renters. In New York, nearly one fifth of all rental units are occupied by the elderly. Since the average income of the vast majority of these city elderly is woefully low, we need hardly guess at the substandard housing facilities they are forced to live in. Researchers who visit the inner-city poor in their dwellings encounter the most indescribable squalor of flea-bag hotels, rodent-infested flop-houses, and filthy tenements (Bogue, 1963). The aged themselves would be the first to agree with these impressions. In fact, these deplorable housing conditions rank first in their complaints about their lot (despite their equally pressing needs in nutrition), and the search for better living quarters is ceaseless. Subjects talk at length about elaborate searches and "deals," listening for the dropped cues that might lead to a favorable move, hunting perpetually for slightly better living arrangements. Sometimes, blessedly, they come, but not without some further cost in loss of social contacts or old proximity to needed services.

The aged themselves value the chance to live with some measure of privacy and autonomy, no matter how dreadful the cost. Inner-city living requires only the most superficial facade of social regularity to act as passport through a few simple, daily routines and, consequently, having "a place of one's own," even in the most turgid of social conditions, can be a positive boost to one's morale. Also, subjects express the feeling that, although they do not care to interact with their neighbors except in the most superficial ways, they consider it a comfort to have someone, anybody, near at hand in case of emergencies. There is no doubt that "a place of one's own" is highly functional for the aged and one could wish that every elderly person, not needing institutional care, could enjoy pleasant, adequate housing. In some perverse ways, the highly inadequate housing facilities of the inner city do manage, ultimately to supply some minimal aid to these people in terms of privacy, individual space, and availability of help. Some cities, like Detroit, have experimented with refurbished downtown hotels for the elderly, recognizing the desires of many to live close to the company of others like themselves. As yet, no assessments of these experiments have been published, but the concept is provocative. In fact, the whole commune movement among the young (especially those communes set up in urban settings) might afford some workable models for elderly groups in the city, suffering from their own varieties of rootlessness and anomie.

MEDICAL SERVICES: There is an illusion in the inner city; there is a belief that medical help is closer than it really is. In fact, the availability of medical help within the inner city may be more distant than in suburban or rural areas (Norman, 1969). A high degree of mobility is necessary to gain transportation to county clinics and many of the poorest elderly, who are often the sickest of all groups of aged, lack both the mobility and the cost of transportation to get to a source of medical help.

The advent of Medicare in 1965 has since helped to alleviate the desperate medical problems of the aged of the inner city to some degree. Unfortunately, the monthly charge (which is matched by the federal government, is still too high for some to pay. Many of this group, especially the male urban nomads, are unaware of these benefits and would even be disinclined to enroll. Their life-style of surly independence from all establishment doings keeps them on the police-prisoner cycle (Spradley, 1970), rather than on the doctor-patient cycle. The code of the inner city is imbued with a profound mistrust of aid programs, especially when emanating from the federal government. Consequently, a hard kernel of our elderly population, we suspect, is still not reached with these grants-in-aid.

Furthermore, we seem to be approaching a new crisis in Medicare. A recent inquiry by a Senate Special Committee on Aging has disclosed that, because of inflation and increased charges, Medicare is now covering only one-half the medical costs of the aged in the United States (*San Francisco Chronicle*, Jan. 11, 1971). The remainder must be paid by the elderly themselves. Clearly, the current Medicare program, while it has so far been a godsend to many of the elderly poor, is not the final answer.

Various "out-reach" programs attempt to keep in contact with the "hidden" aged with medical needs. Some senior centers or old-age clubs employ volunteers to visit the house-bound regularly and provide for professionals a kind of referral service. The Visiting Nurses' Association and public health nurses are also deeply involved in inner-city health care, and, interestingly, some hospitals have become involved in home-care programs that utilize "flying squads" of physicians and nurses. In San Francisco, for example, a geriatric screening unit at the county hospital now provides on-call services for emergencies, treating patients in a home setting wherever possible (Rypins and Clark, 1968).

All in all, it is clear that living in the inner city is a disadvantage to the older person when it comes to procuring much-needed medical services. Very often county medical personnel do not even get to see the ailing aged poor until an acute crisis

arrives. By this time, proper medical treatment is often too late. New ways of bringing medical care to elderly patients before the crisis-point is reached need to be explored.

MOBILITY: It is surprising that this very important factor in the life-support of the aged has been overlooked in gerontological studies until quite recent years. In fact, its importance is evident in every dimension of aging we study. It is strongly related to morale and self-esteem, and for the hospitalized elderly, the ability to move about on one's own volition becomes one of their primary expressed needs (Clark and Anderson, 1967). Its importance for the inner-city aged is clear, once an elderly "loner" loses the ability to move about on his own, he becomes dependent on friends and neighbors to supply him his necessities. If he lacks these, then his loss of mobility might well be the precipitating factor that puts him into the hospital (Lowenthal, 1964). Retaining one's mobility allows for freedom and autonomy; it permits one to remain open to new possibilities and other alternatives in the environment; it allows the older person to reach for the opportunities available in his society. Immobility, on the other hand, is life in an ever-shrinking world, forcing a slow attrition in many other areas of an individual's personal and social system and resulting in an impoverishment of all segments of life.

Urban life has always presented obstacles to the mobility of the elderly. But within the last five years, as civil disorders and street crimes have increased, a sinister, new threat to the mobility of the aged has risen within the city, fears of muggings and assaults which make the elderly prisoners in their own quarters. Most tragically, this situation seems to be beyond remedy, short of a major roll-back of the social deterioration that has been plaguing all American cities within the past decade.

SOCIAL INTERACTION: Cities have always attracted people who either seek a variety of social contacts or prefer to live aloof from others. This wide spectrum of social opportunities has always been a major appeal of city living. One can seek and find deeply personal friendships or a collection of nodding acquaintances. One can build a large network of close friends or one can move about, nameless, never coming too close to others. The point is, in the city, one is *free to make an individual choice.*

The urban elderly share in these advantages of city life. In this environment, they can control the degree of social interaction they desire.

From what we know, the social interaction of the aged poor is simple, seldom intimate, and narrowly circumscribed. One female subject from the San Francisco sample reported that she wanted friends but had trouble making them. Further, it became evident that her real problem was keeping them. "I met this woman in a cafeteria," she said, "She seemed like such a nice person at first, but then I found out that she drank. I can't stand people who do that." Does this coolness and reserve have any functional value for the aged of the inner city? How much of it is the result of sensory loss which, in their poverty, they cannot buy aids for?

It would be especially helpful to know something about the social networks (Bott, 1957; Epstein, 1961) of these people. From the information available, we know they lack personal contact with a variety of other social systems that could be of beneficial help to them. They are, consequently, quite limited in procuring for themselves vital services and must rely on the formal and impersonal systems provided by society for the unfortunate and under-privileged.

With loss of employment and decre-

ments in mobility, the aged individual's social world inevitably shrinks. Yet, we know that social interaction and mental stimulus is of great importance in the mental health of the elderly (Goldfarb, 1958, 1964). We also know that sexuality and sexual needs in individuals in their sixties and seventies are far from extinguished (Rubin, 1965). But research on social and particularly sexual needs is very spotty.

SYMBOLIC VALUES: Cities are the repositories of the most potent symbols of our culture, monuments, cathedrals, skyscrapers, government buildings, technological marvels, fantastic merchandise, memorable landmarks. To live in Boston, New York, Washington, or San Francisco is to live within a symbol of the "best" that our culture has produced. All who live in the city, rich and poor alike, can share in these symbolic values and draw some personal pride from an association with them. Here, in the symbolic realm, the egalitarian dreams of our democracy can become actualized for all.

At one time in our cultural history, an identity as a New Yorker represented the height of sophistication and modernity. No matter how poor one was, status as a New Yorker placed one high above the "hicks" and the "rubes." New York seemed to be the hub of America and the whole universe. Is it possible that any of this old pride in city yet remains or that it has any functional value at all for the elderly, regardless of how poor they are? Have the ethnic and political loyalties so polarized the nation that one's identity as the citizen of a famous, particular city is no distinction anymore? Has the new cynicism so corroded all the old value systems that even the aged, who hold on to them with the greatest tenacity, can only let them fall from their hands in disgust?

Conclusion

The position taken in this paper is that the urban environment, like any other milieu in which aged individuals find themselves, has great potential for promoting both human misery and human survival. One of the more promising approaches to social planning for the inner-city aged is to examine the ways in which the aged poor, when faced with basic problems of physical and psychological survival, develop informal structures for their solution. If planned programs can be constructed to emulate or develop these spontaneous arrangements among people, they are more likely to be acceptable and effective.

REFERENCES

Birren, J. E. The abuse of the urban aged. *Psychology Today*, 1970, *3*, No. 10, *36-38;* 72.

Bogue, D. J. *Skid-row in American cities.* Community and Family Study Center, University of Chicago, 1963.

Bott, E. *Family and social network.* London: Tavistock, 1957.

Brill, N. Q., Weinstein, R., and Garratt, J. Poverty and mental illness: Patients' perception of poverty as an etiological factor in their illness. *American Journal of Psychiatry*, 1969, *125*, 1172-1179.

Canton, M., Rosenthal, K., and Mayer, M. *The elderly in the rental market of New York City.* U.S. Dept. of Health, Education, & Welfare, Administration on Aging, Monogr. 26, n.d.

Clark, M., and Anderson, B. G. *Culture and aging: An anthropological study of older Americans.* Springfield, Ill.: Charles C Thomas, 1967.

Epstein, L. J. The network and urban social organization. *Rhodes-Livingstone Institute Journal*, 1961, *29*, 29-62.

Goldfarb, A. Management of aged patients who are mentally ill. *Roche Report*, 1964, *1*, No. 7.

Goldfarb, A. Patterns in planning a psychiatric program for the aged. *Bulletin of the New York Academy of Medicine*, 1958, *34* (2nd ser.), 811-822.

Harrington, M. *The other America.* New York: Macmillan, 1963.

Howell, S. C., and Loeb, M. B. (Eds.) Nutrition and aging: A monograph for practitioners. *Gerontologist*, 1969, *9*, No. 3, Pt. II.

Koller, M. R. *Social gerontology.* New York: Random House, 1968.

Lowenthal, M. F., and Berkman, P. L. *Aging and mental disorder in San Francisco: A social psychiatric study.* San Francisco: Jossey-Bass, 1967.

Lowenthal, M. F. *Lives in distress: The paths of the elderly to the psychiatric ward.* New York: Basic Books, 1964.

Mumford, L. *The city in history: Its origins, its transformations, and its prospects.* New York: Harcourt Brace, 1961.

New York State Dept. of Mental Hygiene, Mental Health Research Unit. *A mental health survey of older people.* Utica, N.Y.: State Hospitals Press, 1960, 1961.

Norman, J. C. (Ed.) *Medicine in the ghetto.* New York: Appleton-Century-Crofts, 1969.

Rubin, I. *Sexual life after sixty.* New York: Basic Books, 1965.

Rypins, R. F., and Clark, M. L. A screening project for the geriatric mentally ill. *California Medicine*, 1968, *109*, 273-278.

Schwartz, D., Henley, B., and Zeitz, L. *The elderly ambulatory patient: Nursing and psychosocial needs.* New York: Macmillan, 1964.

Spradley, J. P. *You owe yourself a drunk: The ethnography of urban nomads.* Boston: Little, Brown & Co., 1970.

Srole, L., Langner, T., Michael, S., Opler, M., and Rennie, T. *Mental health in the metropolis: The midtown Manhattan Study*, Vol. I. New York: McGraw-Hill, 1962.

Strauss, A. (Ed.) *The American city: a sourcebook of urban imagery.* Chicago: Aldine, 1968.

Chapter 39

WIDOWS AS A MINORITY GROUP

HELENA Z. LOPATA

CUMMING AND HENRY (1961) stated in *Growing Old* that widowhood was less difficult for women than retirement for men, mainly because with widowhood their status in society increased while with retirement the male's decreased. They went even further by claiming that women sometimes look forward to becoming widows, since this event permits them to join "the society of widows." The implication is that husbandless women lead a very pleasurable life, not in interaction with men as Strauss' "Merry Widow," but in sharing prestigeful leisure-time activities with each other.

Other research focused on the life styles of widows indicates that the Kansas City women described by Cumming and Henry may be the exception rather than the rule (Adams, 1969; Berardo, 1967, 1968; Lopata, 1971c; Pihlblad and Rosencranz, 1968). In fact, almost all evidence indicates that most women in modern urbanized, industrialized, complex societies experience a drop in status with the death of their husbands; and they face discrimination, poverty, and related problems precluding a life of recreation (Winch and Blumberg, 1968). The situation of many of them, although by no means of all, resembles that of a minority group as conceptualized by Wirth (1945).

Reprinted by permission from the *Gerontologist*, 1971, *11*, 67-77.

American widows often report that they are being discriminated against simply because they are widows. Of a modified area probability sample of metropolitan Chicago widows 39 percent agree that, "People take advantage of you when they find out you are a widow," and 57 percent that, "widows often feel like a fifth wheel" (Lopata, 1971c). National statistics, particularly those pertaining to urban areas, indicate that widows do not participate fully in the life of the society. Better Business Bureaus report the frequent victimization of widows in the form of unnecessary repairs and inflated prices. Some ballroom dance studios capitalize on their loneliness and sign them up for as much as $10,000 worth of lessons (Lopata and Noel, 1967). Although not required to wear special clothing which would make their marital status physically distinctive, as their counterparts have had to do for centuries in some countries like India (Felton, 1966; Sarasvati, 1888; Thomas, 1964) and Yugoslavia (Smolic-Krkovic, 1970), American widows are visibly different in any situation which requires the presence of a male escort. Their abnormal marital status can be easily discovered by anyone wishing to take advantage of it, and it is known to former friends and associates.

If minority status is based on differences from the dominant group, widows fit into the mold. One of the reasons is that, particularly in American middle- and upper-class society, they are handicapped by not having a mate, in the same way as the never married and the divorced women (Lopata, 1971c). Much of leisure-time activity cannot be entered into by widows, because they lack a male escort or because they disrupt the symmetry of couple companionate socializing. Many of the Chicago area respondents report a reluctance to enter public places alone or with other women and say they are not being invited to the homes of former friends whose husbands are still living. The hardest hit are those who experience widowhood earlier than their associates. Besides feeling like a "fifth wheel," they assume that, "other women are jealous of a widow when their husbands are around" (37% of the Chicago sample), while, "widows are constantly sexually propositioned, even by the husbands of their friends" (19%). This strain in interaction with former friends often results in the widow's withdrawal from the relation, which is not easily replaced, if she wants to associate with married women and their husbands. Respondents often report that they are demeaned by having to limit their socializing to other widows.

A second reason widows feel that they are "second-class citizens" is that friends avoid them in an attempt to ignore the whole subject of death and grief. Gorer (1965) called the American and English way of handling bereavement, "the pornography of death." Lindemann (1944) and several members of the Harvard Medical School team of psychiatrists and sociologists (Maddison, 1968; Parkes, 1965) studying grief report that a major problem of the widowed is that they are not permitted to express their feelings while in the company of others and that their friends even restrict interaction for fear that they might be subjected to tears, talk of the deceased, and confessions of loneliness. Such experiences are so threatening to the living as to interfere with the "grief work" which Lindemann believes to be a necessary process by which the widowed rebuild life without the deceased. Strong emotional problems can result from the blockage of that working-out process, yet Americans do not cooperate with the widowed, rationalizing their avoidance of such situations by saying, "It

is better for them to work it out alone."

A third reason widows could be classified as a minority group is their sex. As Helen Hacker pointed out in 1951 and the various women's liberation leaders proclaimed recently, American, and nearly every, society is male-dominated. Socialization, education, and most social relations have been traditionally designed with the female dependent upon the male, passive in response to his dominance, emotional in contrast to his problem-solving stance, and so forth. The characteristics idealized as feminine by both men and women, especially by psychiatrists following *The Freudian Ethic* (La Pierre, 1959), make it difficult for a widow to exist if she lives alone in a social system which is voluntaristic, demanding initiative and decision making.

In traditional societies, the woman was able to move from the home of her father to that of her husband and after his death to have her eldest son take over the management of the property and her maintenance (Sarasvati, 1888). The situation is now changed, because neither the woman nor her adult children wish to follow those residential customs. Urbanization, industrialization, and increased societal complexity have resulted in personality individualization and neolocal residence. Adult sons move out of the parental household, at least at the time they marry, and they do not want to return when the mother is widowed. Her movement into the home of a married child is very difficult for her, requiring a status drop from mistress of her own place to that of a peripheral and inferior person in another household. Recent research of the aged in many countries (Pihlblad and Rosencranz, 1968; Rosenmayr and Köckeis, 1963; Shanas, Townsend, Wedderburn, Friis, Milhoj, and Stehouwer, 1968) finds most widows refusing to move in with the families of their

children, preferring financial restrictions
and even loneliness to such a situation.
There are several reasons for this stance.
The household of a married child is managed by its housewife, who has her own
system of maintaining it. Adult "assistants"
who have different habits are resented and
even prevented from acting. Thus, the
widow can be made functionless. She is also
frustrated in not being able to do what she
wants to do when she wants to. The children's styles of living are often foreign to
her, due to cultural change and intergenerational social mobility. Their homes are
likely to be located in new suburbs, so that
she lacks peer group relations and the
facilities of her old neighborhood. Finally,
the widow is afraid of living in a three-
generational family over which she has no
control. She expects to disapprove of the
actions of younger people, to be miserable
if she represses her criticism, or in conflict
with others if she expresses it.

Thus, modern older widows do not
want to live with married children but
rather remain alone after the last offspring
leaves. The change in the status of women
is reflected in the fact that they are allowed
by society and by their families to be independent, living alone, and managing their
own property. Of course, this independence
from the kinship group is partly due to the
fact that they have other sources of economic support through their own efforts,
from the society, or thanks to inheritance
laws that permit them to be the main bene-
ficiary. On the other hand, many are not
trained to live independently and to utilize
their resources and they make unwise decisions or become frustrated by not knowing what to do.

A fourth reason widows are prevented
from full participation in the life of the
society is that most of them are older and
thus suffer from the prejudice and discrimination facing older people in youth-
oriented countries, such as America. The
average age at widowhood is fifty-six, when
many new roles are not available. Employment is particularly hard to find in any but
domestic service, as even the retail stores
prefer younger employees. This is particularly true of women who were full-time
housewives prior to the death of their
husbands, because the skills they had obtained prior to marriage are rusty. Other
lines of reengagement in society are also
difficult for older people who are often related to groups which cater to them but
lack significant functionality in a function-
oriented society.

The fifth point is that older widows are
often members of other minority groups,
particularly of ethnic or racial groups. Approximately 1,600,000 of the female elderly
in America are foreign-born, and an additional 1,700,000 are of foreign stock, meaning that one or both of their parents were
foreign-born. Such women face the prejudice and discrimination alloted to all members of their groups. In addition to differential treatment by member of the dominant group and to maladjustment to its
culture, such widows are also likely to have
difficulties in relating even to their own
group. Coming, as most urban migrants
did, from a rural, agricultural background
to urban, industrial centers, they tended to
settle in ethnic communities, isolated from
the American society and culture (Lopata,
1965; Thomas and Znaniecki, 1958). They
were less exposed to opportunities for ac-
culturation than the other members of
their families; the men went out to work,
the children went to school. Their very
foreignness is helping to isolate them from
even their own ethnic community, which
has been acculturating and moving to areas
of secondary settlement.

Widows interviewed in the northwest

section of Chicago are frightened by their community; their property is often destroyed by hostile neighbors and themselves the butt of jokes and pranks by the children. Reared in cultures and times when prejudice against strangers of a different identity was high, they openly hate the Puerto Ricans and blacks who replace the former "urban villagers" with whom they identified (Gans, 1962). These widows are probably the greatest sufferers from minority status; they feel completely deserted by their own ethnics and kin and by an invisible government "out there," which has done nothing to prevent all these changes from happening. The Negro widow, who is likely to have reached this marital status early in life (Lopata, 1970b) must face in addition all the problems of her social race identity.

A further characteristic of widows which helps place them in minority status is their poverty. Although the governments of many nations have started helping their elderly through social security, old age assistance, or some form of insurance, these funds are generally inadequate, particularly if the economy has experienced inflation. Social Security allowances lag far behind the inflated cost of living, so that most of the money received by the elderly goes for food (36.4%) and housing (41.1%), leaving only 22.5% for "incidentals," health services, clothing, transportation, repairs, recreation, etc. (US Department of Labor, 1966). In fact, widows represent a disproportionately large segment of the American poor; one half of the older people living alone, who are mostly women, have less than $1,348 a year (Brotman, 1966). Eighty-eight percent of the Missouri small-town widows and 60 percent of the Chicago respondents live on less than $3,000 a year. Of course, some have hidden assets, such as gifts from children or a paid-up mort-

gage, but many do not, and the total seldom allows for independent movement in a large social life space. Visiting distant relatives or friends and participation in voluntary associations are curtailed because of a lack of money. This is the reason most frequently given for decreasing involvement, followed closely by health. The poor have both problems, because of the harshness of their lives from birth on, the inadequacy of medical care, and their ignorance of preventive measures.

Fear of poverty is also a restriction on life, particularly if the widow is afraid that people will take advantage of her at any opportunity they have. The anxiety over becoming victimized by a close associate can lead to a withdrawal from the relation, preclude overtures of friendship to strangers, and lead to rejection of attempts of others to break down the isolation barriers. Pihlblad and Rosencranz (1968) report that one of their respondents, practically inaccessible behind a high fence guarded by a vicious dog, complained bitterly of being lonely.

Poverty is particularly difficult for widows who had been accustomed to a higher standard of living. Former associates continue on the round of activity enjoyed by the widow in the past but now inaccessible; and the people who could become friends are judged as inferior. Besides closing doors to many if not most aspects of the former life, downward mobility in a society idealizing upward mobility is psychologically difficult. This is a poignant experience for those widows who already feel sorry for themselves because of the death of the husband. Homes are sold, and most of the 50 percent of Chicago area widows who moved after their husband's death entered smaller quarters, many in undesirable neighborhoods. Most older widows do not maintain an automobile, even if they know how to drive, because of the cost of maintaining one. Seventy-five percent of Chicago respondents and 84 percent of the Missouri small town widows do not drive.

Related closely to the factor of poverty is that of ignorance. Modern urbanized and industrialized societies are increasingly voluntaristic in terms of member participation. Entrance into new social roles requires knowledge and well developed skills, and few groups guarantee membership for life. People trained in abstract and ideational thought about the functioning of society and its different components are able to analyze their needs and search for solutions among the resources of an abundant social system. Most older widows were socialized into a restricted world and simply do not understand the society in which they live. For example, some of the Puerto Rican grandmothers in Chicago who were interviewed by Ludwig (1970) had never been in the center of the city or on public transportation. They function in a constricted world consisting of the few blocks surrounding their residence, and even the information presented by mass communication media is viewed as a hodge-podge of items not relevant to them. They often do not take advantage of the financial assistance available through welfare agencies, because they do not know of their existence or are afraid of contact with any governmental agency. The older widows received little formal education. The average year of completed schooling of the Missouri widows was eight years and for the Chicago widows just over eight grades. By modern standards, this level is inadequate to meet the demands of life in urban centers. In addition, many women are functional illiterates, never having absorbed even the little knowledge presented in the poor schools of the past in rural and foreign communities. The content of their knowledge is often irrelevant to modern life, static, and still lodged in the different culture before migration and the cultural change.

The combination of these seven characteristics has made many older widows unsuited for full participation in modern society. They are "urban villagers" without a village; passive females lacking a dominant male; the grieving and the lonely in a society rejecting such emotions; the old in a youth-centered culture; the functionless in a function-oriented nation; the ignorant in a secular, scientifically focused and increasingly educated world; the rural, Negro, or ethnically uprooted in a white-Anglo-Saxon-Protestant urban complex; the single when the ideal is couple companionate; and the poor at a time when such a condition is assumed to be the person's own fault.

Sources of Knowledge about Widows

The author knows of only four sociological studies devoted specifically to the topic of widowhood. The best known of these is Marris' (1958) *Widows and Their Families,* which was limited to women whose husbands died within the $2\frac{1}{2}$ years prior to the interview, at the age of fifty or less. Hutchinson (1954) studied the widowed in Australia, and Berardo (1967, 1968) in both urban and rural areas of the state of Washington. Metropolitan Chicago widows have been studied by Lopata (1971c).

In other than the above mentioned sources, data on life styles of widows is very hard to find. Of special help are ethnographic sources in which anthropologists describe in detail the life of a village or a tribe. Schapera's (1941) *Married Life in an African Tribe* and Freedman's (1965) *Lineage Organization in Southeastern China* are examples of such works.

The Yale Human Relations Area File (HRAF) contains several subjects according to which data are organized which are relevant to widowhood, although this subject is seldom mentioned. A search under the topics of marriage, remarriage, inheritance, funeral rites, residence, etc. brings forth bits of information.

Sociological studies devoted to subjects other than widowhood often contain relevant information. There are three major types of such studies: family, social gerontology, and urban sociology. Of special help have been the crosscultural works, such as Shanas and associates' (1968) *Old People in Three Industrial Countries* and Ward's (1963) *Women of New Asia.* Tunstall's (1966) *Old and Alone* and Townsend's (1957) *The Family Life of Old People* contain much useful information. So does Shanas' (1962) *The Health of Older People.* Secondary analyses made of data collected for other reasons can help in the understanding of life styles of widows. Adams (1969) has just been doing such analyses on the Pihlbiad and Rosencranz study (1968) of *Old People in a Small Town.* Their sample of older people in small towns of Missouri included 707 widows.

The recent attempts of sociologists to generalize about the relation of societal structure to family functions and structures are valuable to a researcher seeking data on widows. Of special significance is Goode's (1963) *World Revolution and Family Patterns* and Winch and Blumberg's (1968) "Societal complexity and family organization."

What We Know About Widows
The Factors Influencing Widowhood

Three sets of factors influence the life style of a particular widow: the social structure and culture of the society and of the community in which she is located; the family institution, especially the norms surrounding the roles of wife, mother, and kin member; and her personal characteristics.

Features of the society and of her community which are relevant include the complexity of the social role system and the availability of different roles to widows; social class and other categorical divisions and differences in life style; the degree to which they are urbanized; the degree of industrialization; the focal institution around which the value hierarchy is organized; religion (especially beliefs concerning after-life); economic institutions (source of livelihood, money economy vs. exchange of services, etc.); recreational facilities (couple companionate vs. sex-segregated; commercial vs. primary); and the educational institutions (formal vs. kin based; restricted to youth vs. continuous).

The characteristics of the family institution which influence the life styles of widows include the legal and social status of women; the form of marriage (monogamy, polygyny); the status of widows; inheritance laws; degree of control by either lateral group; presence or absence of levirate or widow inheritance and the strength of filiation rights; residential customs and facilities; mother-adult child relations; remarriage chances and norms; relations of widows to males; and the form of kin relations (i.e. work group vs. modified services undertaken outside of separate homes).

The personal characteristics of a woman which affect her widowhood include: present age and age at the time of the death of the husband; age, sex, number, and location of children; sources and amount of income and assets; health; capacity to function in society (knowledge and skills); past relations with husband; marital status of friends; degree of involvement in a kin group; employment; friendship patterns; and level of social engagement prior to widowhood.

Research Needs

The dearth of research dealing directly, rather than peripherally, with widowhood has resulted in a real lack of data and generalizations. What are now most needed are longitudinal and cross-cultural studies. Since widowhood does not occur at the same time to everyone, it would be very expensive to follow a group of women who are still married to study changes after death of the husband. In this respect, widowhood differs from retirement which generally comes at the same age, more or less. Probably the most practical way of meeting research needs would be for the study of widowhood to form part of a larger project covering both men and women. For example, a longitudinal project devoted to life changes in aging could devote a major section of the schedule to the anticipation and to the experiences of widowhood.

REFERENCES

Adams, D. Adaptation to widowhood. Columbia, Mo.: University of Missouri, Dept. of Sociology, 1969. (mimeo.)

Berardo, F. Social adaptation to widowhood among a rural-urban aged population. *Washington State College Agricultural Experiment Station Bulletin,* No. 689, 1967.

Berardo, F. Widowhood status in the United States: Perspectives on a neglected aspect of the family life cycle. *Family Coordinator,* 1968, *17,* 191-203.

Brotman, H. B. *Year-end statistical round-up.* Washington: Administration on Aging. Useful facts 16, 1960.

Cumming, E., and Henry, W. *Growing old.* New York: Basic Books, 1961.

Felton, M. *A child widow's story.* New York: Harcourt, Brace, & World, 1966.

Freedman, M. *Lineage organization in South-*
eastern China: New York: Humanities Press, 1965.

Gans, H. *The urban villagers.* New York: Free Press of Macmillan, 1962.

Goode, W. *World revolution and family patterns* New York: Free Press of Macmillan, 1963.

Gorer, G. *Death, grief and mourning.* New York: Doubleday, 1965.

Hacker, H. M. Women as a minority group. *Social Forces,* 1951, *30,* 60-69.

Hutchinson, B. *Old people in a modern Australian community.* Melbourne: Melbourne University Press, 1954.

Kitagawa, E., and Taeuber, K. *Local community fact book, Chicago Metropolitan area.* Chicago: University of Chicago Press, 1963.

La Pierre, R. *The Freudian ethic.* New York: Duell, Sloan, & Pierce, 1959.

Lindemann, E. Symptomology and management of acute grief. *American Journal of Psychiatry,* 1944, *101,* 141-148.

Lopata, H. A re-statement of the relations between role and status. *Sociology & Social Research,* 1964, *49,* 58-68.

Lopata, H. The function of voluntary associations in an ethnic community: Polonia. In E. Burgess and D. Bogus (Eds.), *Contributions to urban sociology.* Chicago: University of Chicago Press, 1965.

Lopata, H. Social relations of widows in black and white urban communities. Paper read at Midwest Sociological Society meetings, St. Louis, April, 1970. (a)

Lopata, H. Social isolation of the lower-class blue collar woman. Paper read at the Ohio Valley Sociological Society meetings, Akron, Ohio, May, 1970. (b)

Lopata, H. Role changes in widowhood: A world perspective. In D. Cowgill and L. Holmes (Eds.), *Aging around the world.* New York: Appleton-Century-Crofts, 1971. (a)

Lopata, H. *Occupation: Housewife.* New York: Oxford University Press, 1971. (b)

Lopata, H. *Widowhood in an American City.* Cambridge, Mass.: Schenkman Publishing Co., 1971. (c)

Lopata, H., and Noel, J. The dance studio: Style without sex. *Trans-action,* 1967, *4,*

Jan.-Feb.

Ludwig, Sister C. Private communication, Loyola University, Chicago, 1970.

Maddison, D. The relevance of conjugal bereavement for preventive psychiatry. *British Journal of Psychology*, 1968, *41*, 223-233.

Marris, P. *Widows and their families*. London: Routledge & Kegan Paul, 1958.

Parkes, R. Effects of bereavement on physical and mental health, a study of the medical records of widows. *British Medical Journal*, 1964, *ii*, 274-279.

Parkes, R. Bereavement and mental illness: A clinical study. *British Journal of Medical Psychology*, 1965, *38*, Pt. 1, 1-12, & Pt. 11, 13-26.

Pihlblad, T., and Rosencranz, H. *Social participation of older people in the small town*. Columbia, Mo.: University of Missouri Dept. of Sociology, 1968.

Rosenmayr, L., and Köckeis, E. Propositions for a sociological theory of aging and the family. *International Social Science Journal*, 1963, *15*, 410-426.

Sarasvati, P. R. *The high-caste Hindu woman*. Philadelphia: James B. Rodgers Printing Co., 1888.

Schapera, I. *Married life in an African tribe*. New York: Scheridan House, 1941.

Shanas, E. *The health of older people*. Cambridge, Mass.: Harvard University Press, 1962.

Shanas, E., Townsend, P., Wedderburn, D., Friis, H., Milhoj, P., and Stehouwer, J. *Old people in three industrial societies*. New York & London: Atherton, Routledge & Kegan Paul, 1968.

Smolic-Krkovic, N. Social relations of widows in the villages of Croatia-Yugoslavia, 1970. (mimeo)

Stehouwer, J. The household and family relations of old people. In E. Shanas, P. Townsend, D. Wedderburn, H. Friis, P. Milhoj and J. Stehouwer (Eds.), *Old people in three industrial societies*. New York & London: Atherton, Routledge & Kegan Paul, 1968.

Thomas, P. *Indian women through the ages*. New York: Asia Publishing House, 1964.

Thomas, W. I., and Znaniecki, F. *The Polish peasant in Europe and America*. New York: Dover Publications, 1958.

Townsend, P. *The family life of old people*. New York: Free Press of Macmillian, 1957.

Tunstall, J. *Old and alone*. London: Routledge & Kegan Paul, 1966.

U.S. Dept. of Commerce, Bureau of the Census. *1960 census of population*, Vol. I. *Characteristics of the population, Pt. 15: Illinois*. Washington: U.S. Government Printing Office, 1963.

Ward, B. (Ed.) *Women of New Asia*. Paris: UNESCO, 1963.

Winch, R., and Blumberg, R. Societal complexity and family organization. In R. Winch and L. Goodman (Eds.), Selected *studies in marriage and the family*. New York: Holt, Rinehart & Winston, 1968.

Znaniecki, F. *Social relations and social roles*. San Francisco: Chandler Publishing Co., 1965.

Section IX

THE INSTITUTIONALIZED AGED

THE DESCRIPTIVE, DEMOGRAPHIC APPROACH OF THE 1930s and early 1950s also characterized the study of the institutionalized aged. For the most part, researchers evidenced concern for the number of persons in institutional contexts as well as the variety of such settings (Fox, 1950; Martin, 1955). As a reflection of this interest, gerontologists devoted much time and energy to amassing data on those factors associated with the institutionalization of older people. In this regard, health, marital status, income, and residential stability proved closely related to the institutional decision. In general, poor health and low income coupled with the loss of spouse and home were primary forces accounting for the move from an independent to a dependent existence.

Along with a desire to explore the dimensions of institutionalization went equal efforts to assess the effect of this experience on the aged. Accordingly, researchers gave attention to the personality characteristics of institutionalized persons (Davidson and Kruglov, 1952; Fox, 1950) as well as the impact of this change on their attitudes and behavior (Martin, 1955; Tuckman and Lorge, 1952). In most respects, institutionalization was viewed negatively. These older persons, for example, proved more depressed and in poorer health than was true of the general population. In addition, they exhibited negative self-images, experienced declines in intelligence and abilities, and seemed more prone to early deaths. By and large, the process of institutionalization was regarded as essentially dehumanizing and productive of a new and generally depreciatory personality type (Davidson and Kruglov, 1952).

It is worthy of note, however, that many of these findings came as a result of *ex post facto* research. That is, efforts were first made to measure a series of social and psychological characteristics of institutionalized older persons. Following this, attempts were made to relate these in a causal fashion to the institutional experience. To make matters worse, these studies frequently employed cross-sectional methodologies and rarely controlled for the type of institutional setting involved. Accordingly, there developed no clear picture of institutionalization as a process involving decision making or exchange. Instead, the institutional context was implicitly regarded as insidious relative to the health and well-being of the aged individual.

Interest in the factors associated with institutionalization remained strong in the late 1950s and early 1960s. The relationship between health, income, marital status, and residential stability to institutionalization was carefully documented during this period (NCHI, 1965; Townsend, 1964). In addition, gerontologists gave greater attention to the range of institutional settings available to older persons (Donahue, 1965). Efforts were also made to explore a host of variables related to one's adjustment to these contexts (Miller and Lieberman, 1965; Bennett and Nahemow, 1965; Bennett *et al.*, 1965). Among those factors associated with good adjustment were a positive self-image (Coe, 1965) and a flexible orientation toward interpersonal relations (Pollack *et al.*, 1962). For the most part, however, adjustment was tied to the nature of the institution and to the quality of relationships found therein.

The focus on adjustment eventually led to a process view of institutionalization. Accordingly, interest shifted to the decisional aspects of this experience. By and large, researchers gave attention to many of the negotiations by family and staff relative to the institutionalization of the aged (Lieberman and Larkin, 1963). As a result, the picture of institutional experience was broadened to consider a series of relationships and decisions formerly ignored by many writers.

On the other hand, the negative view of institutional life remained in the forefront. The dehumanizing factors implicit in these contexts were held to influence one's health, morale, and adjustment. As a result of institutionalization, one could expect to witness a decline in health, an extension in convalescence relative to any disease process or injury, and, usually, an early death (Lieberman, 1961; Fink, 1957; Sommer, 1960; Donahue, 1963). This view went hand in hand with the understanding that institutions were productive of a particular personality type, one characterized by excessive dependence and self-depreciation (Bennett, 1963).

Besides an effort to view institutionalization as a process, another important change in perspective came as a result of methodological improvements. The increasing popularity of the longitudinal format made possible the exploration of the effects of institutional life on the health and well-being of the older person (Bortner, 1962). Although in its seminal phase of development, this emphasis raised a number of questions as to the nature of the institutional experience. Questioned, for example, was the notion that institutionalization meant early or premature death. Similarly, one's self-image and life satisfaction appeared to undergo little change with institutional living. It was becoming apparent that many of the ideas regarding institutions and their effect on the elderly were artifacts of research design.

The process approach described above was to see further development in the late 1960s and early 1970s. The institutional experience was held to be initiated by subtle but significant negotiations between generational and institutional personalities (Brody, 1969; Brody and Spark, 1966; Droller, 1969). So important did this phase of the process become, that it was seen as a major determinate of one's adjustment to the institutional setting (Atchley, 1972). The perception of a choice in this regard also played a decisive role in the individual's morale and satisfaction subsequent to placement.

It is apparent that the concern for institutional adjustment remains strong among gerontologists (Stotsky, 1967; Gelfand, 1968; Jacobs, 1969; Wessen, 1968). To this interest, however, has been added a new dimension. The contemporary focus on institutionalization centers about the concept of *rehabilitation* (Haymes, 1969; Herz, 1968; Szewczuk, 1966; Shanas, 1971; Lawton and Lawton, 1968). Partially the result of developments in several disciplines (e.g. occupational therapy), institutions for older persons have undergone a change in image. No longer stop-overs on the road to death, the modern institutional setting seeks to rehabilitate and return significant numbers of persons to active and independent lives. Although the final chapter has yet to be written as to the effects of institutional living, it is clear that institutions have made many positive contributions to the lives of older people. These accomplishments have included improvements in the quality of institutional care (Bell, 1967). To some extent, these changes help account for the fact that less than 5 percent of older people are presently living in institutions.

Design improvements have also challenged several notions regarding institutions for the aged. While evidence remains generally negative regarding the institutional experience, the longitudinal format and multiple-correlational approaches have shown many of the "effects" of institutionalization to be of statistical or methodological origin (Lieberman, 1969). Biased samples and an *ex post facto* approach to research, for example, give little weight to the character of the individual prior to institutional placement. Contemporary research, on the other hand, has found changes in the attitudes and behavior of institutionalized persons to be less dramatic than initially thought. In addition, the effects of institutionalization are frequently found to be tied to the specific social or cultural setting.

The papers which follow look seriously at the question of institutionalization. Considered, for example, are not only the variety of contexts available to the aged, but also some of the factors making for adjustment and rehabilitation. It is apparent from these writings that institutions for the aged are neither all good nor all bad. To some extent, however, institutional arrangements are preferred over certain patterns of social and residential isolation.

The paper by Reader represents a cataloguing and description of the types of institutions which have been developed both in this country and abroad for geriatric care. While focusing for the most part on the United States, the author makes it apparent that care for the aged has proceeded at a much faster pace in several European and Scandanavian countries. This fact is evidenced by the plethora of institutional forms only recently introduced into this country (e.g. home care agencies, day hospitals, nursing homes, extended care facilities, terminal care homes, and mental and other specialty hospitals). The major impetus to such arrangements in the United States seems to have been the Social Security and Medicare Acts.

The paper by Lieberman examines the literature regarding the effects of institutionalization on the psychological well-being and physical integrity of aged adults. While the author finds essentially negative outcomes regarding the influence of institutionalization on the elderly residing in homes for the aged, domiciliaries, and nursing homes (e.g. poor adjustment, depression and unhappiness, intellectual ineffectiveness, negative self-image, and feelings of isolation and personal insignificance), a closer look at these studies reveals a number of methodological problems.

For Lieberman, "the common stereotype about the destructive influences on the aged of living in institutional settings is overdrawn. Many of the supposed psychological effects are characteristic of the person *prior* to his coming to an institution (and are related in part to the reasons for institutionalization) and some appear to be associated with aspects of *entering* the institution (making a radical change in the environment) which occurred before the individual actually entered the institution. The only long-term effect of living in an institution that can be demonstrated is the increasing difficulty of reentering the community and making appropriate adaptations. There appear to be considerably more destructive effects associated with radical environmental change (*entrance* into institutions) than with residence in an institution."

Turner *et al.* focus their efforts on personality traits as potential predictors of institutional adaptation among the aged. The assumption behind this approach is that, "those aged with preinstitutional personality traits that are congruent with the specific demands of the relocation environment will experience a minimum of distress due to relocation." Such congruent personality traits are felt to facilitate adaptation because the impact of relocation will be reduced when there is a fit between traits and specific adaptive demands of the environment.

Data were obtained from eighty-five elderly persons prior to and one year after moving from the community into homes for the aged in Chicago. The results indicate that for the person undergoing the stress of institutional adaptation, congruent traits facilitate positive adaptation. In addition, the particular trait found to be associated with successful institutional adaptation loaded strongly on activity, aggression, and narcissistic body image. This organization of traits suggests that a vigorous and perhaps combative style of behavior is functional for institutional adaptation.

Markus *et al.* consider still another aspect of the institutionalization picture, the impact of relocation upon mortality rates. The authors focus their attention on 373 older men and women transferring from two homes for the aged in two central city areas to new suburban locations. The impact of relocation is assessed against a control population, "defined as those populations alive in each of the homes taken severally on 15 census dates corresponding to the month and day of the move in each of the past 15 years."

Contrary to expectations, no consistent mortality patterns are revealed in the data. The patterns evidenced include both higher and lower postrelocation mortaility. In general, the authors relate these findings to either chance variability or to different admission policies at the two homes. By so doing, they make clear that, "age, sex, and residency experience *alone* are not sufficient predictors of postrelocation mortality and that factors such as physical and mental status, attitude to change, and degree of hopefulness need to be studied . . ."

Finally, two problems occupy the attention of Curry and Ratliff relative to the institutionalization of the aged, isolation and life satisfaction. Based on a review of previous research as well as an appreciation of phenomenology, the authors suggest an association between nursing home size and the two variables in question. Specifically, they postulate the environment of small institutional structures to be more conducive to the formation of primary relationships. This potential coupled with the confines of a limited physical space suggest less opportunities for social and/or personal isolation. By the same token, as satisfaction is often related to the intimacy and frequency of such primary associations, the authors expect satisfaction to be higher in smaller as opposed to larger institutional contexts.

Data were obtained from twenty-six proprietary nursing homes in a single county in Ohio. The findings indicate that social and personal isolation does increase with the size of the institution. The most dramatic evidence of this difference is seen when the large and small homes are compared with each other. On the other hand, life satisfaction does not evidence a similar pattern relative to nursing home size. That is, satisfaction scores were essentially the same regardless of the size of the home in which these persons were living. Moreover, "general life satisfaction does not appear to be greatly influenced by current isolation."

REFERENCES

Atchley, R. C. *The social forces in later life.* Belmont, California: Wadsworth Publishing Company, 1972.

Bell, T. The relationship between social involvement and feeling old among residents in homes for the aged. *Journal of Gerontology*, 1967, *22*, 17-22.

Bennett, R. The meaning of institutional life. *Gerontologist*, 1963, *3*, 117-125.

Bennett, R., and Nahemow, L. Institutional totality and criteria of social adjustment in residences for the aged. *Journal of Social Issues*, 1965, *21*, 44-76.

Bennett, R., Nahemow, L., and Zubin, J. *The effects on residents of homes for the aged on social adjustment.* USPHS, 1964.

Bortner, R. W. Test differences attributable to age, selection, processes, and institutional effects. *Journal of Gerontology*, 1962, *17*, 58-60.

Brody, E. M. Follow-up study of applicants and nonapplicants to a voluntary home. *Geontologist*, 1969, *9*, 187-196.

Brody, E. M., and Spark, G. M. Institutionalization of the aged: a family crisis. *Family Process*, 1966, *5*, 76-90.

Coe, R. M. Self-conception and institutionalization. In A. M. Rose and W. A. Peterson (Eds.), *Older people and their social world.* Philadelphia. F. A. Davis, 1965.

Davidson, H. H., and Kruglov, L. Personality characteristics of the institutionalized aged. *Journal of Consulting Psychology*, 1952, *16*, 5-12.

Donahue, W. Rehabilitation of long-term aged patients. In R. H. Williams, C. Tibbitts, & W. Donahue (Eds.) *Processes of aging.* New York: Atherton Press, 1963.

Donahue, W. Impact of living arrangements on ego development in the elderly. In *Patterns of living and housing of middle aged and older people*, USPHS, 1965.

Droller, H. Institutionalization. In M. F. Lowenthal and A. Zilli (Eds.), *Colloquium on health and aging of the population.* New York: S. Karger, 1969.

Fink, H. The relationship of time perspective to age, institutionalization, and activity. *Journal of Gerontology,* 1957, *12,* 414-417.

Fox, C. The intelligence of old indigent persons residing within and without a public home for the aged. *American Journal of Psychology,* 1950, *63,* 110-112.

Gelfand, D. E. Visiting patterns and social adjustment in an old age home. *Gerontologist,* 1968, *8,* 272-275.

Haymes, D. E. Psychological factors in rehabilitation of the elderly. *Gerontologia Clinica,* 1969, *11,* 126-129.

Herz, K. G. New patterns of social services for the aging and the aged. *Journal of Jewish Community Service,* 1968, *44,* 236-245.

Jacobs, R. H. One-way street: an intimate view of adjustment to a home for the aged. *Gerontologist,* 1969, *9,* 268-275.

Lawton, M. P., and Lawton, F. G. Social rehabilitation of the aged: some neglected aspects. *Journal of the American Geriatrics Society,* 1968, *16,* 1346-1363.

Lieberman, M. A. The relationship of mortality rates to entering a home for the aged. *Geriatrics,* 1961, *16,* 515-519.

Lieberman, M. A. Institutionalization of the aged: effects on behavior. *Journal of Gerontology,* 1969, *24,* 330-340.

Lieberman, M. A., and Larkin, M. On becoming an aged institutionalized individual. In W. Donahue, C. Tibbitts, and R. H. Williams (Eds.), *Social and psychological processes of aging.* New York: Atherton Press, 1963.

Martin, D. Institutionalization. *Lancet,* 1955, *269,* 1188-1190.

Miller, D., and Lieberman, M. A. The relationships of affect state and adaptive capacity to reaction to stress. *Journal of Gerontology,* 1965, *20,* 492-497.

National Center for Health Statistics. Characteristics of residents in institutions for the aged and chronically ill, United States, April-June, 1963. *Vital and Health Statistics,* Washington, D.C.: USGPO, 1965.

Pollack, M., Karp, E., Kahn, R. L., and Goldfarb, A. I. Perception of self in institutionalized aged subjects. *Journal of Gerontology,* 1962, *17,* 405-408.

Riley, M. W., and Foner, A. *Aging and society, Vol. I, an inventory of research findings.* New York: Russell Sage Foundation, 1968.

Shanas, E. Measuring the health home needs of the aged in five countries. *Journal of Gerontology,* 1971, *26,* 37-40.

Sommer, T., and Osmond, H. Symptoms of institutional care. *Social Problems,* 1960, *3,* 244-253.

Stotsky, B. A. A controlled study of factors in a successful adjustment of mental patients to a nursing home. *American Journal of Psychiatry,* 1967, *123,* 1243-1251.

Szewczuk, W. Rehabilitation of the aged by means of new forms of activity. *Gerontologist,* 1966, *6,* 93-94.

Townsend, P. *The last refuge.* New York: Rutledge, 1964.

Tuckman, J., and Lorge, I. The effect of institutionalization on attitudes toward old people. *Journal of Abnormal and Social Psychology,* 1952, *47,* 337-344.

Wessen, A. F. Some sociological characteristics of long-term care. *Gerontologist,* 1968, *8,* 72-75.

Chapter 40

TYPES OF GERIATRIC INSTITUTIONS

GEORGE G. READER

IN EACH CULTURE and each country, people develop their own ways of caring for the elderly. Patterns of care are distinct between industrialized and developing countries usually because of technological variations, but availability of trained personnel and total costs are also important determinants everywhere.

Included herein is a description of types of institutions that have been developed for geriatric care, leaning heavily on the United States as an example but pointing to principles that may be applicable in other societies. It concludes with a statement of future expectations and some recommendations for a suitable pattern of care, at least for the industrialized nations.

RANGE OF TYPES

Institutions in the United States for medical care of the elderly constitute a spectrum based on intensity and complexity of care that includes home care, day care, day hospital, infirmary care in homes for the aged or retirement communities, nursing homes, extended care facilities, chronic disease hospitals and terminal care homes, mental and other specialty hospitals, and acute general care hospitals.

Home Care

Shanas (1971) estimates from her studies of Denmark, Britain, the United States,

Reprinted by permission from the *Gerontologist*, 1973, *13*, 290-294.

Israel, and Poland that from 8 to 15 percent of those over sixty-five are either bedfast or housebound but living in their own homes. An additional 6 to 16 percent are able to go outdoors only with difficulty. These people all presumably need health care in the home on a regular basis. In addition, episodic home care is required by one fourth to one half of all old people, depending on country, who spend at least one day a year in bed because of an episode of illness. Yet in these five countries, one out of five bedfast sick is not visited by a physician. Evidently, those who receive health services, and many apparently do not receive them, do so from others than physicians.

In the United States, organized home care has developed in large part as a reaction to the stimulus of the Medicare Act. Since the passage of Medicare, home health agencies have increased from about 1,200 in 1966 to about 2,800 in 1970. As of 1971 there were 2,333 home health agencies certified for Medicare reimbursement, being approved to provide both skilled nursing care for patients at home and at least one other therapeutic service, for example, physical therapy. Fifty-seven percent of these are sponsored by official health agencies such as health departments, 24 percent by visiting nurse associations, 3 percent by combined government and voluntary agencies, and 9 percent by hospitals. In the Northeast, visiting nurse associations account for 53 percent of all home health agencies, compared with 6 percent in the South, while official health agencies account for only 28 percent in the Northeast compared with 77 percent in the South. Many parts of the United States are not served by organized home health agencies.

Prior to 1965, and still today in the United States, visiting nurse associations provide a good part of the service to the elderly sick at home, but not as home health agencies. The nurse visits on a doctor's order or, as in New York City, will make one visit to the house without an order but will not continue to visit unless a physician is officially in attendance on the patient.

Hospital-based home care projects hospital standards on to the delivery of services in the home. The Home Care Service is considered a regular section of the hospital, and patients are transferred and readmitted as they would be between services such as Medicine and Surgery.

Day Care

Centers where the elderly may obtain social services and opportunities to carry on an active group life have been known for some time. Many of these have paid attention to physical health through counseling and referral, health education, and provision of adequate nutrition. Day Care, as distinct from Senior Centers, are new on the United States' scene and are to be sparsely found. The geriatric day hospital is an even newer phenomenon, quite rare as yet in many countries, including the United States, but flourishing in the United Kingdom. The first day hospital for this purpose opened at Cowley Road Hospital, Oxford, in 1958. By the end of 1970 there were at least 119 day hospitals in Great Britain. The aim of the geriatric day hospital is to provide active care to elderly patients during the day. Besides treatment, the day hospital offers relatives relief from strain and provides emotional support to patients. Most authorities believe the day hospital should be supplemented by a day care center so that progressive patient care is possible.

Brocklehurst (1970) found in his survey of geriatric day hospitals in Great Britain that physical rehabilitation was the most important function, with physical maintenance therapy second. Social care of the mentally confused was rated lowest in importance by the consultants he queried. The day hospitals, on the average, provided between thirty and fifty places daily. Fifty-seven percent of patients attended once weekly; only 5 percent came four or five times weekly; 37 percent attended for over one year. Sixty-one percent received physiotherapy, and all but 1 percent had occupational therapy. Stroke was the commonest reason for attendance in those under eighty. Over that age, chronic brain syndrome and arthritis were more common. Fifteen percent of the patients discharged themselves, almost one half of these in the first two weeks. They tended to be older and more of them suffered from cardiovascular or respiratory rather than neurological or locomotor diseases. Over 20 percent of patients had second or subsequent periods of attendance. Following a second admission, more of the patients were admitted to hospital, became ill at home, or died than after the first admission.

Infirmary Care

Most homes for the aged have beds available for infirmary care either in their own buildings or in adjacent medical facilities. These may be fairly elaborate in terms of care offered and may even be a place where terminal care is given. Usually they are minimally staffed. Any patient with a serious condition is immediately transferred to a local hospital.

A variation on this arrangement can be seen in the large number of retirement communities springing up in the United States. A community of several thousand households, as in Leisure Village at Sea Beach, California, will have a well-ordered clinic that serves the residents. For minor illnesses, patients may stay at home and services are organized through neighbors or visiting nurses. Those more severely affected are hospitalized in one of several nearby hospitals. Because of the *esprit* of the community and the free time available to the residents, it is possible to provide excellent attention to those who are ill. The clinic staff holds a regular sick call, carries out diagnostic examinations, and provides a high-quality health maintenance service.

Nursing Homes

Prior to the 1930s few nursing homes existed in the United States. The sick elderly were cared for by relatives, sometimes in an eleemosynary home for the aged or in almshouses. Enactment of the Social Security Act, in 1935, provided some support funds for the aged, and nursing and boarding homes began to develop. Since then there has been a growing demand for nursing home beds, especially with prolongation of life because of improved medical technology and increasing government support of medical care for the aged, blind, and disabled.

The Medicare Act gave impetus to the development of nursing homes, and at the same time changed the concept and standards of what a nursing home should be. Because organized medicine waged a long and arduous campaign to prevent social legislation from emerging from the deliberations of the Congress, the lawmakers who framed the 1965 amendments to the Social Security Act had little help from the medical profession. They, therefore, proceeded to develop many of the concepts on their own.

Title XVIII of Medicare defined an extended care facility as including provisions for twenty-four-hour nursing service, a nursing care plan based on per-

sonalized needs of individual patients, and proper dietary and medical supervision. Patients were to be admitted only after a three-day stay in a hospital, where presumably they would be properly studied and diagnosed. The intent was to reduce the overall length of hospital stay and provide for a convalescent period under supervision and at a reduced cost compared with the hospital. The legislators conceived of an elderly patient's falling ill, entering the acute hospital, convalescing in the extended care facility, and then returning home to receive services from an accredited home health agency. This completely neglected the elderly population who are chronically ill and require long-term institutional care.

Chronic Disease Hospitals

Shanas, Townsend, Wedderburn, Friis, Milhoj, and Stehouwer (1968) in their comparisons of health care of the elderly point up the difficulties of classifying types of institutions. They found in 1967 that the United States had close to 30,000 beds (38,144 in 1971) listed as chronic, while Britain had 65,000 with another 20,000 "geriatric" beds. They point out that this does not mean that there are more chronically sick patients in Britain than in the United States. Nursing homes are relatively scarce in Britain and relatively numerous in the United States, but nursing home means different things in different countries. Some American nursing homes resemble British hospitals for the chronically sick in staff and facilities but are not so classified.

Chronic disease hospitals in the United States are often closely associated with acute general hospitals or may even be contiguous. Many municipal and county hospitals that offer care to the general population may have bed-stays of over sixty days for some patients, and in that sense have a large proportion of chronic patients. In fact, the definition of an acute patient is not clear-cut. Elderly people, particularly, may have several chronic diseases and a number of episodes requiring hospitalization in the course of their latter years. Each episode may be acute but should be considered in the perspective of the medical management available. High-quality ambulatory care may reduce the number and length of hospitalizations for the chronically ill so that for these people the requirement is for acute hospital beds and not chronic ones.

Some countries in Western Europe, particularly Great Britain, have developed the geriatric hospital as an entity in itself. This often is a combination of home for the aged, infirmary, and chronic disease hospital, catering to the needs of the elderly who cannot live at home, and is staffed by geriatricians. As has been noted, some homes for the aged in the United States closely resemble the British geriatric hospital but are not so designated.

Terminal care homes are found in many countries, where the aim is to make the patient's last days as comfortable as possible rather than to continue efforts to halt or reverse the course of illness. In the Western World many of these are operated by religious orders. They are generally not counted as separate in-bed statistics but are lumped with chronic disease hospitals, so it is difficult to know what proportion of the population needing them is served. An outstanding example of a hospital of this type is St. Christopher's Hospice in London. It was opened in 1967 and has fifty-four beds for the care of patients with advanced or terminal malignant or neurological disease and supports approximately the same number at home. Some 400 patients die each year in St. Christopher's, and between 10 and 15 percent of that number are discharged home to their families, at least for a short time. It provides a pleasant and supportive environment for the patient and his family at the end of life.

Mental Hospitals and Other Specialty Hospitals

Fewer than 10 percent of the 20 million persons aged sixty-five and older in the United States are in mental hospitals. A significant number, however, of those in other types of institutions are psychiatrically impaired to a greater or lesser degree. Again it is a problem of classification of degree of disability and availability of services. Many of those in institutions because of what is labeled mental illness might be living in the community if supportive services were available to them. On the other hand, the report prepared for the White House Conference on Aging—1971 estimates that a little less than one million elderly living in the community suffer from such severe psychiatric impairment as to make them as sick as many of those who are hospitalized.

Besides mental hospital care, there have developed, particularly in the Netherlands, home care services for the mentally ill. These served to reduce the need for mental hospital beds even before the impact of the psychotropic drugs was felt. In the United States, community mental health centers have also begun to provide services since the passage of enabling legislation in 1964, 1965, and 1966. By mid-1969 more than 200 of these centers were in operation. According to this concept, a catchment area is designated and all those living in a particular geographic area are eligible to be served by a community mental health center. One professional person is usually named as the coordinator of mental health services for the elderly. Community mental health centers work in close cooperation with general hospitals and state mental hospitals, with the private sector of mental health care, and with various full-care and part-care facilities. When a patient leaves a mental hospital to return to the community, a coordinator or advocate is available locally to see that follow-up is available, including psychiatric, social work, nursing, rehabilitative, and supportive services.

Short-Term General Care Hospitals

During 1968 and 1969, in the United States the rate of discharge from short-stay hospitals was 232.6 per 1,000 for those over sixty-five, almost twice that of all ages combined. Average length of stay in days was 15.3 for the over sixty-five, compared with 9.1 for all ages combined. This clearly indicates that the elderly utilize hospital beds in the United States more than any other group in the population.

Shanas and her colleagues found, too, that more of the aged in the United States are hospitalized during a year (13%) than in Denmark (11%) or Britain (8%). Bed-stay, however, was much shorter for the aged in the United States compared with Britain; that is, hospitals in the United States tend to be used more intensively than those in Britain. At the same time, however, Shanas *et al.* (1968) found that physicians visit the incapacitated, the bed-fast, and the housebound more often in Britain than in the United States. There are a number of explanations for these differences, but probably the most important factor is that British general practitioners are closer to their patients geographically and perhaps emotionally. Also,

insurance reimbursement in the United States favors the hospitalization of patients rather than emphasizing either ambulatory care or home care.

In the United States the types of geriatric institutions are at least in part due to the fragmentation of services to the elderly ill. Costs of care are probably higher in the United States than anywhere else in the world, although Sweden is rapidly approaching proportionate budgetary levels. But services for the elderly are neither as available, nor can patients find access to them as readily, as in many poorer and less-developed societies. The point is that a profusion of types of institutions is probably less important than a system of health care that reaches those in need.

Future Expectations

As infectious diseases and other causes of early death come under control in most of the world, the population of the world may expect to change in the direction of having an ever enlarging component of persons over sixty-five. Although much may yet be done through prevention, most of the illnesses of this age group are likely to increase as people live long enough to develop arteriosclerosis, arthritis, and senility. More and more social institutions will have to be invented to provide appropriate support and protection, but the obvious aim should be to keep people in their own homes and functioning as long as possible. To accomplish this, health systems that emphasize ambulatory and domiciliary care will be needed. Hard choices may be necessary when it comes to deciding how far technology should be carried to prolong life as an end in itself rather than to allow human beings to function in a self-sufficient and productive way.

The neighborhood health center as it

has grown under federal auspices may be a first step in the direction of improving availability of services and access for the elderly where they live. This, combined with the suggestions for health care corporations encompassing a highly specialized referral center with satellite general care hospital and chronic care beds serving an insured population, may be the best present answer for the United States.

REFERENCES

Brocklehurst, J. C. *The geriatric day hospital.* London: King Edward's Hospital Fund, 1970.

Shanas, E. Measuring the home health needs of the aged in five countries. *Journal of Gerontology,* 1971, *26,* 37-40.

Shanas, E., Townsend, P., Wedderburn, D., Friis, H. Milhoj, P., and Stehouwer, J. *Old people in three industrial societies.* New York: Atherton Press, 1968.

Chapter 41

INSTITUTIONALIZATION OF THE AGED: EFFECTS ON BEHAVIOR

Morton A. Lieberman

T HE EFFECTS OF institutionalization on the psychological well-being and physical integrity of aged adults has been a question of humanitarian interest since the late nineteenth century and of scientific inquiry for thirty years. This paper assesses current knowledge and research strategies regarding the effects of institutional living on the elderly and delineates the contributions future research might make to policy formation.

For the purpose of this review, institutions are defined as residential facilities providing one or more central services that meet some particular need of the client and/or society. Studies of geriatric centers, nursing homes, domiciliaries, and chronic disease units are included, as well as facilities that serve a large number of aged but are not exclusively oriented toward them, such as mental hospitals. Such settings imply permanent or indefinite residence involving a major change from a community living pattern. Temporary institutionalization (such as brief hospitalizations) or settings which do not provide multiple centralized services (such as retirement villages) are not included. Empirical studies on the institutionalization of children and of psychiatric patients are discussed to illu-

Reprinted by permission from the *Journal of Gerontology*, 1969, *24*, 330-340.

strate gaps in knowledge regarding the aged.

Effects of Institutionalization

It is commonly believed that most institutions have deleterious effects caused by the "dehumanizing" and "depersonalizing" characteristics of institutional environments.

Such a veiw has been associated with the contention that institutions for the aged are often "dumping grounds," housing many who need not live there. This view is countered by Shanas (1961) and others who suggest, on the basis of survey data, that the majority of institutionalized aged have real needs they are attempting to solve via the institution. Whether alternatives exist to meet these needs is unknown, and whether, in fact, alternatives are needed depends at least in part on whether institutionalization really does have deleterious effects and, if so, to what extent and in what ways.

The common sense view that institutions have deleterious effects on the psychological well-being and physical survival of aged adults appears to be supported by a host of empirical studies.

A representative compilation of studies of the elderly residing in homes for the aged, domiciliaries, and nursing homes suggests that they share the following characteristics: poor adjustment, depression and unhappiness, intellectual ineffectiveness because of increased rigidity and low energy (but not necessarily intellectual incompetence), negative self-image, feelings of personal insignificance and impotency, and a view of self as old. Residents tend to be docile, submissive, show a low range of interests and activities, and to live in the past rather than the future. They are withdrawn and unresponsive in relationship to others. There is some suggestion that they have increased anxiety, which at times focuses on feelings of death (Ames, 1954; Chalfen, 1956; Coe, 1967; Davidson and Kruglov, 1952; Dorken, 1951; Eicker, 1959; Fink, 1957; Fox, 1950; Lakin, 1960; Laverty, 1950; Lepkowsky, 1954; Lieberman and Lakin, 1963; Mason, 1954; Pan, 1950; Pollack, Karp, and Goldfarb, 1962; Shrut, 1958; Swenson, 1961; Tuckman and Lorge, 1952). Other investigators (Camargo and Preston, 1945; Kay, Norris, and Post, 1956; Lieberman, 1961; Roth, 1955; Whittier and Williams, 1956) have reported marked increases in mortality rates for aged persons entering mental institutions or homes for the aged.

These studies clearly demonstrate that aged persons residing in a variety of institutional settings are psychologically worse off and likely to die sooner than aged persons living in the community. Without additional information all of this research is worthless, however, in determining whether life in the institution induces such effects. Difference between institutional and community residents does not of itself mean that institutionalization is the essential variable that created the differences. Before such a conclusion can be entertained, aged persons in institutions and aged persons living in the community must be shown comparable, differing only in respect to where they live. It must also be shown that the characteristics of institutional life, *per se,* and not other factors associated with becoming institutionalized, induce these deleterious effects.

Selection Biases

How many of the effects attributed to living in institutions can be explained on the basis of population differences between those living in the community and those residing in institutions? Such an approach

might explain the negative psychological characteristics of institutionalized aged as a product of disease (physical or mental), or as a product of personality characteristics associated with resolving crises of old age by seeking institutional settings, or as a product of certain life crises that brought about institutionalization. Three types of evidence are relevant to this issue: (*a*) population survey data, (*b*) longitudinal or follow-up studies of institutionalized aged, and (*c*) studies that attempt to identify the particular populations from which specific institutions draw their residents.

POPULATION SURVEYS: Since the turn of the century the proportion of aged residing in institutions has steadily increased. This trend, coupled with increased longevity, has meant that institutions have been used more and more to cope with major incapacitating physical or mental illness. It would be reasonable to conclude, therefore, that aged residing in institutions are physically and mentally different from community aged.

Studies of particular samples of institutionalized aged, however, in contrast to simple population statistics, show that significant proportions of the elderly residing in institutions do not differ physically or mentally from their community counterparts. Gitlitz (1956), utilizing morbidity, mortality, and psychiatric disorder statistics from a large home for the aged, suggests that the incidence of specific types of morbidity may not differ from the community aged. These apparent discrepancies between population statistics and studies carried out on particular small samples stem to some extent from the underestimation of psychiatric and physical morbidity in community samples and the relative overestimation in the institutional samples because of better diagnostic techniques.

The occurrence of physical illness among the institutionalized aged takes on added significance because of the suggestive evidence (Birren, 1959; Coe, 1962) that physical illness, even at preclinical levels, affects psychological status. If it could be shown that logical characteristics attributed to institutionalization were significantly related to physical illness, the evidence for selective factors would be appreciably strengthened. To date there is no strong empirical evidence demonstrating this relationship.

It has also been shown (Goldfarb, 1962) that in particular types of institutions, such as homes for the aged, the incidence of chronic brain syndrome varies, ranging from rates of one percent or less to rates that parallel those found in state mental hospitals. Such variations, even among a limited group of institutions for the aged, lend further weight to the probability that some of the effects attributed to living in an institution may be associated with other than institutional factors.

LONGITUDINAL STUDIES: As yet, few longitudinal studies of the aged exist which include data about the period before actual residence in the institution. One study, however, (Lieberman, Prock, and Tobin, 1968) revealed considerably less psychological deterioration when institutionalized aged were measured relative to their own preinstitutional characteristics than cross-sectional comparisons of institutional to noninstitutional populations would suggest. This adds to the evidence that some of the effects attributed to institutionalization environment might more appropriately be accounted for by selection.

STUDIES ON SELECTION: Who come to institutions and why they come is an exceedingly complex issue that no single study answers. There are several studies that are directly applicable. Unfortunately most (Bortner, 1962; Fogel, Swepston, Zintek, Vernier, Fitzgerald, Marnocha, and Weschler, 1956; Webb, 1959) represent highly specialized populations among the institutionalized aged (VA domiciliaries). Although utilizing different methods, these investigators attribute psychological differences between institutionalized and community aged to selection processes. For example, Webb (1959) found that the type of individual who applies and resides in such institutions differs in specific socioeconomic factors as well as personality variables, rigidity, stereotyped thinking, apathy, resignation, ego-eccentricity, passivity, strong needs for love, affection, and care. Many of these factors identifying the persons who apply are the same characteristics as those of "institutionalized populations." Lowenthal (1964) investigating pathways to mental institutions among the aged, found a particular type of interpersonal relationship differentiating those who enter from those who do not enter such institutions. These studies, although few in number and covering a limited range of institutions, point to an association between entering an institution and certain psychological or social characteristics. In contrast, a study comparing community residents, applicants for old age homes, and long-term residents of such homes (Lieberman, Prock, and Tobin, 1968) did not show personality characteristics or occurrences of crises events distinguishing those who entered institutions from those who remained in the community.

Population survey data can at best be suggestive; it cannot offer positive evidence that selection plays a role. Other studies, focused more directly on the selection issue, are limited in number and scope. There are, however, sufficient data to indicate that the differences between institutionalized and noninstitutionalized aged are significantly influenced by the factor of selection. Institutionalized aged share some characteristics because of *who* they are and not *where* they are. On the other hand, the evidence for selection is not sufficient to explain all of the noxious effects associated with living in an institution.

Environmental Change

A number of investigators have studied the effects of radical environmental changes on the psychological well-being and physical survival of the aged. Many of these studies have involved changes from community living to life in an institution; others have studied relocation from one institutional setting to another. Some have investigated environmental changes that involve movement from one community setting to another. These studies are particularly relevant to the consideration of the effects of living in institutional settings. They suggest that the conditions associated with *moving* into an institution create many of the effects attributed to *living* in an institutional setting. The majority of these studies (Aldrich and Mendkoff, 1963; Blenkner, 1967; Goldfarb, Shahinian, and Turner, 1966; Jasnau, 1967; Lieberman, 1961) showed that changing the environment of elderly persons sharply increased the death rate.

While the studies of Lawton and Yaffe (1967) and Miller and Lieberman (1965) failed to show increased mortality, other negative effects were observed. In Lawton and Yaffe's study, the relocated group was judged to have declined more frequently on measures of health compared to the control group; in the Miller and Lieberman study, one half the *Ss* declined either psychologically (occurrences of confusion, memory defects, bizarre behavior) or physically (hospitalization, restrictions of activity, health failures). A recent study (Lie-

berman *et al.*, 1968) showed that many of the effects (on self-image, interpersonal relationships, mood-tone, etc.) ascribed to living in an institution were set in motion by the *decision to enter* an institution and occurred with maximum intensity prior to actual entrance. Fried (1963), in studying relocation forced by urban renewal, noted that many persons suffered serious depressive reactions subsequent to such relocation. He explained these effects in terms of a fragmentation of spatial and group identity. Friedsam (1961), who studied reactions to disaster, showed that events which markedly changed living patterns created profound psychological distress and were particularly destructive for the aged.

Although, overall, the evidence suggests that radical environmental change for the aged leads to destructive physical processes and has noxious psychological effects, some investigators present data which suggest that more precision is required in understanding which conditions and what types of aged will experience such environmental changes as severe crises.

Dobson and Patterson (1961), Epstein and Simon (1967), and Stotsky (1967) studied elderly mentally ill moved for "therapeutic" purposes to nursing homes, boarding homes, or homes for the aged. Here, relocation (many of these *Ss* had lived in institutions most of their adult lives) did not produce massive death rates or increased psychological or physical disabilities. Carp's study (1967) of elderly persons moving into apartment dwellings showed an increase in satisfaction and adjustment. Goldfarb *et al.* (1966) and Donahue (1965) have suggested that under certain conditions (which are at this juncture mostly unknown) some individuals entering or being relocated from one institution to another experienced positive (ego-enhancing) effects.

This pattern of negative and positive findings suggests a number of potentially fruitful hypotheses that are beginning to gain investigative attention. Such studies can add significantly to knowledge about the noxious effects associated with institutionalization and, more important, to specifying the conditions associated with negative effects.

Data are also beginning to accumulate about the characteristics of people who are vulnerable to environmental change. A number of investigators have found that psychiatric disturbance and cognitive malfunctioning (Aldrich and Mendkoff, 1963; Goldfarb, 1966) are positively associated with risk. Studies investigating personality patterns, depression, etc. have also suggested associations with risk (Aldrich and Mendkoff, 1963; Miller and Lieberman, 1965). Goldfarb *et al.* (1966) have suggested that cognitive intactness is associated with improvement under relocation.

Evidence concerning the conditions which affect reactions to change is only beginning to appear in the literature, and the multiplicity of theoretical propositions and technical problems makes the findings presently rather tentative. Voluntary or involuntary change (Lawton and Yaffe, 1967) and the adequacy of preparation are associated with vulnerability to change. Jasnau (1967) suggests that "massed" relocations without adequate "warning" are destructive. The meaning of institutionalization for the individual may affect his reactions. The attitudes of the elderly toward institutional arrangements closely parallel the common societal stereotypes about such institutions. Kleemeier (1960) suggested that older persons exhibit a generalized negative feeling toward all special settings for the aged. Montgomery (1965), studying rural aged, found a consistent desire to remain in the present residence and

equated this with highly-valued independence. Shanas (1961) found aged adults associated moving with loss of independence, prelude to death, rejection by the children. Lieberman and Lakin (1963) found aged awaiting institutionalization attached symbols of fear, rejection, and dread to the event. Tobin (1968) found thema of extreme loss in a group facing institutionalization.

Although data are not available which bear directly on the relationships of such feelings of loss to subsequent effects of institutionalization, studies in other areas on the effects of loss are highly suggestive (Yarrow, Blank, Quinn, Youmans, and Stein, 1963). Research on the sequelae of widowhood has shown some of the same patterns as for institutionalization: increased mortality, incidence of physical disorder, withdrawal, and depression. A number of investigators have associated psychological loss with the onset of physical illness. Research on childhood hospitalization supports the view that the feeling of loss is a major contributor to the upsetting aspects of institutionalization. Inquiry based on the psychology of loss may offer a more effective framework for identifying factors leading to noxious effects of institutionalization than analyses of institutional characteristics. Unfortunately, the state of current research on the psychology of loss makes it impossible to determine if all losses are psychologically equivalent. The degree of specificity such a model would offer is unknown, e.g. whether loss associated with widowhood is analogous in detail to loss surrounding institutionalization.

Characteristics of environmental change have also been studied in terms of "overload." To what extent change is disruptive and destructive depends upon the relationship between the characteristics of the two environments, a question that is currently being investigated. The larger the difference between old and new situations, the greater the possibility that the aged individual will need to develop adaptive responses often beyond his capacity. In this light, the effect of an institution can be viewed less as a product of its quality or characteristics than of the degree to which it forces the person to make new adaptive responses or employ adaptive responses from the previous environment. It is possible that some of the current trends aimed at "deinstitutionalizing" institutions, e.g. making them more open to the outside community, less congregant, etc. are effective because they permit the use of prior adaptive responses.

This review of the effects of selection and degree of environmental change suggests that these two factors may explain many of the deleterious effects on aged which are associated with living in an institution.

Institutional Effects—Studies of Institutional Samples

Another group of studies which bear on the effects of institutionalization are not subject to selection biases created by comparing institutional to noninstitutional populations or to the unknown effects of radical environmental change itself. These studies have used one of three design strategies: study of the psychological well-being of institutional persons as a function of alterations made in the structure of the institution; study of the effects on behavior of the length of time spent in an institution; and comparison of the effects on individuals of residence in various institutional settings. Although these strategies minimize some methodological pitfalls inherent in the previously discussed studies, they raise some new problems.

Alteration in Institutional Structure

The view that certain characteristics of institutionalized persons (which were previously thought part of a disease process, such as the withdrawal and apathetic behavior of schizophrenics) were associated with life in an institution has in large measure been supported by evidence from studies of institutional change. A large body of descriptive anecdotal material and some controlled studies in mental hospitals, beginning with the classic descriptions of Stanton and Schwartz (1954) suggest that hospital structure has an impact upon the inmates and that certain changes in such structures may be ameliorative. Much of this change has been directed toward therapeutic goals, e.g. the change from custodial to therapeutic care in mental hospitals. Although studies specific to the aged are less frequent, the findings agree with the broad findings in the field, that certain types of alteration in the social-physical world have ameliorative effects and that such changes are toward "deinstitutionalizing" the institution (Greenblatt, York, and Brown, 1955).

Some current works (Gottesman, 1963; Kahana, 1968) are illustrative. Kahana experimented with age-segregated and age nonsegregated environments and found that the nonsegregated environment led to an increase in social interaction and emotional responsivity and toward improvement in mental functioning. Her samples were composed mainly of new admissions, thus making the results for the purpose of this review only suggestive. Gottesman's study also suggested that alterations in the physical or social structure of institutions for aged mental patients can mitigate negative behavior.

Despite such results that indicate a positive association between environmental qualities and psychological functioning, a research strategy based only on alterations in the environment cannot make the critical contribution to the central questions on delimiting the general psychological effects of living in an institutional environment. The characteristics of the institutionalized mental patient, apathy, withdrawal, etc., may be a product of the disease which is ameliorated or changed by alterations in the environment. However, changes in behavior do not demonstrate that a *particular* institutional environment was directly associated with those maladaptive behaviors. Moreover, the generally positive results produced by most therapeutic millieu programs in hospitals for the mentally ill strongly suggest the possibility of a "Hawthorne" effect. These considerations, in addition to the pragmatic problems of making salient alterations in many institutional structures, suggest that this research strategy has limited usefulness in determining whether in general an institution for the elderly has noxious effects and which of its characteristics can be associated with such effects.

Length of Institutionalization

Several investigators have attempted to isolate the effects of living in an institution by measuring behavior of *Ss* who live in a particular institution for varying amounts of time. Although potentially offering a reasonable method for specifying the noxious effects of institutional living, the yield from this method has been limited. Townsend (1962) found that those residing less than a year in an institution did not differ from residents of ten years or more. Webb (1959), on the other hand, suggested that those who had lived in institutions for long periods of time indicated more concern about re-entry into the community and less willingness to attempt it. Ongoing work (Lieberman, Tobin, and Slover, 1969)

suggests a relationship between emotional responsivity and length of residence in institutions; however, most analyses reported in the literature have yielded few positive associations between length of time and psychological effects. As is all too often, a characteristic of research in the general area of institutional effects, "negative" results are often noncontributory. The methodological errors make such results too ambiguous for use. For example, the lack of significant findings may be associated with difficulties in method; length of time in an institution is associated with a biased population (discharge or death) and some investigators have not taken this factor into account. Given the relatively homogeneous populations in institutions, the need for sensitive measurement is increased, and most studies have reported results based upon crude data that may not discriminate existing differences.

Comparative Analysis

Studies comparing a variety of institutions offer the best potential for isolating specific effects on the psychological behavior of the aged and for determining the environmental characteristics associated with these effects. Overall, the promise of this approach has not as yet been fulfilled. Townsend (1962) compared various types of institutions in a sample of 173 institutions. Utilizing scales based on adequacy ratings of physical facilities, staffing and services, mobility, freedom in daily life and social provisions, he suggested that differences in occupations, the number of visitors received, and the amount of mobility occurred between "good" and "bad" institutions. Townsend's evidence unfortunately did not provide information associating the quality of institutions and psychological characteristics attributed to institutional living, nor is it possible to determine from this study how much these institutions differed in populations served.

Dobson and Patterson (1961) compared geriatric mental patients living in nursing homes to patients living in state mental hospitals. Their analysis of behavioral ratings suggested no difference between the two groups. In a similar study, Epstein and Simon (1967) compared nursing homes and state hospital patients and found results comparable to those of Dobson and Patterson.

Coe (1962), using a model for assessing institutional structure, found some association between the degree of depersonalization of environment and the effects on self-imagery. Bennett, Nahemow, and Zubin (1964), using Goffman's framework (1961), suggested that the more total the institution (based on such items as orientation of activities, scheduling of activities, provisions for dissemination of rules and standards of conduct, provisions for allocation of staff time and observation of the behavior of inmates, types of sanction system, how personal property is dealt with, decision-making about the use of private property, pattern of recruitment, voluntary-involuntary and residential pattern, congregate versus private) the greater its depersonalizing effects. Shrut (1958) compared sixty *Ss,* thirty living in "apartment-like" dwellings associated with old age homes and thirty living in the more central "institutional" home, found that the *Ss* living in the apartments (more like their previous living arrangements) showed less anxiety about their health and less fear or preoccupation with death than *Ss* living in the central facility.

The studies in this area that have produced positive findings (an association between institutional characteristics and effects on persons living in those institutions) have had two common characteristics: (*a*)

the different institutions were compared using a conceptual framework for measuring differences among institutions rather than making comparisons based upon types of institutions, and (*b*) the effects on the psychological well-being of the residents were measured by instruments that were apparently more sensitive than the more commonly used rating scale approach.

None of the studies surveyed has met the problem of differences in population found among different institutions of a similar type [for example, Goldfarb's (1962) report of extreme ranges in cognitive impairment among homes for the aged]. Thus, it is unknown how many of the positive findings can be attributed to population differences. To make the method of comparative analysis effective, the population characteristics of institutions must be taken into account, perhaps by the use of multivariate statistical procedure (use of complex statistical methods is rare in research on institutionalization).

An overview of the findings available to date suggests the tentative conclusion that, despite the appearance of what seem to be "good" and "bad" institutions, those characteristics that are instrumental in influencing the behavior of the individuals residing in them are shared by all institutions, and these common characteristics may be more salient in producing negative influences than those characteristics that differentiate one institution from another.

Summary and Recommendations for Future Research

The common stereotype about the destructive influences on the aged of living in institutional settings is overdrawn. Many of the supposed psychological effects are characteristics of the person *prior* to his coming to an institution (and are related in part to the reasons for institutionalization) and some appear to be associated with aspects of *entering* the institution (making a radical change in the environment) which occurred before the individual actually entered the institution. The only long-term effect of living in an institution that can be demonstrated is the increasing difficulty of reentering the community and making appropriate adaptations. There appear to be considerably more destructive effects associated with radical environmental change (*entrance into institutions*) than with residence in an institution.

REFERENCES

Aldrich, C. K., and Mendkoff, E. Relocation of the aged and disabled: A mortality study. *Journal of the American Geriatrics Society,* 1963, *11,* 185-194.

Ames, L. B., Learned, J., Metraux, R., and Walker, R. *Rorschach responses in old age.* New York: Hoeber-Harper, 1954.

Bennett, R., Nahemow, L., and Zubin, J. The effects on residents of homes for the aged on social adjustment. USPHS Grant No. 0029, mimeographed progress report, 1964.

Birren, J. E. (Ed.) *Handbook of aging and the individual.* Chicago: University of Chicago Press, 1959.

Blenkner, M. Environmental change and the aging individual. *Gerontologist,* 1967, *7,* No. 2, Pt. I, 101-105.

Bortner, R. W. Test differences attributable to age, selection, processes, and institutional effects. *Journal of Gerontology,* 1962, *17,* 58-60.

Camargo, O., and Preston, G. H. What happens to patients who are hospitalized for the first time when over sixty-five? *American Journal of Psychiatry,* 1945, *102,* 168-173.

Carp, F. M. The impact of environment on old people. *Gerontologist,* 1967, *7,* No. 2, Pt. I, 106-108.

Chalfen, L. Leisure-time adjustment of the aged: II. Activities and interests and some factors influencing choice. *Journal of Genetic Psychology,* 1956, *88,* 261-276.

Coe, R. M. Institutionalization and self-conception. Unpublished PhD dissertation, Washington University, St. Louis, 1962.

Davidson, H. H., and Kruglov, L. Personality characteristics of the institutionalized aged. *Journal of Consulting Psychology,* 1952, *16,* 5-12.

Dobson, W. R. and Patterson, T. W. A behavioral evaluation of geriatric patients living in nursing homes as compared to a hospitalization group. *Gerontologist,* 1961, *1,* 135-139.

Donahue, W. Impact of living arrangements on ego development in the elderly. In *Pattern of living and housing of middle aged and older people.* PHS No. 1496, 1965.

Dorken, H., Jr. Personality factors associated with paraplegia and prolonged hospitalization: A clinical note. *Canadian Journal of Psychology,* 1951, *5,* 134-137.

Eicker, W. F. Age-related differences in behavioral rigidity, level of aspiration, and administration domiciliary population. Unpublished PhD dissertation, University of California, Los Angeles, 1959.

Epstein, L. J., and Simon, A. Alternatives to state hospitalization for geriatric mentally ill. Langley Porter Neuropsychiatric Clinics, San Francisco, 1967, dittoed paper.

Fink, H. The relationship of time perspective to age, institutionalization, and activity. *Journal of Gerontology,* 1957, *12,* 414-417.

Fogel, E. J., Swepston, E. R., Zintek, S. S., Vernier, C. N., Fitzgerald, J. F., Marnocha, R. S., and Weschler, C. H. Problems of aging: Conclusions derived from two years of interdisciplinary study of domiciliary members in a veterans administration center. *American Journal of Psychiatry,* 1956, *112,* 724-730.

Fox, C. The intelligence of old indigent persons residing within and without a public home for the aged. *American Journal of Psychology,* 1950, *63,* 110-112.

Friedsam, H. J. Reactions of older persons to disaster-caused losses: An hypothesis of relative deprivation. *Gerontologist,* 1961, *1,* 34-37.

Fried, M. Grieving for a lost home. In L. J. Duhl (Ed.), *The urban condition.* New

York: Basic Books, 1963.

Gitlitz, I. Morbidity and mortality in old age. Parts I-VIII. *Journal of the American Geriatrics Society,* 1956, *4,* 543-559, 708-721, 805-822, 896-908, 975-997; 1957, *5,* 32-48, 299-305.

Goffman, E. Asylums: *Essays on the social situation of mental patients and other inmates.* Garden City, N. Y.: Doubleday, 1961.

Goldfarb, A. I. Prevalence of psychiatric disorders in metropolitan old age and nursing homes. *Journal of the American Geriatrics Society,* 1962, *10,* 77-84.

Goldfarb, A. I., Shahinian, S. P., Turner, H. Death rates of relocated nursing home residents. Paper presented at the 17th annual meeting of Gerontological Society, New York, Nov., 1966.

Gottesman, L. E. Two treatment programs for the hospitalized aged. University of Michigan, Division of Gerontology, 1963, mimeographed.

Greenblatt, M., York, R. H., and Brown, E. L. (in collaboration with R. W. Hyde) *From a custodial to a therapeutic patient care in mental hospital: Exploration in social treatment.* New York: Russell Sage Foundation, 1955.

Jasnau, K. F. Individualized versus mass transfer of nonpsychotic geriatric patients from mental hospitals to nursing homes, with special reference to the death rate. *Journal of the American Geriatrics Society,* 1967, *15,* 280-284.

Kahana, E. The effects of age segregation on elderly psychiatric patients. Unpublished PhD dissertation, University of Chicago, 1968.

Kay, D., Norris, V., and Post, F. Prognosis in psychiatric disorders of the elderly. *Journal of Mental Science,* 1956, *102,* 129-140.

Kleemeier, R. W. Attitudes toward special settings for the aged. Paper presented at the International Seminar on the Social and Psychological Aspects of Aging, Berkeley, Calif., Aug., 1960.

Lakin, M. Formal characteristics of human figure drawings by institutionalized aged. *Journal of Gerontology,* 1960, *15,* 76-78.

Laverty, R. Nonresident aid—community versus institutional care for older people. *Journal of Gerontology,* 1950, *5,* 370-374.

Lawton, M., and Yaffe, S. Mortality, morbidity and voluntary change of residence. Paper presented at the meeting of the American Psychological Association, Washington, Sept., 1967.

Lepkowsky, J. R. The attitudes and adjustments of institutionalized and noninstitutionalized Catholic aged. Unpublished PhD dissertation, 1954. Abstracted in *Dissertation Abstracts,* 1955, *15,* 287-288.

Lieberman, M. A. The relationship of mortality rates to entering a home for the aged. *Geriatrics,* 1961, *16,* 515-519.

Lieberman, M. A., and Lakin, M. On becoming an aged institutionalized individual. In W. Donahue, C. Tibbitts, and R. Williams (Eds.), *Social and psychological processes of aging.* New York: Atherton Press, 1963.

Lieberman, M. A., Prock, V. N., and Tobin, S. S. Psychological effects of institutionalization. *Journal of Gerontology,* 1968, *23,* 343-353.

Lieberman, M. A. Adaptation and survival under stress in the aged. USPHS Grant No. HD-00364, University of Chicago in progress.

Lieberman, M. A., Tobin, S. S., and Slover, D. Effects of relocation on long-term geriatric patients. State of Illinois, Dept. of Mental Health Project No. 17-328, University of Chicago, in progress.

Lowenthal, M. F. *Lives in distress: The paths of the elderly to the psychiatric ward.* New York: Basic Books, 1964.

Mason, E. P. Some correlates of self-judgments of the aged. *Journal of Gerontology,* 1954, *9,* 324-337.

Miller, D., and Lieberman, M. A. The relationship of affect state adaptive reactions to stress. *Journal of Gerontology,* 1965, *20,* 492-497.

Montgomery, J. E. Living arrangements and housing of the rural aged in a central Pennsylvania community. In *Patterns of living and housing of middle aged and older people.* PHS No. 1496, 1965.

Pan, J. A comparison of factors in the personal adjustment of old people in the Protestant church homes for the aged and the old people living outside of institutions. Unpublished PhD dissertation, University of Chicago, 1950.

Pollack, M., Karp, E., Kahn, R. L., and Goldfarb, A. I. Perception of self in institutional aged subjects. I. Response patterns to mirror reflection. *Journal of Gerontology*, 1962, *17*, 405-408.

Roth, M. The natural history of mental disorders in old age. *Journal of Mental Science*, 1955, *101*, 281-301.

Shrut, S. D. Attitudes toward old age and death. *Mental Hygiene*, 1958, *42*, 259-266.

Shanas, E. *Family relationships of older people.* National Opinion Research Center, University of Chicago, Health Information Foundation, Series No. 20, Oct., 1961.

Stanton, A. H., and Schwartz, N. S. *The mental hospital.* New York: Basic Books, 1954.

Stotsky, B. A. A controlled study of factors in a successful adjustment of mental patients to a nursing home. *American Journal of Psychiatry*, 1967, *123*, 1243-1251.

Swenson, W. M. Attitudes toward death in an aged population. *Journal of Gerontology*, 1961, *16*, 49-52.

Tobin, S. S., and Etigson, E. C. The effects of stress on the earliest memory. *Archives of General Psychiatry*, 1968, *4*, 435-444.

Townsend, P. *The last refuge—a survey of residential institutions and homes for the aged in England and Wales.* London: Routledge & Kegan Paul, 1962.

Tuckman, J., and Lorge, I. The effect of institutionalization on attitudes toward old people. *Journal of Abnormal (& Social) Psychology*, 1952, *47*, 337-344.

Webb, M. A. Longitudinal sociopsychologic study of a randomly selected group of institutionalized veterans. *Journal of the American Geriatric Society*, 1959, *7*, 730-740.

Whittier, J. R., and Williams, D. The coincidence of constancy of mortality figures for aged psychotic patients admitted to state hospitals. *Journal of Nervous & Mental Diseases*, 1956, *124*, 618-620.

Yarrow, M. R., Blank, R., Quinn, O. W., Youmans, E. G., and Stein J. Social psychological characteristics of old age. In J. E. Birren, R. N. Butler, S. W. Greenhouse, L. Sokoloff, and M. R. Yarrow (Eds.), *Human aging.* Washington: U. S. Govt. Print. Office, 1963, PHS Publ. No. 986.

Chapter 42

PERSONALITY TRAITS AS PREDICTORS OF INSTITUTIONAL ADAPTION AMONG THE AGED

BARBARA F. TURNER, SHELDON S. TOBIN, AND MORTON A. LIEBERMAN

HEIGHTENED MORBIDITY and mortality rates have been associated with the entrance of aged into institutions (Aldrich and Mendkoff, 1963; Blenkner, 1967; Jasnau, 1967; Lawton and Yaffe, 1967; Lieberman, 1961; Miller and Lieberman, 1965; Shahinian, Goldfarb, and Turner, 1966). The interpretation of these adverse effects has usually related to preinstitutional characteristics of the aged that increase their vulnerability to the impact of relocation. Thus, the focus has been on psychological qualities, such as deficits in cognitive ability, denial of the impending event, or psychiatric illness. These are traits, therefore, that reduce the capacity of the aged individual to adapt to the stress-inducing qualities associated with relocation from community to institutional environments. This approach has, as an underlying assumption, that in any relocation experience, deficits in adaptive potential will predict vulnerability.

A different approach, however, is proposed in the present investigation which

Reprinted by permission from the *Journal of Gerontology*, 1972, *27*, 61-68.

will relate psychological qualities to the specificity of the environment to which the aged person is relocated. The assumption in this approach is that those aged with preinstitutional personality traits that are congruent with the specific demands of the relocation environment will experience a minimum of distress due to relocation. Such congruent personality traits may facilitate adaptation because the impact of relocation is lessened when there is a fit between traits and specific adaptive demands of the environment. In this approach the unit of analysis becomes the person-environment relationship in which situational demands determine the predictive power of personality traits.

A relationship between personality traits and situational demands has been reported for several settings. For example, in a report of adaptation to concentration camp internment, Wolf and Ripley (1947) suggested that a predisposition toward psychopathological ruthlessness (evidenced especially by former criminals who became inmates) maximized the chances for survival. Gunderson (1964) found that gregarious, active men showed better adjustment to Antarctic isolation in large stations where recreational facilities and many teammates were available than in stations where such opportunities and company were lacking. In general, a predisposition toward task-orientation facilitated adaptation in Antarctic isolation, whereas orientations toward social interaction and physical activity were maladaptive. In a discussion of types of prison inmates, Jackson (1966) suggested that chronic convicts whose criminal and noncriminal careers outside of prison are marked by persistent failure often find the prison to be the only place they can settle in some comfort. It is notable that many psychological attributes associated with favorable adaptation in special settings are not necessarily functional in everyday community living. The specific adaptive demands of the relocation environment may determine, therefore, the value of particular prerelocation personality traits.

To study this relationship between personality traits and institutional adaptation, a group of aged were studied who were in the process of moving from the community into homes for the aged. The specific hypothesis in this study was that those aged who were successfully adapted one year after institutionalization would have had at preadmission those traits identified as congruent with institutional living.

Materials and Methods

THE EXPERIMENTAL SAMPLE: The experimental sample consisted of eighty-five elderly persons who had placed themselves on waiting lists for three homes for the aged maintained by the Jewish Federation of Chicago and who were subsequently admitted. The age range was sixty-three to ninety-one years old (mean age was 78); there were twenty-four men and sixty-one women. At the time they were selected for study, all respondents were ambulatory, free of major incapacitating illnesses, and showed no gross signs of altered brain function (as defined by poor performance on several cognitive measures, Mental Status Questionnaire, Bender-Gestalt Test, Paired Associate Word Learning, Face-Hand). None was so incapacitated as to be unable to tolerate several hours of interview and tasks when on the waiting list. Personality traits were assessed when on the waiting list at three to twelve months before admission to one of the three homes (Md=4 months). Approximately twelve months after admission, assessment was made of adaptation to institutionalization. Of these eighty-five

aged, twenty-three (or 27%) were not interviewed at one year after admission because of death (13), morbidity (7), and refusals (3).

THE MEASURE OF ADAPTATION: The effort was made to develop a two-way classification of those who maintained a *status quo* over the period of institutionalization and of those who became seriously deteriorated compared to their initial status. The procedure used for classification consisted of first using change in functioning from preadmission to one year after institutionalization to place each respondent into one of four categories: (1) no change, or enhancement of physical, mental, or behavioral functioning; (2) some negative change in physical, mental, or behavioral functioning; (3) extreme negative change; and (4) death within the first year of institutionalization. Two members of the interviewing team, who had worked on the development of this classification system and made all judgments, selected three "hard to rate cases" for each other to rate. For all six cases there was exact agreement. The four levels were then collapsed to form the two-way classification of an intact survivor group from those placed in levels one or two, and of a vulnerable, or nonintact morbid-dead, group from those placed in levels three and four. Of the eighty-five aged, forty-four were thus placed into an intact survivor group and forty-one into a vulnerable group.

THE INSTITUTIONAL ENVIRONMENT: The three Jewish homes for the aged are quite similar (Pincus, 1968), varying primarily in size, 142 to 286 beds, and in birthplace of residents, one home attracting German and American born and the other two homes attracting Eastern European Jews. The relocation environment is one of congregate living with other chronically ill aged in a hospital-type environment.

Among available institutions for the aged, these homes are considered excellent and efforts are made to reduce their totality through unrestricted visiting hours and opportunities for trips into the community, if the resident is not too physically impaired. Strong efforts are made by staff to keep residents engaged in activities and interaction, and there is tolerance of complaining and individuality within the limits of institutional rules and regulations. Interaction, even if combatative at times, becomes a criterion of adjustment, whereas disengagement is viewed as deleterious. Residents quickly become aware of the reward system, attempting to define themselves as engaged and as unlike their more debilitated peers who, like themselves, are preoccupied with physical integration. Fear of decline and enforced living with other ill aged not of one's own choosing, as well as dependency on a custodial staff, eventuate in peer relationships that tend to be distant and conflictful.

SELECTION OF PERSONALITY TRAITS CONGRUENT WITH ADAPTATION TO INSTITUTIONALIZATION: Previous literature on institutionalization (Goffman, 1961; Martin, 1955; Sommer and Osmond, 1960; Townsend, 1962) had suggested several dimensions of potential importance for adaptation, such as activity-passivity and trust-mistrust of others. Additional dimensions were suggested by a previous study of thirty-seven residents of the homes for the aged; the homes that comprise the relocation environments for the eighty-five aged in the experimental sample (Lieberman, Prock, and Tobin, 1968). This earlier sample of thirty-seven was a highly select group of aged who had "made it in the homes," having managed to weather the assumed disruptive impact of institutionalization and retaining a level of functioning rather similar to the level that they had at

admission to the homes three to five years previously. Also they were comparable to the experimental sample when on the waiting list on such variables as marital status, number of living children, and level of cognitive deficit. For these thirty-seven institutionalized aged, the earlier study suggested that "old-timers" could be characterized in terms of preoccupation with the body and its functioning, distrust of other residents and a "distancing" (or lack of engagement) with other residents. For example, when these "old-timers" were asked for their advice to a new resident, many recommended that the new resident avoid interaction with the other residents because interaction would only prove unrewarding and lead to interpersonal conflict. As shown in Table 42-I adopting a distrustful stance, as well as avoiding interpersonal contact with other residents, may indeed facilitate institutional adaptation by diminishing noxious and conflictful interaction with other residents.

A further clinical analysis of extensive data on these thirty-seven "old-timers" suggested additional dimensions to those outlined in the literature or suggested in the earlier study by Lieberman, *et al.* (1968). The portrait that was then developed from this clinical analysis encompassed nine traits that seemed of particular importance in describing the "old-timers." As shown in Table 42-I, these nine traits are activity-passivity, aggression, narcissistic body image, authoritarianism, status drive, distrust of others, nonempathy, extrapunitive, and nonintrapunitive. Of importance is that the traits assumed to relate to successful institutional adaptation, as is shown in Table 42-I are not traits uniformly considered characteristic of adaptive potential or competence in coping with stress.

Five-point scales were developed for each of the nine personality traits, using different portions of the data for each assessment (Lieberman and Tobin, 1968). Each scale was rated separately, and each was constructed to distribute the sample evenly among the five points. Interjudge reliability on twenty interviews ranged from .78 to .90 across the nine traits. To verify an earlier assumption that "old-timers" defined the high end of each scale, a subsample of nine respondents from the institutional sample of thirty-seven was rated by a rater who was not aware of the assumption that these respondents were hypothesized to be high on congruence. Seventy percent of these ratings were toward the congruent end of the scale suggesting the appropriateness of the earlier assumption.

Results

The correlations among the traits, as shown in Table 42-II ranged from $-.28$ to $+.54$; with an interquartile range of $-.09$ to $+.27$. Because of this relative independence of the individual traits, a total congruence score was generated by summing the scores for all nine traits, range nine to forty-five. Of the nine traits, only nonintrapunitiveness was not significantly correlated with the total congruence score, which correlated from .34 to .66 with the other traits. This total congruence score was considered to assess the level of general fit between the personality pattern of an aged respondent and the optimal congruence pattern.

To further specify the nature of the relationship between outcome after one year of institutionalization and congruence scores that were assessed at preadmission, the nine congruence traits were submitted to a principal component factor analysis with orthogonal varimax rotations. This procedure produces factors that are independent of each other. The factor analysis

produced four independent congruence factors. To ascertain the meaning of each factor, the congruence traits that loaded more than .40 on a given factor were inspected, as shown in Table 42-III where the factors are named and briefly described. Because the factors are zero-order correlated with each other, their individual correlations with total congruence, as shown also in Table 42-III, reflect their relative importance in the interpretation of the total score. While total congruence is positively correlated with each factor, high scores on the total congruence measure are more related to (1) authoritarian and extrapunitive tendencies, and to (2) preoccupation with appearance and physical functioning, combined with high activity and considerable aggressiveness; than to (3) an unreflective, even bland stance, with little blame of self and low capacity for empathy with others, and to (4) high distrust of others in combination with tendencies to blame others and relative disinterest in status striving.

The total congruence score was then correlated, for the eighty-five aged, with other available scores that were assumed to measure adaptive potential. As shown in Table 42-IV the total congruence score was independent of cognitive functioning $(r = -.09)$. However, congruence was inversely related to denial of impending institutionalization $(r = -.29)$, suggesting that those with higher congruence tend to deny less, but as suggested by the correlation with the mental health measure $(r = -.32)$ to have more psychopathology. Consistent with the negative relationship with mental health, congruence is negatively associated with feelings of well-being $(r = -.21)$ and positively associated with anxiety $(r = .26)$. The presence of psychopathology and a dysphoric mood, however, does not appear to become manifest in the

TABLE 42-I

THE RELATIONSHIP OF NINE CONGRUENT CHARACTERISTICS TO SUCCESSFUL ADAPTATION TO INSTITUTIONAL LIFE

Variable	Characteristics Congruent with the Institutional Setting	Relationship of Congruent Characteristics to Successful Institutional Adaptation
Activity-Passivity	High activity	Institutional staff rewards residents who are active participants in institutional functions and penalizes more passive, withdrawn residents.
Aggression	High aggression	In a setting in which many residents are physically and/or mentally incapacitated to some degree an aggressive resident is best able to meet his needs because he is able to assertively reach out for himself.
Narcissistic body image	High narcissistic	Because sick, physically unattractive residents tend to be avoided by other residents, an orientation toward projecting an attractive appearance is rewarded by overtures and admiration from other residents. This tangible differentiation of the self from unattractive residents enhances self-esteem.
Authoritarian	Authoritarianism rather than equalitarianism	Orientation toward dominance-submission is facilitated by the need to differentiate the self from debilitated residents; even "helping" other residents confers a dominant position. Identification with strength and scorn for weakness, or egocentric focus, may be helpful in obtaining one's "share" of available resources.
Status drive	High status drive	Orientation toward identification with staff rather than residents, by means of superordination over other residents, is encouraged by the staff-resident status differentiation; staff hierarchy within the staff; and explicit efforts by staff to develop and reward resident "leaders." Staff controls more rewards and are more attractive than other residents who are often debilitated and personally unattractive.
Distrust of others	High distrust of others	Distrust may be functional for institutional living because the debilitation of many residents decreases their ability to respond to interpersonal overtures, so that one may often be disappointed about not receiving "appropriate" responses from such overtures if one does not soon learn to distrust others. "Old-timers" suggest that most other residents should be avoided because interpersonal contacts are likely to be conflictful. Distrust of others may thus reduce interpersonal conflict and diminish unrealistic expectations of pleasant and rewarding interchange.

Nonempathy	Disinterest or disregard for the viewpoint of others is enhanced by efforts to avoid identification with illness and debilitation.
Extrapunitive	A tendency to blame others increases engagement with others and focuses staff attention on the self.
Nonintrapunitive	High self-blame further diminishes self-esteem within the institutional setting and causes a reduction in the type of outer-directed interpersonal activity that is rewarded by the other residents and institutional staff.

TABLE 42-II
CORRELATIONS AMONG CONGRUENCE TRAITS AND BETWEEN TOTAL CONGRUENCE AND TRAITS

	Act.	Aggr.	Narc. Body Image	Auth.	Stat. Drive	Dis-trust	Non-emp.	Extra-punit.	Non-intrapunit.
Component Traits:									
Activity	1.00								
Aggression	.26	1.00							
Narc. body image	.36	.35	1.00						
Authoritarianism	.04	.19	.04	1.00					
Status drive	.25	.40	.27	.28	1.00				
Distrust of others	−.09	.04	−.01	.33	−.13	1.00			
Non-empathy	−.14	−.13	−.21	.36	−.28	.33	1.00		
Extrapunitive	−.02	.18	−.06	.54	.21	.52	.27	1.00	
Nonintrapunitive	−.14	−.12	−.03	−.09	−.26	−.08	.26	−.13	1.00
Total Congruence	.40	.55	.45	.66	.44	.46	.34	.61	.14

TABLE 42-III
CONGRUENCE FACTORS

Factor	Primary Loadings		Salient Characteristics	Correlation with Total Congruence
Punitive-authoritarian	Authoritarian	.84	High is authoritarian and punitive as well as somewhat competive	.69
	Extrapunitive	.68		
	Status drive	.59		
Aggressiveness	Other-directed body image	.84	High is active, outgoing, dominant and interested in activities of others	.59
	Activity	.72		
	Aggression	.59		
Nonreflective	Nonintrapunitive	.87	High is unreflective; tends to be bland and meek in appearance	.23
	Nonempathy	.64		
Unfriendly	Distrust	.91	High is unfriendly, introverted, extrapunitive and disinterested in interpersonal contact	.32
	Extrapunitive	.50		
	Status drive	−.41		

quality of interpersonal relationships as reflected in the positive association between congruence and quality of relations (r = .29). On the other hand, while the quality of relations may tend toward positive for those with high congruence, they do not necessarily describe themselves as dominant (r = .04) but do describe themselves as less loving (r = −.29) or more cold and distant, which is consistent with the direction of the traits that comprise the total congruence score. The modest association (r = .15) with adequacy of examples for the Self-Sort Task suggests an ability to use the environment for feedback in the present.

The intact and vulnerable groups after one year of institutionalization were compared on congruence scores that were assessed at preadmission. As shown in Table 42-V, these two outcome groups were significantly different on the total congruence score (t = 4.32, p<0.01) with the positive outcome group, the intact, having a mean score of 30.1 and the negative outcome group, the vulnerable, having a mean score of 25.6. Comparing the two outcome groups for each of the four independent congruence factors revealed that, for each of these factors, the intact group had more congruent scores than the vulnerable group. The outcome groups were significantly different on only one of the congruence factors, aggressiveness (t = 4.89, p<0.01), with the intact group having a mean score of +.46 and the vulnerable group having a mean score of −.49. Aggressiveness remained as a statistically significant predictor when variables such as cognitive adequacy and expectations were removed in a step-down analysis (Lieberman, 1971).

Discussion

A group of aged that had successfully adapted to the relocation-stress of institutionalization, therefore, were found to be different from a group that was more vulnerable to this stress on those personality traits that had been generated by the congruence approach. These traits, based on the fit between the person and the specific environment of relocation, would not typically be those considered indices of adaptive potential, an impression that was confirmed by the correlations between the total congruence score and other measures for these eighty-five aged. The traits identified as congruent with adaptive demands, however, would tend to vary from one relocation situation to another because relocation environments vary in their adaptive demands. Also, for any specific relocation situation some of these congruent traits, as was found in this study, may be inversely related to dimensions, or measures, that typically comprise adaptive potential. Furthermore, congregate-living environments often make adaptive demands that reward coping styles that are dysfunctional for everyday community living.

These data suggest that for the individual undergoing the stress of institutional adaptation, congruent traits facilitate positive adaptation. Most likely the initial impact of the stressor event is less a psychological stressor for these congruent individuals. If, however, the adaptational style of the person undergoing a radical environmental change is consistent with the style rewarded in the new environment, then for this person it may be less of a radical psychological change; and thus there would be less of a subjective experience of the potentially stressful event, as well as less adverse psychological effects.

To explore such a relationship in this study between congruent traits and the subjective experience of initial institutional impact, impact ratings were generated from reports by interviewers and institutional staff of the aged respondents' reac-

TABLE 42-IV

TOTAL CONGRUENCE AND ADAPTIVE POTENTIAL

(CORRELATIONS ABOVE r = ± .21 ARE SIGNIFICANT AT $p<0.05$)

ADAPTIVE POTENTIAL

Dimension	Measures	Description of Measure	Correlation With Total Congruence
I Cognitive functioning	Impairment	Defect level established for six tasks, and a respondent's score is the number of tasks on which the defect level is reached; range 0—6. Tasks; Mental Status Questionnaire (Kahn, Pollack, and Goldfarb, 1961); Paired-Word Association Test (Inglis, 1959); Clock-Time Estimate of One Minute; Bender-Gestalt Design Copying scored by Pascal and Suttell (1951) System; Murray TAT Cards 1, 2, 6BM, 7BM, 10 and 17BM scored by Dana (1955) System; Reitman Stick Figures (Reitman and Robertson, 1950) scored for number of different responses (Slover, 1967).	—.09
II Unrealistic expectations	Denial of impending institutionalization	Four Institutional TAT Cards (Lieberman and Lakin, 1963), each scored on three-point scale for denial of latent content (Turner, 1969).	—.29
III Mental health	Q-sort description	The 100-item Personality Q-Sort was developed by Block (1961) and used by Alt (1968) in describing behavior of each respondent. By sorting the 100 items into nine piles, from low to high descriptive, a score of one to nine is generated for each of the 100 items. In correlating these 100 scores with the "optimum" profile, the coefficient becomes the score for each respondent, where higher scores reflect a greater similarity with the optimum profile.	—.32
IV Affect states	Life Satisfaction Rating (LSR)	LSR development by Neugarten, Havighurst, and Tobin (1961) consists of the sum of five-point rating scales: Zest, Resolution, Congruence between Desired and Achieved Goals, Self-concept, and Mood.	—.21
	Cattell Anxiety	Cattell's (1962) 16PF self-report form consists of ninety items, six items for each of Cattell's fifteen traits (omitting Intelligence, which was not appropriate for this sample). Anxiety is a global factor, computed by summing traits.	.26
	Experiencing Scale	Gorney (1966) scoring of responses to items on eight feelings, or affect states, such as loneliness and happiness, using Gendlin and Tomlinson (1967) seven-point Experiencing Scale for responses to each affect state; and then summing across all eight states.	.17

V Interpersonal	Quality	Interviewers' judgments of respondent interaction during interviews. Sum of five-point scales for each of five areas: depth, warmth, motivated, cooperative, and spontaneous.	—.29
VI Self-system	Dominance	Lieberman-Rosner Self-Sort Task consists of forty-eight self-descriptive items, using the Leary (1957) system to develop three items for each of the sixteen dimensions. Task is first to select from the forty-eight items those that describe self, which generate dominance-love scores. Then the respondent is asked to give an example in the present for each of the selected items, usually about thirty of the forty-eight. Judgment is made of each example as to adequacy in meeting the task requirement for example-in-present, and then total score computed from percentages of types of examples (whether in present, from past, conviction of self, "wished for" description, or distortion) (Rosner, 1968).	.04
	Love		.29
	Adequacy of examples		.15

TABLE 42-V

CONGRUENCE COMPARED FOR THE INTACT AND VULNERABLE GROUPS

Congruence Measure as Assessed at Preadmission	The Intact (N = 44)		The Vulnerable (N = 41)		Mn Diff.	t	p
	Mn	SD	Mn	SD			
Total congruence	30.1	4.7	25.6	5.0	4.5	4.32	<0.01
Component traits							
Activity-passivity	3.4	1.0	2.4	1.3	1.0	3.92	<0.01
Aggression	3.5	1.3	2.4	1.4	1.1	3.66	<0.01
Narcissistic body image	3.6	1.2	2.7	1.3	.9	3.24	<0.05
Authoritarianism	3.3	1.4	2.9	1.2	.4	1.57	NS
Status drive	3.4	1.2	3.0	1.4	.4	1.26	NS
Distrust of others	3.3	1.4	3.2	1.3	.1	0.35	NS
Nonempathy	3.3	1.3	3.2	1.2	.1	0.46	NS
Extrapunitive	3.2	1.2	2.9	1.3	.3	1.19	NS
Nonintrapunitive	3.1	1.3	2.9	1.4	.2	0.81	NS
Factor 1. Punitive-authoritarian	.16	1.00	—.17	1.00	.33	1.50	NS
Factor 2. Aggressive	.49	1.00	—.46	.81	.95	4.89	<0.01
Factor 3. Non-reflective	.12	.92	—.13	1.01	.26	1.19	NS
Factor 4. Unfriendly	.04	1.01	—.05	1.01	.09	.42	NS

tions in the first days and weeks of institutional life. Respondents' "stress reactions" were of several types: both interviewer and staff reported disturbances in affect, disturbances in behavior, and physiological changes. The assumption was made that these reports reflected the severity or degree of stress of the initial institutional impact. However, congruent traits were found to be unrelated to impact ratings. The best explanation of this finding is that data for the impact ratings were gathered after the end of the impact phase (mean = 9.53 weeks postadmission), so that the subjective experience of the initial impact was not captured. On the other hand, congruent traits were found to be related to an index of physical decline at nine weeks postadmission, suggesting that for the aged person without such congruent traits, the initial distress and disorganization can be particularly destructive because of physical fragility that may lead to consequent morbidity and death.

The particular trait factor found to be associated with successful institutional adaptation in this study loaded highly on activity, aggression, and narcissistic body image. This cluster of traits suggests that a vigorous, if not combatative, style is facilitory for adaptation. It is a style of being intrusive into the environment: of actively seeking interaction, of aggressively relating, and of insisting on responsivity from others regarding physical attractiveness. At a more covert level, it suggests a narcissistic-hostile and controlling orientation toward the institutional environment.

Summary

Adaptation to institutional life, or vulnerability as measured one year after admission, was related to personality traits of elderly persons awaiting entrance into homes for the aged. These were traits that were generated by a congruence approach which assumed that the fit between the person's coping style and the demands of the specific relocation environment facilitate adaptation. An assessment of long-term institutionalized aged who had successfully adjusted to institutional life indicated nine personality traits to be characteristic. Interviews with eighty-five aged awaiting institutionalization were then rated on the nine variables. One year after institutionalization, these aged were then placed into an intact group (N = 44) or a vulnerable group (N = 41). These groups were significantly different on the total congruence score; and, while all four independent factors generated by a factor analysis of the nine component traits were in the hypothesized direction only one, that of aggressiveness, reached the .05 level of significance.

These results suggest the need to consider adaptive demands of the specific relocation environment in the prediction of vulnerability. In focusing on the varying demands of different environments, congruent traits may be identified that are not typically considered as having adaptive potential. The congruent traits identified as predictive for the present relocation environment suggest that a vigorous, if not hostile-narcissistic, preadmission style is related to intactness one year after institutionalization.

REFERENCES

Aldrich, C. K., and Mendkoff, E. Relocation of the aged and disabled: A mortality study. *Journal of the American Geriatric Society,* 1963, *11*, 185-194.

Alt, S. Personality as measured by Q-sort as a predictor of adaptation to institutionalization in the aged. Unpublished MA dissertation, Committee on Human Development, University of Chicago, 1968.

Blenkner, M. Environmental change and the aging individual. *Gerontologist,* 1967, *7*, 101-105.

Block, J. *The Q-sort method in personality assessment and psychiatric research.* Springfield, Ill.: Charles C Thomas, 1961.

Cattell, R. B. *Handbook supplement for Form C of the sixteen personality factor test* (2nd ed). Champaign, Ill.: Institute for Personality and Ability Testing, 1962.

Dana, R. H. Clinical diagnosis and objective TAT scoring. *Journal of Abnormal Psychology,* 1955, *50*, 19-25.

Gendlin, E. T., and Tomlinson, T. M. The process conception and its measurement. In C. Rogers (Ed.), *The therapeutic relationship and its impact.* Madison: University of Wisconsin Press, 1967.

Goffman, E. *Asylums.* New York: Doubleday, 1961.

Gorney, J. E. The function and correlates of experiencing among the aged. Unpublished MA dissertation, Committee on Human Development, University of Chicago, 1966.

Gunderson, E. K. E. Personal history characteristics of Antarctic volunteers. *Journal of Social Psychology,* 1964, *64*, 325-332.

Inglis, J. A paired-associate learning test for use with elderly psychiatric patients. *Journal of Mental Science,* 1959, *105*, 440-443.

Jackson, B. Who goes to prison: Caste and careerism in crime. *Atlantic Monthly,* 1966, *1*, 52-57.

Jasnau, K. F. Individualized versus mass transfer of nonpsychotic geriatric patients from mental hospitals to nursing homes, with special reference to the death rate. *Journal of the American Geriatric Society,* 1967, *15*, 280-284.

Kahn, R. L., Pollack, M., and Goldfarb, A. I. Factors related to individual differences in mental status of institutionalized aged. In P. H. Hoch and J. Zubin (Eds.), *Psychopathology of aging.* New York: Grune & Stratton, 1961.

Lawton, M. P., and Yaffe, S. Mortality, morbidity, and voluntary change of residence by older people. Paper presented at Annual Meeting of the American Psychological Association, Washington, Sept. 5, 1967.

Leary, T. *Interpersonal diagnosis of personal-*

ity. New York: Ronald Press, 1957.

Lieberman, M. A. Relationship of mortality rates to entrance to a home for the aged. *Geriatrics*, 1961, *16*, 515-519.

Lieberman, M. A., and Lakin, M. On becoming an institutionalized person. In R. H. Williams, C. Tibbitts. and W. Donahue (Eds.), *Processes of aging*. Vol. I. *Social and psychological perspectives*. New York: Atherton, 1963.

Lieberman, M. A., Prock, V. N., and Tobin, S. S. Psychological effects of institutionalization. *Journal of Gerontology*, 1968, *23*, 343-353.

Lieberman, M. A., and Tobin, S. S. Adaptation and survival under stress in the aged. Memo on file with the Committee on Human Development, University of Chicago, 1968.

Lieberman, M. A. Some issues in studying psychological predictors of survival. In F. C. Jeffers and E. Palmore (Eds.), *Prediction of life span*. Lexington, Mass.: Heath, 1971.

Martin, D. Institutionalization. *Lancet*, 1955, *269*, 1188-1190.

Miller, D., and Lieberman, M. A. The relationship of affect state and adaptive capacity to reactions to stress. *Journal of Gerontology*, 1965, *20*, 492-497.

Neugarten, B. L., Havighurst, R. J., and Tobin, S. S. The measurement of life satisfaction. *Journal of Gerontology*, 1961, *16*, 134-143.

Pascal, G. R., and Suttell, B. J. *The Bender-Gestalt Test; quantification and validity for adults*. New York: Grune & Stratton, 1951.

Pincus, A. M. Toward a conceptual framework for studying institutional environment in homes for the aged. Unpublished doctoral dissertation, School of Social Work, University of Wisconsin, 1968.

Reitman, F., and Robertson, J. P. Reitman's Pin-Man Test; a means of disclosing impaired conceptual thinking. *Journal of Nervous & Mental Disorders*, 1950, *112*, 498-510.

Rosner, A. Stress and the maintenance of self-concept in the aged. Unpublished doctoral dissertation, Committee on Human Development, University of Chicago, 1968.

Shahinian, S. F., Goldfarb, A. I., and Turner, M. Death rate in relocated residents of nursing homes. Paper presented at the 19th Annual Meeting of Gerontological Society, New York, Nov. 4, 1966.

Slover, D. The relationship between rigidity and adaptation to the stress of institutionalization in the aged. Unpublished MA dissertation, Committee on Human Development, University of Chicago, 1967.

Sommer, T., and Osmond, H. Symptoms of institutional care. *Social Problems*, 1960, *3* 244-253.

Townsend, P. *The last refuge—a survey of resi dential institutions and homes for the aged in England and Wales*. London: Routledge & Kegan Paul, 1962.

Turner, B. F. Psychological predictors of adaptation to the stress of institutionalization in the aged. Unpublished doctoral dissertation Committee on Human Development, University of Chicago, 1969.

Wolf, S., and Ripley, H. A. Reactions among Allied prisoners of war subjected to three years of imprisonment and torture by the Japanese. *American Journal of Psychiatry* 1947, *104*, 180-193.

Chapter 43

THE IMPACT OF RE-LOCATION UPON MOR-TALITY RATES OF INSTITUTIONALIZED AGED PERSONS

Elliot Markus, Margaret Blenkner, Martin Bloom, and Thomas Downs

STUDIES BY Aldrich and Mendkoff (1963), Aleksandrowiscz (1961), Killian (1970), and Kral, Grad, and Berenson (1968) have suggested that relocation of aged persons has negative effects and for some people is accompanied by increased morbidity and mortality. A dissenting note is sounded by Miller and Lieberman (1965), who were unable to discover any significant differences between postrelocation mortality and that of the control group (see especially Blenkner, 1967, for an overview of these studies). Markus, Blenkner, Bloom, and Downs (1970) found relocation to have differential effects, negative for some persons and positive for others.

In an attempt to hold constant the effects of institutionalization so as to study relocation effects *per se* on mortality rates, Markus *et al.* (1970) studied the transfer of an already institutionalized population from one building to another in a recent move of a home for the aged. Relocation of this type had a clear, although differential, association with mortality in the sample

Reprinted by permission from the *Journal of Gerontology*, 1971, *26*, 537-541.

studied: (*a*) significantly greater mortality than expected for males and persons of both sexes admitted to the home under age seventy-five, and (*b*) significantly less mortality than expected for females above admission-age eighty. (Admission-age equals age at time of admission; in general, admission-age is less than true age, i.e. age at last birthday.)

The present report is based upon the transfer of the entire populations of two homes for the aged from old downtown buildings to new suburban plants with modern facilities.

Institutional moves such as those studied here are often accompanied by huge inputs by the staff of stress-alleviating efforts and are capped off by the conveniences of an ultramodern plant and equipment. Some aged will be particularly stressed by the relocation, others may soon get over that stress and delight in the extra attention and new facilities, and others may actually benefit from the break in routine and boredom which relocation offers. Whatever the reasons, we may expect variations in postrelocation mortality, both greater and lesser than the expected mortality rate had relocation not occurred.

The Two Samples

The samples included the entire populations of the Jewish Orthodox Home for the Aged, Cleveland (JOHA) and the Hebrew Home of Greater Washington, Washington, DC (HHA), a total of 105 males and 268 females, who were relocated on April 9, 1968, and May 20, 1969, respectively. HHA was picked as the second sample, as it seemed to match JOHA closely in age-sex-race and geographic structure and was undergoing an essentially similar relocation.

Relocatees ranged in age (age at last

TABLE 43-I

AGE AND SEX DISTRIBUTION FOR TWO SAMPLES, BY PERCENTAGE OF TOTAL
SAMPLE

Age	Males		Females	
	JOHA N 59 (%)	*HHA* N 46 (%)	*JOHA* N 144 (%)	*HHA* N 124 (%)
<70	2.5	3.0	6.4	4.7
70 — 74	1.5	2.4	6.9	7.1
75 — 79	5.9	6.5	19.2	19.5
80 — 84	9.4	6.5	24.6	21.3
85 — 89	7.4	5.3	14.3	13.6
>90	2.5	3.0	3.9	7.1
Total	29.1	26.6	70.9	73.4

birthday) at time of move from sixty-four to ninety-nine at JOHA and from fifty-seven to ninety-nine at HHA, with the age and sex distribution as presented in Table 43-I. Table 43-I shows remarkable similarity in the age-sex structure of the two samples. The proportion of all males to all females is on the order of three to seven with proportionately more females in the higher age group for both samples.

The two samples were similar with respect to both age and years of residence in the home (Table 43-II).

TABLE 43-II

MEAN AGES AND RESIDENCY EXPERIENCE
BY SEX OF TWO SAMPLES

	Mean Years	
	Males	Females
Age		
JOHA	81.2	79.7
HHA	79.7	80.7
Residency experience		
JOHA	3.2	3.3
HHA	3.0	3.7

Postrelocation Mortality Rates

The impact of relocation was judged against a control population, defined as those populations alive in each of the homes taken severally on fifteen census dates corresponding to the month and day of the move in each of the past fifteen years. The mortality experience of these populations was examined from the records of the home and used to estimate the expected mortality, had relocation *not* occurred. Breakdown of the control population and the sample to be studied into age-sex-residency categories yields relatively small subsamples. *Death rates either greater or lesser than those in fourteen of the fifteen control years were considered as significantly different from the expected rates.*

There are some differences in the baseline mortality rates for the two samples. To compare the impact of relocation upon mortality rates, standardization of rates is appropriate. This is easily done by dividing the *observed mortality rate following relocation (O)* by the *expected mortality rate had relocation not occurred (E)*, i.e. O/E (E, the expected mortality rate had relocation not occurred, is estimated by the mean mortality rate for the 15 control years).

Whereas the expected mortality rate for JOHA males, in the first six months following relocation, was .128, the actual observed rate was .182, almost $1\frac{1}{2}$ times as high. For HHA males the ratio 1.22 is somewhat less but in the same direction (Table 43-III). Female rates show differences in direction across samples with HHA females having the greatest proportionate increase in mor

TABLE 43-III

RATIO OF OBSERVED TO EXPECTED MORTALITY FOR SIX MONTHS, BY SEX, FOR TWO SAMPLES

	Males		Females	
	Obs/Exp	*Ratio*	*Obs/Exp*	*Ratio*
JOHA	.182/.128	1.42	.083/.107	0.78
HHA	.156/.128	1.22	.116/.071	1.63

tality (1.63) and JOHA females showing a decrease (0.78), following relocation, the only group with such a decrease. Female rates in every case were lower than male rates, reflecting general superiority in longevity.

Although the mortality ratio, O/E, provides a useful way in which to compare postrelocation mortality across samples, it may be grossly biased by chance variability in postrelocation mortality rates.

Significant deviations from the estimated (adjusted mean) probability of death were derived from the yearly fluctuations of the fifteen control years. Death rates *either greater* or *smaller* than those in fourteen of the fifteen control years were considered significant, not solely due to chance. In effect, this test requires simple rank ordering of the mortality rates of each of the fifteen control years and that of the sixteenth year following relocation. If postrelocation mortality ranks either first or second, i.e. *greater* than that of the other fifteen or fourteen years, respectively, that rate is considered significantly *greater*. If the rank of the postrelocation mortality is fifteen or sixteen, i.e. *smaller* than that of the other fourteen or fifteen years, respectively, that rate is considered to be significantly *smaller*.

Table 43-IV illustrates this statistical test with findings from the total samples.

The observed postrelocation mortality rates of JOHA males and HHA females each had the rank order of *one* when compared to the mortality rates for the same

groups over the fifteen control years. These postrelocation mortality rates are considered significant and are likely due to factors beyond chance. Analysis of all males and all females as a group yielded conflicting results between the replicates; postrelocation mortality was significantly greater following relocation for JOHA males but not for HHA males and significantly greater following relocation for HHA females but not for JOHA females. Partialization by age and residency experience helps to expose some patterns.

TABLE 43-IV

RANK OF SIX-MONTH POSTRELOCATION MORTALITY RATES BY SEX FOR TWO SAMPLES

	Males	Females
JOHA	1*	12*
HHA	5	1*

*Significant ($p<0.13$).

Age

Table 43-V presents the ratio of observed to expected mortality rates by age and sex.

Among males, high mortality ratios occur in the age group seventy-five through seventy-nine for both JOHA and HHA (1.9 and 1.5, respectively). Consistently high ratios occur for males over eighty (1.2 and 1.8, respectively) and postrelocation mortality rate of HHA males over eighty is significant. For males under seventy-five years of age, no consistent pattern emerges.

TABLE 43-V

RATIO OF OBSERVED TO EXPECTED MORTALITY AND RANK OF OBSERVED
MORTALITY BY AGE AND SEX, FOR TWO SAMPLES

	JOHA			HHA		
Age[a]	Ratio	Rank	N[b]	Ratio	Rank	N[b]
Males						
Under 75	1.4	6	8	0.0	16*	9
75 — 79	1.9	3	12	1.5	4	11
80 — over	1.2	8	35	1.8	2*	25
Females						
Under 75	0.8	8	27	2.5	1*	20
75 — 79	2.3	1*	39	1.9	3	33
80 — over	0.6	15*	78	1.0	10	69

[a]Age equals age at last birthday. The apparent inconsistencies between data presented in this table and the data in text derive from the different definitions of age. Admission-age equals age at date of admission.

[b]N equals number of relocated persons.

*Significant.

TABLE 43-VI

MORTALITY RATIOS AND RANKS FOR UNDER 75s, BY SEX, FOR TWO SAMPLES

	JOHA			HHA		
Age	Ratio	Rank	N[a]	Ratio	Rank	N[a]
Males						
Under 70	2.6	2[b]	5	0.0	15[b]	5
70 — 74	0.0	5	3	0.0	15.5*	4
Females						
Under 70	0.0	5	13	2.1	2*	8
70 — 74	1.6	3.5	14	2.7	2*	12

[a]N equals number of relocated persons.

[b]Not significant due to ties.

*Significant.

TABLE 43-VII

MORTALITY RATIOS AND RANKS BY SEX AND RESIDENCY EXPERIENCE, FOR
TWO SAMPLES

Res. exp.	JOHA			HHA		
(Years)	Ratio	Rank	N[a]	Ratio	Rank	N[a]
Males						
Under 1	1.1	6	13	0.6	10	10
1 through 5	1.7	1.5*	30	2.1	1*	28
6 or more	1.3	6	12	0.0	2[b]	7
Females						
Under 1	1.0	9.5	32	1.5	6	32
1 through 5	0.7	13.5	81	1.3	4	55
6 or more	0.8	11.5	31	2.1	2*	35

[a]N equals number of relocated persons.

[b]Not significant due to ties.

*Significant.

Among females, consistently high ratios occur among the same age groups as males, where mortality for those seventy-five through seventy-nine following relocation is relatively high (2.3 and 1.9, respectively) and for those over eighty years of age where mortality is relatively low (0.6 and 1.0, respectively). Of these, JOHA females aged seventy-five through seventy-nine had significantly *greater* mortality, and JOHA females aged eighty and over significantly *less* mortality following relocation. For females less than seventy-five years of age, no consistent pattern emerges.

Although a closer look at the "under seventy-five" age group (Table 43-VI) yields cells too small for inferences, the consistent pattern appears to continue among seventy- through seventy-four-year-olds, lower postrelocation male mortality and higher female mortality. The inconsistencies seem to occur among the residents of the youngest age group, under seventy years of age.

In general, there is great variability of illness and infirmity among the younger admissions to old age homes, and this variability may help explain the rather erratic results among this under-seventy group, particularly at JOHA. Typically, in the month or two preceeding relocation, admissions are curtailed; it is likely that HHA cut back on convalescent admissions, i.e. low risk females and high risk males.

Table 43-VII presents the mortality ratios and ranks by residency experience. Postrelocation mortality is relatively high for all JOHA males and HHA females. Among newly admitted persons, HHA females have the highest ratio; it is to be noted that this ratio is based upon a relatively low expected mortality rate, .081. If, indeed, the HHA admission policies were more selective prior to relocation, with fewer low risk females, then the 1.5 ratio can

be interpreted as a result of the interaction effect of relocation and the newly admitted females of relatively higher risk. Conversely, the curtailment of high risk male admissions would serve to explain some portion of the low postrelocation mortality among newly admitted HHA males.

Males with one through five years' residency experience at both JOHA and HHA have significantly greater postrelocation mortality, as do females of six or more years' residency experience at HHA.

Summary

Several patterns and several inconsistencies have been noted between the two samples (105 males and 268 females), with the inconsistencies possibly due to chance variability and/or possibly related to different admission policies at the two homes. The patterns which have been replicated include both higher and lower postrelocation mortality.

The data in this study indicate that age, sex, and residency experience *alone* are not sufficient predictors of postrelocation mortality and that factors, such as physical and mental status, attitude to change, and degree of hopefulness need to be studied for possible inclusion in a multivariate discriminate model which might make for sufficient predictability.

REFERENCES

Aldrich, C., and Mendkoff, E. Relocation of the aged and disabled: A mortality study. *Journal of American Geriatric Society*, 1963, *11*, 185-194.

Alesksandrowicz, D. Fire and its aftermath on a geriatric ward. *Bulletin Menninger Clinic*, 1961, *25*, 23-32.

Blenkner, M. Environmental change and the aging individual. *Gerontologist*, 1967, *7*, 101-105.

Killian, E. C. Effect of geriatric transfers on

mortality rates. *Social Work,* 1970, *15,* 19-26.

Kral, V., Grad, B., and Berenson, J. Stress reactions resulting from the relocation of an aged population. *Canadian Psychiatric Association Journal,* 1968, *13,* 201-209.

Markus, E., Blenkner, M., Bloom, M., and Downs, T. Relocation stress and the aged.

Interdisciplinary Topics in Gerontology, 1970, *7,* 60-71.

Miller, D., and Lieberman, M. The relationships of affect state and adaptive capacity to reactions to stress. *Journal of Gerontology,* 1965, *20,* 492-497.

Chapter 44

THE EFFECTS OF NURSING HOME SIZE ON RESIDENT ISOLATION AND LIFE SATISFACTION

TIMOTHY J. CURRY AND
BASCOM W. RATLIFF

THE PROBLEMS OF isolation and life satisfaction of residents in homes for the aged are of considerable current concern (Townsend, 1971). However, research is lacking which directly compares different size nursing and rest homes in regard to these phenomena. Presumably, the size of the home should play an important role in determining friendships within the home. Moreover, the size of the home may also have a direct influence on the life satisfaction of individuals residing in the home. These are topics of obvious practical and theoretical importance.

Several investigators have investigated phenomena relating to friendship roles and life satisfaction of elderly, institutionalized residents (Beattie and Bullock, 1964; Townsend, 1962). The work of Greenwald and Linn (1971) in particular suggested that as homes for the aged get larger, patient satisfaction, activity, and communication decline. But Greenwald and Linn's study concentrated mostly on the physical aspects of nursing home size. They did not

Reprinted by permission from the *Gerontologist*, 1973, *13*, 295-298.

examine in great detail the social consequences of increased size. Indeed, their attempt to rate patient satisfaction and interaction was based on the overall impressions of the researchers rather than on the self-reports of the residents of the nursing homes. As Henley and Davis (1967) point out, life satisfaction or dissatisfaction is a subjective process of evaluation. One cannot "assume dissatisfaction on the part of clients either on the basis of objective criteria alone, nor on the basis of what would affect the practitioner himself." Consequently, it seems necessary to obtain self-reports from the residents of nursing homes in order to determine resident satisfaction.

There are some theoretical reasons for predicting that nursing home size may influence directly (and independently) the resident's isolation and life satisfaction. Henley and Davis (1967) argue that a person's life satisfaction is "likely to be influenced by certain aspects of his or her current environment." If a person is prevented from living as he is accustomed to, then this should create some dissatisfaction with this area of his life. Since smaller nursing homes generally have a more home-like atmosphere than do larger, more institutionalized nursing homes, smaller homes may therefore also create fewer disruptions in accustomed living arrangements. Presumably, this should increase resident satisfaction. Bennett (1963) posits also that as institutions for the aged become more "total," several types of regimentation occur. Not only may the residents lose their personal identity, but primary relations with other residents and the staff become less likely. The end result may be increased feelings of isolation, dependency, powerlessness, and old age on the part of the residents of total institutions. Although the size of a nursing home does not necessarily reflect its totality, it would seem that the two are correlated to some extent. As size of the institution increases, the size of the staff does not increase in proportion to the number of residents, more formal procedures are devised to handle the reoccurring problems of resident care, and less personal accommodations can be made between resident and staff member, and even between resident and resident. Consequently, we expect that resident isolation will be greater in the larger nursing home and also that the residents of larger nursing homes will have greater dissatisfaction with their lives than will residents of smaller nursing homes.

Study Design and Interview Schedule

Since nursing home size is the chief variable of this study, an effort was made to select nursing homes and the residents in those homes that were as comparable as possible. Rather than to attempt to achieve comparability by the matching of individual residents, demographic, economic, and social status variables were employed as the chief control variables.

Only licensed proprietary nursing homes from the same county in Ohio were studied. Of the large (over 100 beds) homes, seven of the eight in the county agreed to cooperate with the study; of the seven intermediate-sized (between 50 and 99 beds) homes, all but one agreed to cooperate; and of the twenty-eight small (up to 49 beds) homes, all but two agreed to cooperate. A random sample was drawn of thirteen of the remaining twenty-six of these homes. The sample, then, consisted of seven large homes, six intermediate-sized homes, and thirteen small homes. Nonproprietary nursing homes were excluded from the sample, as were a few small proprietary homes that specialized in the care of extremely senile or terminally ill residents.

In order to insure comparability, the residents who were selected for interviewing within the homes had the following social and economic characteristics in common: (1) all were Aid for the Aged (AFA) recipients; (2) all were sixty years of age or older; (3) all had been residents of the county in question at least five years; (4) and all were mentally competent.

Over 90 percent of the residents of the small homes who met these criteria were interviewed, and 60 to 75 percent of the residents of the large and intermediate-sized homes who met these criteria were interviewed. A random sampling procedure was used to determine which residents of those eligible would be interviewed. The final sample included sixty residents of small homes, seventy residents from intermediate sized homes, and seventy residents from large homes, a total sample of 200.

Data were collected by two researchers who conducted oral interviews (lasting approximately 30 minutes) inside the selected nursing homes during the summer of 1972.

Havighurst-Neugarten's Life Satisfaction Index (LSI) was used to determine the level of life satisfaction among the residents of the different homes (Adams, 1969; Havighurst, Neugarten, and Tobin, 1961, 1964). For analysis purposes, the LSI scores were ordered into three levels of satisfaction; residents scoring below twenty were felt to be dissatisfied, residents scoring between twenty and forty were felt to be satisfied, and residents scoring over forty were felt to be highly satisfied (the range of LSI is 0–60).

Questions concerning isolation of individuals were scored according to the monthly contact the resident had with friends or relatives. If a person indicated that he or she saw a friend or relative on the average of once a month they received a score of one, if the contact was on the average of once a week the score was four, and so forth. Persons were then simply given numerical scores to represent the total number of contacts they had with friends and relatives.

The control variables we selected did produce a homogeneous sample. The residents of the three different sized homes did not differ significantly among themselves in terms of their average age, social class, sex distribution, education, racial characteristics, religious affiliation, and years of residence in the county or home. Some of the similar background factors are as follows: the average Social Class position was low (60 on Hollingshead's Two-Factor Index; Haug, 1972; Hollingshead, 1957); women outnumbered men almost two to one (64 and 36%, respectively); the average age of the sample was seventy-five years; average education was 8.4 years; the majority (80%) were Protestant (i.e. 16% were Catholic, 4% were Jewish or none); 84 percent were white, 16 percent were black; the average residency was forty-four years in the county; the average length of nursing home residency was 2.5 years; and the marital statuses were 65 percent widowed, 7 percent married, 17 percent single, and 11 percent divorced or separated. Finally, the residents were relatively healthy, over 90 percent were in good to fair health (although all residents did have chronic health conditions requiring medication).

Effect of Nursing Home Size on Isolation and Life Satisfaction

Turning now to the effects of nursing home size on the isolation of these residents, substantial differences in the amount and type of isolation were experienced in the different sized homes. To begin with, only 5 percent of the residents sampled from the smaller homes were totally isolated from contact with friends or relatives,

but 23 percent of the residents sampled from intermediate sized homes and 22 percent of the residents sampled from the large homes were totally isolated from friends and relatives. Differences this large between the small and larger homes are statistically significant at the .01 level.

Checking to see if substantial numbers of these isolated individuals had no living relatives or friends (which would explain some of their isolation) revealed that only one person from the intermediate sized home and five persons from the large homes indicated that they had no living friends or relatives. Clearly, then, the isolation of these individuals results from a lack of contact from relatives and friends from outside the home as well as the failure to develop friendships within the home.

When the total isolation index is broken down into its component parts, a more detailed indication of the isolation differences is shown. The residents of the smaller homes have significantly ($p<.05$) more friends within the home and significantly ($p<.01$) more monthly contacts with those friends within the home. Moreover, for all three sized homes, contact with friends outside the home is minimal. This suggests that friendships developed within the home are of paramount importance.

Interestingly enough, the residents of the intermediate and larger homes have more living relatives and a significantly higher ($p<.01$) monthly contact with those relatives. This difference does not offset the larger differences found for the contact with friends, however. As the figures for the average number of total monthly contacts indicate, the residents of the smaller homes have significantly more ($p<.05$) total monthly contacts. Differences between the intermediate and large homes are not that great or consistent, indicating that the effect of nursing home size on isolation is not linear.

Turning now to the life satisfaction of the residents within the homes, the Havighurst-Neugarten "Life Satisfaction Index" does not indicate significant differences in life satisfaction attributable to nursing home size. The average Life Satisfaction score for residents in the small homes was twenty-four, for the intermediate homes it was also twenty-four, and for the large homes it was twenty-three. This similarity remained even when the relative number of high, middle, and low scores were compared among each institutional group. The majority of the nursing home residents we sampled were moderately satisfied with their life, irrespective of the size of the home they were living in.

Moreover, general life satisfaction does not appear to be greatly influenced by current isolation. Some residents who were highly satisfied were also severely isolated, similarly there were residents who were dissatisfied but not isolated. The product moment correlation between isolation and life satisfaction was only a low .237.

Concluding Comments

The reason that small nursing homes facilitate the development of a greater number of friendships within the institution may not be just the result of their small physical size. As a variety of studies of propinquity and attraction have shown (Berscheid and Walster, 1969), the hindering effects of physical size can be overcome through time. As Bennett (1963) has suggested, administrators themselves in large institutionalized homes may tend to discourage close relationships between nursing home residents and to foster a feeling of dependence and inactivity in their patients. Additionally, the fact that smaller homes are usually converted into nursing homes from large private residences may

give these homes a more "residential" tone, where friendships are felt to be socially appropriate. The long corridors and more hospital-like appearance of the larger homes may create just the opposite social psychological feeling among the residents. These reasons apply also to the nonlinear nature of the influence of size on isolation. Beyond a certain small size, homes begin to take on a more institutional flavor. Increases of size beyond this point do not have the same critical influence on primary relations.

The reason that the residents of the smaller homes sampled in our study had fewer relatives and, consequently, less contact with these relatives can only be speculated on at this point. We suspect that there is a self-selection bias operating. Persons who have more living relatives may be less likely to enter small nursing homes. For one thing, persons with more relatives may be able to wait until there is room to move into the nursing home of their (or their relatives') choice. Since small homes seemingly have the reputation (e.g. Townsend, 1971) of being less able to care for the physical and medical needs of their patients, persons with more relatives to depend upon may wait until they can be assured of a spot in a larger home. Once the individual has moved into the larger home, the greater continued contact with relatives outside the home may be due in part to the isolation from friendships within the home itself. The relatives may attempt to keep the person from becoming too isolated. Relatives of persons inside small homes may not feel the necessity of frequent visitation is as great.

The results pertaining to life satisfaction were a bit surprising. Although substantial numbers of the residents were dissatisfied with their lives, the majority were not. However, the failure of the LSI to correlate highly with isolation may be due in part to the fact that the LSI measures general life satisfaction. While the isolated residents may be very lonesome and unhappy with their current isolation, they may still be relatively satisfied with other areas of their life.

REFERENCES

Adams, D. L. Analysis of a life satisfaction index. *Journal of Gerontology*, 1969, *24*, 470-474.

Beattie, W. M., and Bullock, J. Evaluating services and personnel in facilities for the aged. In M. Leeds and H. Shore (Eds.), *Geriatric institutional management*. New York: Putnam's, 1964.

Bennett, R. The meaning of institutional life. *Gerontologist*, 1963, *3*, 117-125.

Berscheid, E., and Walster, E. H. *Interpersonal attraction*. Reading, Mass: Addison-Wesley, 1969.

Greenwald, S. R., and Linn, M. W. Intercorrelation of data on nursing homes. *Gerontologist*, 1971, *11*, 337-340.

Haug, M. An assessment of inequality measures. In G. W. Theilbar and S. D. Feldman (Eds.), *Issues in social inequality*. Boston: Little, Brown, 1972.

Havighurst, R. J., Neugarten, B. L., and Tobin, S. S. The measurement of life satisfaction. *Journal of Gerontology*, 1961, *16*, 134-143.

Havighust, R. J., Neugarten, B. L., and Tobin, S. S. Disengagement, personality, and life satisfaction in the later years. *Age with a future*. Copenhagen: Munksgaard, 1964.

Henley, B., and Davis, M. S. Satisfaction and dissatisfaction: A study of the chronically-ill aged patient. *Journal of Health and Social Behavior*, 1967, *8*, 65-75.

Hollingshead, A. B. Two-factor index of social position. New Haven: Yale Univ., 1957. (mimeo).

Townsend, C. *Old age: The last segregation*. New York: Grossman Publishers, 1971.

Townsend, P. *The last refuge*. London: Routledge & Kegan Paul, 1962.

CONTEMPORARY RESEARCH STRATEGIES

No one methodological tradition or approach can be said to characterize the time dimensions considered in the present text. Instead, it is necessary to sketch in rather general terms the methodological features of each era. In so doing, the reader should keep in mind that many divisional characteristics frequently overlap one another. Nevertheless, it is appropriate to comment briefly on the more dominant contributions of each time frame.

The era of the 1930s through the early 1950s can be characterized by a number of discrete methodologies. In general, however, this period of time saw a number of anthropological studies of aging (Simmons, 1945, 1946; Moore, 1950). Although basically descriptive in nature, these early efforts were such as to force the consideration of age and aging beyond the narrow focus of national interest. On the other hand, these contributions made little use of either descriptive statistics or correlational techniques.

In addition to a lack of statistical sophistication, these early studies relied upon cross-sectional research designs. Such designs, although productive of aging data, did not allow a thorough examination of aging as a process in its own right. Similarly, the lack of a sound theoretical base did not permit the integration of subsequent findings.

The late 1950s and early 1960s witnessed an influx of sociologists and psychologists into the field of aging. Accordingly, the research topics and methodologies of this period reflect a strong empirical bias (Birren and Botwinick, 1955; Birren, 1959; Cattell and Gorsuch, 1956; Dana, 1957; Maddox and Eisdorfer, 1963; Neugarten et al., 1961). For the most part, concern was given to the perfecting of methodologies, the creating of measurement devices, and the training of methodologically sophisticated gerontologists.

The interest in cross-cultural and cross-national research did not wain during this era. Instead, efforts were made to perfect this approach from the standpoint of national comparisons (Burgess, 1960; Hudson, 1959; Kaplan, 1961; Schaie, 1959; Townsend, 1964). Nevertheless, efforts reminiscent of the previous period continued in the cross-cultural domain (Arth, 1965; Talmon-Garber, 1961).

From the standpoint of research design, on the other hand, the cross-sectional model remained dominant. Nonetheless, the value of the longitudinal or panel approach was fast being recognized (Cumming and Henry, 1961). Only an approach offering the continual measurement of a single group of persons would permit of theory construction or verification. In addition to the change over to a longitudinal model, descriptive statistics began to give way to inferential measures. Correlation, factor, and regression analyses came more and more to characterize the literature of social gerontology.

Going hand in hand with design and methodological changes were theoretical developments. As indicated previously, a variety of theories began to emerge during this period of time. The work of the gerontologist was becoming both theoretically and methodologically precise. As a consequence, "isolated" inquiries now became the basis for an integrated and viable body of knowledge concerning age.

As in the case of the development of theory in gerontology, the era of the late 1960s and early 1970s can be seen as a time of refinement. The previous impetus to methodological sophistication has continued apace (Atchley, 1969; Damon, 1965; Kuhlen, 1968; Simpson and McKinney, 1966). In addition, a number of innovative methodologies have been employed to explore the phenomena of age (Martel, 1968; Neugarten and Gutmann, 1968).

Cross-cultural and cross-national efforts, however, have by no means gone out of vogue. On the contrary, these efforts have been expanded to include such phenomena as patterns of social interaction (Bengston, 1967; Shanas *et al.*, 1968), personality development (Holtzmann, 1965), and adjustment to retirement (Havighurst *et al.*, 1966; Havighurst *et al.*, 1969; Lehr and Bigot, 1966). In a similar fashion, attention has been directed toward cultural migrants as well as toward minority segments of the larger culture (Jackson, 1971; Kalish and Yuen, 1971; Kent, 1971; Lawton *et al.*, 1971).

The focus on the cross-cultural dimensions of age has also stimulated a greater appreciation for the longitudinal research design. The present period has been productive of significant findings in many areas chiefly through the use of this technique. (See the findings reported by the researchers at the Duke University Center for the Study of Aging and Human Development.) Concomitantly, measuring instruments and statistical applications have increased in sophistication. *Multiple regression, factor analysis, partial correlation,* and *path coefficient* are now words in the working vocabulary of the contemporary gerontologist. Through the use of these techniques, he is free to explore areas and problems heretofore closed to investigation.

Finally, the methodology utilized by today's gerontologist is carefully built upon a sound theoretical foundation. For the most part, theory tends to guide rather than to emerge from contemporary research. As such, the scholar is in a position not only to describe the problem at hand, but is also able to integrate the findings of his work into a predictive format. This development has made possible a significant linkup between the pure and applied perspectives of social science.

The papers to follow illustrate many of the above-mentioned trends. They have been selected with an eye toward the imagination and creativity of the writer. All three selections stress the care to be taken in even the most innovative designs. In addition, they argue an interactive model of aging and suggest the necessity for a theoretical as well as applied perspective in social gerontology.

The paper by Glenn and Zody offers an alternative methodology to the time and expense of longitudinal designs as well as the artificial character of cross-sectional studies. The methodology in question involves a cohort analysis utilizing national survey data. The authors point to the wealth of unused social information collected by such organizations as the Survey Research Center at the University of Michigan, the National Opinion Research Center, and the American Institute of Public Opinion, as inexpensive and valuable data sources for the gerontologist.

The authors illustrate the use of this methodology by indicating a substantial increase in the percentage of nondrinkers in the cohort that matured beyond middle age from 1945 to 1960. They also demonstrate that this increase cannot be attributed to influences that would have increased nondrinking in the population as a whole.

The paper by Sherman is illustrative of the care taken by the contemporary gerontologist in his research endeavors. The work in question describes the methodology utilized in a longitudinal study of residents of housing facilities for the well elderly. The author reports on a total of 600 interviews conducted at six retirement housing sites, a retirement hotel, three retirement villages, an urban high-rise, and a life-care home. These interviews are then compared to interviews with 600 matched controls living in conventional age-integrated housing in an effort to determine the impact of residence in retirement housing.

In the paper, the author gives careful consideration to describing site and resident selection for the study, construction of the interview instrument, and the various methods used to minimize attrition. Considerable emphasis is also given to the assemblage of the dispersed sample as well as to the matching procedures employed. Finally, Sherman presents an analysis of comparability between the test and control groups following attrition.

Schwartz and Proppe sound a challenge for the future course of gerontological research. The authors lament the fact that much of the carefully conducted research in the field bears little apparent relation to the everyday needs of the elderly. The issue at point concerns the pure versus the applied perspective in social gerontology.

The authors argue that an interactional or "transactional" dimension is perhaps the most useful to describe the behavior and/or personality of the older person. For them, the "degredation spiral" of age is more a matter of the individual's transactions with his physical, social, and psychological environment, than with biological changes *per se*. As such, they suggest that most of the so-called old age deficits and degredations presently described in the literature can be subsumed under the rubric, "loss of control and effectiveness with the environment."

The authors draw upon the social psychological literature to emphasize the dual character of their approach. They insist that the behavior of the aged not be viewed as occurring in front of the backdrop of a fixed environment. The contemporary gerontologist must "take into account how individual behavior contributes to the environment and is in turn influenced by it."

REFERENCES

Arth, M. *The role of the aged in a west African village.* Paper read at the annual meeting of the Gerontological Society, Los Angeles, California, November, 1965.

Atchley, R. C. Respondents vs. refusers in an interview study of retired women: an analysis of selected characteristics. *Journal of Gerontology,* 1969, *24,* 42-47.

Bengston, V. L. A cross-national study of patterns of social interaction in aged males. Unpublished doctoral dissertation, *Committee on Human Development,* University of Chicago, 1967.

Birren, J. E. Principles of research on aging. In J. E. Birren (Ed.), *Handbook of aging and the individual.* Chicago: University of Chicago Press, 1959.

Birren, J. E., and Botwinick, J. Speed of response as a function of perceptual difficulty and age. *Journal of Gerontology,* 1955, *10,* 433-436.

Burgess, E. W. *Aging in western societies.* Chicago: University of Chicago Press, 1960.

Cattell, R. B., Gorsuch, R. L. The definition and measurement of national morale and morality. *Journal of Social Psychology,* 1956, *67,* 77-96.

Cumming, E., and Henry, W. E. *Growing Old.* New York: Basic Books, 1961.

Damon, A. Discrepancies between findings of longitudinal and cross-sectional studies in adult life: physique and physiology. *Human Development,* 1965, *8,* 16-22.

Dana, R. H. A comparison of four verbal subtests on the wechsler-bellevue form I, and the wais. *Journal of Clinical Psychology,* 1957, *13,* 70-71.

Havighurst, R. J., Munnichs, J. M. A., Neugarten, B. L., and Thomae, H. *Adjustment to retirement: a cross-national study.* Assen, The Netherlands: Van Gorcum & Co., 1969.

Havighurst, R. J., Neugarten, B. L., and Bengston, V. L. A cross-national study of adjustment to retirement. *Gerontologist,* 1966, *6,* 137- 138.

Holtzmann, W. H. Cross-cultural research on personality development. *Human Development,* 1965, *8,* 65-86.

Hudson, B. B. (Ed.) Crosscultural studies in the Arab middle east and the United States. *Journal of Social Issues,* 1959, *15,* 1-70.

Jackson, J. J. Negro aged: toward needed research in social gerontology. *Gerontologist,* 1971, *11,* 52-57.

Kalish, R. A., and Yuen, S. Americans of East Asian ancestry: aging and the aged. *Gerontologist,* 1971, *11,* 36-47.

Kaplan, B. *Studying personality cross-culturally.* Evanston, Illinois: Row & Peterson, 1961.

Kent, D. P. The elderly in minority groups: variant patterns of aging. *Gerontologist,* 1971, *11,* 26-29.

Kuhlen, R. G. Age and intelligence: the significance of cultural change in longitudinal vs. cross-sectional findings. In B. L. Neugarten (Ed.), *Middle age and aging: a reader in social psychology.* Chicago: University of Chicago Press, 1968.

Lawton, M. P., Kleban, M. H., and Singer, M. The aged Jewish person and the slum environment. *Journal of Gerontology,* 1971, *26,* 231-239.

Lehr, U., and Bigot, A. A cross national study of adjustment to retirement: a first report on retired steel workers. In *Proceedings of the 7th International Congress of Gerontology,* 1966, *6,* 101-102.

Maddox, G. L., and Eisdorfer, C. Some correlates of activity and morale among the elderly. Social Forces, 1963, *40,* 254-260.

Martel, M. U. Age-sex roles in American magazine fiction. In B. L. Neugarten (Ed.), *Middle age and aging: a reader in social psychology.* Chicago: University of Chicago Press, 1968.

Moore, W. E. The aged in industrial societies. In M. Derber (Ed.), *The aged and society.* Champaign, Illinois: Industrial Relations Research Association, 1950.

Neugarten, B. L., and Gutmann, D. L. Age-sex roles and personality in middle age: a thematic apperception study. In B. L. Neugarten (Ed.), *Middle age and aging: a reader in social psychology.* Chicago: University of Chicago Press, 1968.

Neugarten, B. L., Havighurst, R. J., and Tobin, S. S. The measurement of life satisfaction. *Journal of Gerontology,* 1961, *16,* 134-143.

Schaie, K. W. Cross-sectional methods in the study of psychological aspects of aging. *Journal of Gerontology,* 1959, *14,* 208-215.

Shanas, E., Townsend, P., Wedderburn, D., Friis, H., Hilhoj, P., and Stehouwer, J. *Old people in three industrial societies.* New York: Atherton Press, 1968.

Simmons, L. W. *The role of the aged in primitive society.* New Haven: Yale University Press, 1945.

Simmons, L. W. Attitudes toward aging and the aged: primitive societies. *Journal of Gerontology,* 1946, *1,* 72-95.

Simpson, I. H., and McKinney, J. C. *Social aspects of aging.* Durham, North Carolina: Duke Univerisity Press, 1966.

Talmon-Garber, Y. Aging in Israel, a planned society. *American Journal of Sociology,* 1961, *3,* 284-295.

Townsend, P. The place of older people in different societies. *Lancet,* 1964, *1,* 159-161.

Chapter 45

COHORT ANALYSIS WITH NATIONAL SURVEY DATA

NORVAL D. GLENN AND RICHARD E. ZODY

IT IS HARDLY NECESSARY to remind the reader of the limitations of cross-sectional data for the study of changes in attitudes, behavior, and social relations that occur as people grow older. Furthermore, every serious student of social gerontology is aware of the paucity of good longitudinal data dealing with many kinds of attitudes and behavior. Panel studies that can adequately demonstrate how people change as they grow older take at least several years, and the academic reward system discourages researchers from spending a great deal of time and money on projects that will lead to publications only in the distant future. In view of this fact, a surprising number of good panel studies have been conducted, but there is no prospect that there will soon be enough such studies to answer all the important questions about the behavioral, attitudinal, and social correlates of aging.

Fortunately, existing national survey data can yield much information to the student of aging who is adept at secondary analysis, and the research may be done in weeks rather than years and may cost only a few hundred rather than several thousand dollars. To be sure, the researcher is never

Reprinted by permission from the *Gerontologist*, 1970, *10*, 233-240.

able to ask of these data all the questions he wishes to ask; the research design must be drawn to fit the existing data. Furthermore, there are pitfalls in this kind of research for those inexperienced in the secondary analysis of survey data. But the potential utility of existing survey data to students of aging is considerable, and the failure of gerontological research to exploit this potential fully is wasteful.

The Survey Research Center at the University of Michigan, the National Opinion Research Center, the American Institute of Public Opinion (the Gallup Poll), and several of the Gallup organizations outside the United States have each repeated a number of questions, with identical or nearly identical wording, at intervals of several years. This enables one to trace reported attitudes and behavior within cohorts as they grow older. The Gallup and NORC data are available at reasonable cost from the Roper Public Opinion Research Center in Williamstown, Massachusetts, and data may be obtained directly from the SRC. Access to these data, and to information about them, is greatly facilitated if one's college or university has membership in the International Survey Library Association (sponsored by the Roper Center) and the SRC sponsored Inter-University Consortium For Political Research.

We do not attempt to report here all the variables that can be studied with cohort analysis of existing national survey data, nor have we discovered just how many questions have been repeated at intervals of several years. However, we know from experience that a considerable number of variables can be subjected to cohort analysis. Furthermore, the American Institute of Public Opinion has agreed to add to its surveys occasional questions suggested by researchers in colleges and universities that are members of the International Survey Library Association. Hopefully, some of the questions will follow the wording of earlier ones, and it is likely that the AIPO could be persuaded to repeat many of the questions it asked once or a few times during the 1940s, 1950s, and early 1960s.

It is our purpose here to draw attention to this resource for social gerontologists and to review the methods that must be followed in cohort analysis of survey sample data in order to avoid erroneous conclusions. We also provide an example of a cohort study with Gallup poll data.

The Basic Procedures

The discussion that follows is concerned primarily with American Gallup data, because these offer the greatest opportunities and also pose the greatest problems. Unfortunately, age is not coded in the NORC data in a way that facilitates cohort analysis. Whereas both the Gallup and the more recent SRC surveys record the exact age of the respondent, the NORC surveys record age by broad intervals. Unless questions are repeated at time intervals that coincide in years with these age intervals, it is impossible to trace cohorts with precision. The SRC has most consistently used a good area probability sample, and, therefore, cohort analysis with SRC data is not plagued with difficulties growing out of changes in sampling techniques. Furthermore, the SRC questions are carefully worded, and in almost all respects the surveys exemplify high quality, academic research. However, the SRC surveys have repeated relatively few questions at intervals of several years, and rarely have surveys conducted within a few months of one another gathered the same information so that several samples can be combined to form the large N's that are desirable for cohort studies. Therefore, the data from the American and the various

foreign Gallup Polls are a somewhat greater resource for gerontological research than either the NORC or the SRC data.

The unwary researcher could easily perform cohort analyses with Gallup data that would lead to erroneous conclusions. Until 1952, Gallup used quota samples exclusively, and it is well known that most such samples systematically underrepresent the lower social strata. After 1952, the American Gallup samples were progressively refined and improved, so that by the 1960s the lower social strata of the noninstitutionalized population were adequately represented. The result is that if one traces a cohort from the mid-1950s or earlier into the 1960s, the reported average educational status within the cohort becomes progressively lower. An example is shown in Table 45-I. In fact, we know that average amount of education within a cohort increases slightly as the cohort grows older, because a few people will complete additional schooling, and mortality is higher among the older members, who are somewhat less educated on the average than the younger members. Therefore, if a dependent variable is appreciably associated with amount of education, a cohort analysis without controls for education will show a change in the variable as the cohort ages, even if in fact no change has occurred. Or, a real change can be masked by this bias in the data.

It is apparent, then, that any cohort study with Gallup data gathered before 1960 requires rather precise controls for amount of education. However, inconsistent coding of the data at the different dates usually precludes making distinctions within the broad level of from zero to eight years of school so no more than five educational levels can be used. Since respondents with college training are a small percentage of the samples, and since most dependent

TABLE 45-I

YEARS OF SCHOOL COMPLETED BY A COHORT OF WHITE MALES, AS SHOWN
BY AMERICAN GALLUP SAMPLES[a], 1945 THROUGH 1965

Years of School Completed	Year: (Ages):	1945 (50 — 59)	1949 (54 — 63)	1953 (58 — 67)	1957 (62 — 71)	1961 (66 — 75)	1965 (70 — 79)
0 — 8		43.5	51.0	50.3	57.5	60.9	65.1
1 — 3 of high school		18.7	15.6	21.0	19.2	15.2	7.9
4 of high school		16.0	16.3	16.1	15.9	15.7	16.7
At least some college		21.9	17.1	12.6	7.4	8.2	10.2
Total		100.0	100.0	100.0	100.0	100.0	100.0
(N)		(771)	(812)	(366)	(365)	(440)[b]	(430)[b]

[a]The data for 1945 are from Gallup surveys 353, 360, 364, and 377; those for 1949 are from surveys 432, 433, 434, and 435; those for 1953 are from surveys 521, 522, 523, and 524; those for 1957 are from surveys 578, 580, 582, and 587; those for 1961 are from surveys 639, 647, and 649; and those for 1965 are from surveys 702, 706, 709, and 712.

[b]These samples are inflated by about 100 per cent by a weighting procedure used by Gallup to increase representativeness. Therefore, the reported N's are about twice the number of respondents represented.

variables do not differ greatly within the college level, little is to be gained by distinguishing between the college graduates and the college-educated respondents without degrees. Therefore, we recommend use of the four educational levels shown in Table 45-I. When these controls are applied, the sample size at each educational level is usually quite small, especially if the data for each year are from only one survey, and little confidence can be placed in the data for any one educational level. This problem can be minimized by converting the percentages for the four educational levels into a standardized percentage for the entire cohort. For some purposes, it is satisfactory simply to compute the mean of the percentages at the four educational levels (Glenn and Grimes, 1968), but a preferable procedure is to standardize the percentages from the earlier survey or surveys to the educational distribution shown for the cohort by the later survey.

A disadvantage of percentages adjusted in this manner is that their standard error is not exactly the same as that of raw percentages and cannot be precisely determined. Therefore, strictly speaking, tests of significance are not applicable to the corrected percentages. However, the senior author has found that the variance of percentages from Gallup quota samples that are corrected for the systematic underrepresentation of the lower educational levels is usually very similar to, although often slightly greater than, the variance of raw percentages from the same samples (Glenn, 1970). Consequently, tests of significance may be useful for estimating sampling variability *if* one interprets the results with caution and requires a slightly greater difference for statistical significance than he would with raw percentages. Increasing the difference required for significance by 15 to 30 percent, depending upon whether or not both of the compared percentages are adjusted, should be sufficiently conservative.

Readers familiar with national survey samples know that the textbook formulae for tests of significance, which are designed for simple random samples, cannot be applied to national survey data. The variance of percentages from quota samples is often as great as 1.6 times the variance of percentages from simple random samples (Stephan and McCarthy, 1958), although the variance of percentages from the quota samples used by Gallup during the 1940s seems usually to have been somewhat less than that magnitude (Glenn, 1970). The variance of percentages from the area probability samples used by Gallup during the 1960s is, on the average, around 1.3 times the variance with simple random samples. Therefore, when raw percentages from recent and early Gallup polls are being compared, it is reasonably safe to assume that the variance of the difference between percentages is between 1.4 and 1.5 times the variance with simple random samples. If one of the compared percentages is adjusted, the factor should be about 1.6, and if both are adjusted, the cautious researcher may wish to use a factor as great as 1.8. If both percentages are from quota samples and are adjusted, a factor of at least 2.0 seems advisable.

Another word of caution is needed concerning the use of tests of significance in comparing percentages from recent and early Gallup polls. Since 1960, most of the Gallup samples have been inflated by about 100 percent by a weighting procedure used as a substitute for callbacks. Use of both the original sample and the weighting cards should usually result in percentages more representative of the universe, but the N of the original sample should be used for statistical tests.

Controls of sex should be routinely applied in all cohort studies, regardless of the source of data, because the greater mortality of males reduces the sex ratio in an aging cohort. Of course, this demographic change brings about real changes

in the attitudes and behavior of the surviving portion of a cohort, considered as a whole, but the student of aging is usually interested in what typically happens to the aging individual rather than to the aggregate characteristics of the surviving portion of the cohort. Therefore, insofar as possible, he should separate the effects of differential mortality from those of changes in the attitudes and behavior of individuals.

In cohort analysis with census data, the age span covered by each cohort is often equal in years to the time between dates for which data are presented. In such cases, the data can be arranged in a matrix that facilitates comparisons within and among cohorts. When the cross-sectional data by age for each date are presented in the columns, cohorts can be compared as of the time each was in a certain age range by reading across the rows, and each cohort can be traced from one date to the next by reading diagonally across and down the matrix.

Unfortunately, cohort data from survey samples can rarely be presented in such convenient form. The time between dates is dictated by the available data, over which the researcher doing a secondary analysis has no control, and the need for adequate sample sizes usually dictates use of cohorts whose age span is greater in years than the time between dates. In these cases, the most convenient presentation of the data is in a table in which each cohort can be traced through time by reading across a row, as in Tables 45-II through 45-IV. Furthermore, the age span of the cohorts usually must be greater than that needed to determine precisely at what age or ages an indicated change in attitudes or behavior has occurred. If data from only one poll are available for each date, at least a fifteen-year cohort is usually required for reasonably adequate sample sizes. However, if change is continuous and in one direction from young adulthood to old age, the imprecision caused by use of broad cohorts is of little importance.

If the same question has been asked by several polls during a period of a few months, the data from the polls can be pooled and the problem of sampling variability largely overcome (Glenn and Grimes, 1968). Unfortunately, only a few questions, such as those on voter turnout and political party preference, have been repeated with such frequency. However, several questions have been asked by Gallup polls once every year, every other year, or every few months for ten years or longer. These include questions on church attendance, drinking of alcoholic beverages, and the like, and cohort analyses with these variables can provide very nearly conclusive evidence on changes that have occurred within aging cohorts. For instance, if data for a cohort for each of twenty successive years are examined, sampling variability can account for considerable year-by-year fluctuation but is not likely to obscure any long-range trends or stability in the variable under study.

Even if a question has been repeated at intervals of five years or so and asked no more than four or five times, the problem of sampling variability can be largely overcome if one is willing to assume that changes within a cohort as it passes through an age range are similar to changes that have occurred in earlier cohorts in that age range and that will occur in later ones. In such cases, one can trace three or more cohorts through a given age range, and consistency of results among the cohorts provides evidence that the apparent changes did not result from sampling error. Lack of consistency, on the other hand, could reflect sampling error or could mean that the assumption that all cohorts experience

the same change in a given age range is incorrect. If one also assumes that change is continuous and in one direction from young adulthood to old age, the problem of sampling variability is further reduced, because there are data on at least three cohorts for each time span. Again, however, unambiguous evidence is provided only by consistency among the cohorts, since inconsistency could reflect either sampling error or lack of monotonic change through the adult stages of the life cycle.

An Illustration

An example of a set of data that allows rather confident conclusions about the direction of change that has occurred within aging cohorts is presented in Tables 45-II and 45-III. Even more nearly conclusive evidence of changes in drinking within aging cohorts could be amassed, because Gallup has asked a question about drinking at least once a year since the mid-1940s. However, such extensive data are available for very few variables, and, therefore, we use data from only four polls to illustrate the kind of conclusions that can be drawn from the more limited data with which one must usually work.

Cross-sectional data for 1960 (or any recent date) on percentage of persons who say they drink alcoholic beverages show a negative monotonic relationship between age and percentage of reported drinkers. If one has data for only one date, he cannot very confidently choose among an "aging," a "generational," or a "demographic" interpretation of these data, although he may refine his analysis of them to provide some fairly good clues (Glenn, 1969). According to the "aging" interpretation, fewer old people drink because many individuals stop drinking as they grow older; according to the "generational" interpretation, each successive cohort that has matured into adulthood during recent decades has been more prone to drink than those before it; and according to the "demographic" interpretation, fewer old people drink because there has been greater mortality among the drinkers. The "demographic" interpretation does not necessarily assume that drinking itself leads to early death. Rather, certain kinds of people, such as males, may have higher rates of both death and drinking even though the two are not causally related. Of course, the lower percentage of drinkers at the older ages could have resulted from two or all three of these possible causes.

If one has data for two or three earlier dates, he may be able to rule out the generational explanation without doing a cohort analysis. In the case of our illustration, if the percentage of drinkers had not declined within aging cohorts, and if each successive cohort that matured into adulthood had been more prone to drink than those before it, then the percentage of drinkers in the total adult population would necessarily have increased. Since

Gallup poll data show little change in the percentage of drinkers from 1945 to 1960, the generational hypothesis is rather conclusively discredited. However, we need to proceed with a cohort analysis in order to decide between, or estimate the relative importance of, the aging and demographic interpretations.

Since the sex ratio declines within an aging cohort, and since a smaller percentage of females drink, demographic change undoubtedly leads to some decline in drinkers at the older ages. However, the data in Table 45-II show a rather steep decline in drinkers among both males and females. It is possible, of course, that higher mortality among the drinkers of both sexes reduced the percentage of drinkers, but a few quick calculations reveal that differential mortality of drinkers and nondrinkers could hardly have accounted for most of the apparent decline. In recent American cohorts, of every 100 persons alive at age twenty, fewer than twenty died by age sixty. Since about 30 percent of the people in their twenties were nondrinkers, only

TABLE 45-II

PERCENTAGE OF RESPONDENTS WHO SAID THEY WERE DRINKERS, IN THREE FIFTEEN-YEAR COHORTS, BY SEX, 1945, 1950, 1955, AND 1960[a]

(N'S ARE IN PARENTHESES)

Cohort No. 1 — ages:	*23 — 34*	*25 — 39*	*30 — 44*	*35 — 49*
Males	80.9 (407)	78.3 (198)	78.2 (289)	74.2 (244)
Females	66.8 (530)	54.6 (301)	58.9 (297)	65.1 (195)
Mean	73.9	66.5	68.6	69.7
Cohort No. 2 — ages:	*35 — 49*	*40 — 54*	*45 — 59*	*50 — 64*
Males	77.0 (539)	70.4 (210)	68.2 (212)	65.1 (195)
Females	59.4 (510)	39.8 (170)	49.6 (202)	49.1 (177)
Mean	68.2	55.1	58.9	57.1
Cohort No. 3 — ages:	*50 — 64*	*55 — 69*	*60 — 74*	*65 — 79*
Males	68.3 (371)	54.6 (150)	52.8 (123)	56.5 (138)
Females	46.1 (305)	38.0 (103)	25.5 (84)	33.7 (83)
Mean	57.2	46.3	39.2	45.1

[a]Percentages for all dates except 1960 are standardized to the educational distribution in the cohort as shown by the 1960 data.

The data for 1945 are from Gallup survey 360, those for 1950 are from survey 450, those for 1955 are from survey 543, and those for 1960 are from survey 622.

TABLE 45-III

PERCENTAGE OF RESPONDENTS WHO SAID THEY WERE DRINKERS, IN TWO
ELDERLY FIFTEEN-YEAR COHORTS, BY SEX, AT FIVE-YEAR INTERVALS[a]
(N'S ARE IN PARENTHESES)

Cohort No. 1:	*1945 — ages 60 — 74*	*1950 — ages 65 — 79*
Males	58.7 (209)	38.6 (70)
Females	32.9 (170)	36.5 (63)
Mean	45.8	37.6
Cohort No. 2:	*1950 — ages 60 — 74*	*1955 — ages 65 — 69*
Males	41.4 (107)	46.0 (100)
Females	40.9 (96)	30.9 (68)
Mean	41.2	38.5

[a]The percentages for the earlier dates for both cohorts are standardized to the educational distributions shown by the data for the later dates.

The data for 1945 are from Gallup survey 360, those for 1950 are from survey 450, and those for 1955 are from survey 543.

about six nondrinkers in the original 100 people died before age sixty if nondrinkers experienced their proportional share of deaths. Let us assume that the nondrinkers experienced only one-half their proportional share of deaths and that only three died. In that case, seventeen drinkers would have died, effecting a reduction in percentage of drinkers from about 70 to around 66.2, a reduction of less than 4 percentage points. Even if all twenty deaths were to occur among the drinkers, the percentage of drinkers would decline by only 7.5 points. In contrast, we can infer from the data in Table 45-II, by a procedure described below, that the percentage of drinkers in recent cohorts has actually declined by about 15 points from the twenties and early thirties to the late forties and the fifties. The indication is clear: the primary reason for the smaller percentage of drinkers at the older ages is that many people stop drinking after early adulthood.

Although the decline in drinkers appears to occur in both the early and late stages of the adult life cycle, it may well not be continuous from young adulthood to old age. There are some apparent plateaus at which little or no change occurs,

but these may have resulted from sampling error.

Table 45-II reveals only one apparent increase in percentage of drinkers large enough to warrant further examination, and that was in Cohort No. 3 from ages sixty through seventy-four to ages sixty-five through seventy-nine. This apparent increase might well have resulted from sampling error, since neither the difference for males nor that for females approaches statistical significance, or it could reflect a tendency for elderly exdrinkers to begin drinking again to alleviate the boredom, loneliness, and physical discomfort that many very old people experience. In order to decide between these two explanations, we can derive additional evidence from the same polls used for the data in Table 45-II. The apparent increase probably was not real if other cohorts that reached the late seventies recently did not experience it, and, therefore, in Table 45-III we trace two other fifteen-year cohorts from ages sixty through seventy-four to ages sixty-four through seventy-nine. In both cohorts, the mean of the male and female percentages *decreased;* therefore, there is no convincing evidence that exdrinkers who have become very old in recent years tended to resume drinking.

If one has data for only two dates, rather than for four as in the illustration above, he is much less likely to be able to arrive at confident conclusions. To illustrate how one might arrive at an incorrect conclusion from data from only two polls, we present data in Table 45-IV from two of the polls used for Tables 45-II and 45-III. In each of the three cohorts, the mean of the male and female percentages is greater at the later date, although none of the differences is very large and none of the differences for each of the sexes is statistically significant. In spite of the lack of statistically significant differences, one might conclude on the basis of the consistency among the three cohorts that in recent years there has been an accumulation of drinkers within aging cohorts. However, we have already presented evidence that rather conclusively demonstrates that this

TABLE 45-IV
PERCENTAGE OF RESPONDENTS WHO SAID THEY WERE DRINKERS, IN THREE FIFTEEN-YEAR COHORTS, BY SEX, 1950 AND 1960[a]
(N'S ARE IN PARENTHESES)

	1950	1960
Cohort No. 1 — ages:	*20 — 34*	*30 — 44*
Males	69.7 (172)	79.4 (233)
Females	58.1 (274)	57.5 (280)
Mean	63.9	72.5
Cohort No. 2 — ages:	*35 — 49*	*45 — 59*
Males	75.1 (335)	67.3 (246)
Females	35.8 (230)	49.5 (290)
Mean	55.5	58.4
Cohort No. 3 — ages:	*50 — 64*	*60 — 74*
Males	57.6 (175)	57.0 (165)
Females	37.3 (116)	43.9 (130)
Mean	47.5	50.5

[a]The percentages for 1950 are standardized to the educational distribution in the cohort as shown by the 1960 data.

The data for 1950 are from Gallup survey 450 and those for 1960 are from survey 622.

conclusion is incorrect. The lesson is clear: when data from only two polls are available, all conclusions should be very tentative unless there are large, consistent, and statistically significant differences.

Cohort analysis is useful not only to study the correlates of aging but also to throw light on the nature of long-term trends in attitudes and behavior (Ryder, 1965). Even when the primary purpose of the analysis is to study the aging process, examining the data to assess trends in the total adult population aids the interpretation. If aging individuals change in the same direction as the total population, the interpretation should be different than if the two changes are in opposite directions. For instance, a given change in attitudes within an aging cohort cannot very well be considered a consequence of the aging process if the total adult population changes to a greater extent in the same direction. Rather, the two changes can be attributed to the same influences. Therefore, in spite of sampling difficulties, a cohort study with national survey data can usually provide more nearly conclusive evidence on the effects of aging than a panel study with a local or otherwise restricted sample, in which changes in the sample cannot be related to changes in the total population. Obviously, a panel study cannot use a control group that is not subjected to the aging process, whereas in cohort studies with national data, the total adult population serves roughly the same function as a control group. It is subjected to many of the same influences as the aging cohort but usually does not experience marked change in its age characteristics during the period covered. However, the total adult population is never a totally satisfactory substitute for a control group, since it may change under the impact of influences, such as changes in preadult socialization and in the age structure, that do not directly affect the older cohorts. There is usually no way to identify and isolate the effects of changes in preadult socialization on the trend in the frequency of a dependent variable in the total adult population, but the effects of changes in the age structure can be identified. In order to deal only with changes in the dependent variable not attributable to changes in the age structure, one can trace the trend in the dependent variable in successive cohorts that mature into adulthood, and this is the trend that should be compared with the trend within aging cohorts.

As we point out above, if one studies N-year cohorts at N-year intervals and arranges the data into the usual matrix, he can compare different cohorts as of the time they were in the same age range by reading across the rows, and the same matrix can be used to trace each cohort through time and to compare the cohorts. However, since our data are not in such convenient form, we must compile separate data for the needed intercohort comparison. These are reported in Table 45-V. In order to maintain adequate samples sizes, we use overlapping cohorts (Zody, 1969). For instance, in the national population (but probably not in the samples), the cohort that was twenty through thirty-four in 1945 contained many of the pepole who were in the same age range in 1950. Still, examining the data for people in a given age range at successive points in time reveals how successive cohorts have differed.

The data provide no strong evidence for either an increase or a decrease in percentage of drinkers in successive cohorts. Although the differences between 1945 and 1960 are not statistically significant, some approach significance, and each of these suggests a downward trend in successive cohorts in percentage of drinkers. However, this trend, if real, seems to have been very small in relation to the downward trend within aging cohorts, and, therefore, whatever influences account for the former trend seem hardly sufficient to account for the latter. It seems very likely, therefore, that the aging process and/or passage through the life cycle are causally related to the decline in percentage of drinkers

TABLE 45-V

PERCENTAGE OF RESPONDENTS WHO SAID THEY WERE DRINKERS, AGES 20 — 34 AND 35 — 49, BY SEX, 1945, 1950, 1955, AND 1960[a]

(N'S ARE IN PARENTHESES)

Ages	1945	1950	1955	1960
20 — 34				
Males	80.9 (407)	69.7 (172)	77.9 (217)	74.3 (167)
Females	66.8 (530)	68.1 (274)	62.0 (254)	62.7 (225)
Mean	73.9	68.9	70.0	68.5
35 — 49				
Males	77.0 (539)	75.1 (539)	72.1 (279)	67.3 (246)
Females	59.4 (510)	35.8 (230)	57.7 (297)	49.5 (290)
Mean	68.2	55.5	64.9	58.4

[a]Percentages for all dates except 1960 are standardized to the educational distribution in the cohort as shown by the 1960 data.

The data for 1945 are from Gallup survey 360, those for 1950 are from survey 450, those for 1955 are from survey 543, and those for 1960 are from survey 622.

within aging cohorts. Of course, it is possible, and even likely, that the influences on drinking of aging and of passage through the life cycle are dependent on conditions that vary from one society to another and from time to time in any one society.

REFERENCES

Glenn, N. D. Aging, disengagement, and opinionation. *Public Opinion Quarterly,* 1969, *33,* 17-33.

Glenn, N. D. Problems of comparability in trend studies with opinion poll data. *Public Opinion Quarterly,* 1970, *34,* 82-91.

Glenn, N. D., and Grimes, M. Aging, voting, and political interest. *American Sociological Review,* 1968, *33,* 563-575.

Ryder, N. B. The cohort as a concept in the study of social change. *American Sociological Review,* 1965, *30,* 843-861.

Stephan, F. F., and McCarthy, P. J. *Sampling opinions.* New York: John Wiley, 1958.

Zody, R. E. Cohort analysis: some applicatory problems in the study of social and political behavior. *Social Science Quarterly,* 1969, *50,* 374-380.

Chapter 46

METHODOLOGY IN A STUDY OF RESIDENTS OF RETIREMENT HOUSING

Susan R. Sherman

THE RESEARCH DESCRIBED in this paper is the second part of a large-scale study of retirement housing. The first phase of the study was a survey of all retirement housing in the state of California and is reported in detail in Walkley, Mangum, Sherman, Dodds, and Wilner (1966). In the first phase, over 600 housing facilities, of several different types, for the well-elderly were surveyed with mail questionnaires sent to the housing managers. This provided virtually a complete census of all such retirement housing in the state.

The second phase of the research, the major focus, is a longitudinal study of residents at selected retirement housing facilities. Interviews with 600 persons (test subjects) residing in special housing for the well-elderly were compared to interviews with matched controls living dispersed throughout conventional age-integrated communities in order to observe the effects of residence in retirement housing. Two interviews were completed with each respondent. This was not strictly a before-after design, as the first interview did not take place until after the move into retirement housing. All respondents were rein-

Reprinted by permission from the *Journal of Gerontology*, 1973, *28*, 351-358.

terviewed approximately two years after the first interview in order to assess change and stability.

The interviews with tests and controls focused on a number of controversial issues in the field of housing for the elderly, such as integration vs. segregation of the elderly (Mumford, 1956; Rosow, 1967); provision of leisure activities vs. fears of community pressures and loss of privacy (Carp, 1966; Donahue, 1960; Sherman, 1971); provision of supportive services vs. encouragement of premature dependency; rental vs. purchase of housing (Walkley *et al.*, 1966). Other sections of the interview were devoted to motivation and pathways into retirement housing, morale and psychological well-being, physical health, and demography.

The present paper is devoted to a description of the methodology used in this study. Particularly emphasized will be descriptions of matching, and methods used to minimize attrition. Other areas to be described include interview construction and selection of the particular test sites and residents therein.

Since one purpose of the study (Wilner and Walkley, 1963) was to measure the effect of the retirement housing setting on behavior and attitudes, it was necessary to choose control groups who were as much like the test residents as possible, differing only according to where they lived. This was particularly important as it became apparent that the site residents were not typical of the general aged population of the state, although they were typical of those living in (relatively large) retirement housing settings. That is, we had to ensure that the data we would analyze could not be attributed, for example, to a higher than average income among site residents rather than to residency in retirement housing. Throughout the study we endeavored to verify that the test and control groups were well matched.

The design of the study cannot overcome completely the problem of self-selection. That is, the test residents were persons who chose to move into special housing, while the controls were persons who chose not to, for the most part. We did not attempt to interview, for example, persons who were on the waiting lists for the sites, and would thus have been matched on desire to move in (Carp, 1966). We did attempt to lessen the importance of self-selection by matching on variables of socioeconomic status and household composition. Substantive interest could be found in the issue of choice itself (Sherman, 1971). Because of such considerations, it was particularly critical to interview those persons who moved, between interviewing waves, to the opposite type of housing from that in which they were initially found.

In any longitudinal study there are problems of sample attrition between waves. Although the elderly are not as mobile as some younger age groups, the losses through death and illness can be presumed to be higher. This paper will describe the various approaches used in the second wave to locate any respondents not at the original address. Finally, we will assess the differences, if any, between those who were interviewed (at the same address) at both waves and those who were not interviewed at the second wave or who were interviewed, but at a new address.

Interview Construction

Pilot interviews, conducted with managers and residents at approximately thirty sites, were used to generate the research instrument. The interview was pretested with seventy-two residents at four sites similar to the test sites and a parallel control form was pretested with fifty dispersed residents.

The final interview schedule required on the average $1\frac{1}{4}$ hours to complete.

Interviews with Test (Site) Respondents

Selection of the Six Test Sites

As mentioned above, in an earlier phase of the study, over 600 sites for the well-elderly in the state were identified, and information was obtained on the number of residents, their age, facilities provided, costs and financial arrangements, and the type of dwelling unit. These data were used in selecting six prototypical sites in which to interview residents. The criteria for selection included variety and frequency. That is, it was desired to represent the range of retirement housing then available (of a size large enough for sampling purposes) catering to different socioeconomic groups, and to select the modal types. This variety and modality would make generalizations from the data more justifiable.

Table 46-I gives a summary description (as of the first interviewing wave) of the six test sites, listed in increasing order of socioeconomic status. Included are a retirement hotel, an urban apartment tower, three retirement villages, and a life-care home. Fuller descriptions of the six sites appear elsewhere (Sherman, 1971).

Systematic Probability Sample

Having selected the six sites and obtained permission to interview, a systematic probability sample was chosen for each site. Only one person in a dwelling unit was to be interviewed. From rosters of residents, 100 possible respondents were selected by denoting every nth individual (where n = total number of site residents/100) following a random start. Strenuous attempts were made to interview these 100 persons, with numerous call-backs. Only in cases

TABLE 46-I

CHARACTERISTICS OF THE RETIREMENT HOUSING SITES

	Retirement Hotel	Rental Village	Apartment Tower	Purchase Village	Manor Village	Life-Care Home
Location in California	Downtown Southern	Suburban Central	Downtown Southern	Suburban Southern	Suburban Northern	Urban Southern
Year construction began	1923	1960	1964	1962	1964	1960
Sponsorship	Private enterprise	"League" Senior Citizens (FHA) 231)	Church (CFA 202)	Private enterprise	Private enterprise	Church (FHA 231)
Cost	$103 — 145 per month 2 meals daily	$75 — $101 per month	$66 — 111 per month	$13,900 — 27,290	$12,000 — 32,500	$5,000 — 25,000 initial; $175 — 200 per month, per person
Type(s) of Dwellings	Rooms	Apartments	Apartments	Houses and apartments	Apartments	Rooms, apartments, cottages
Number of residents	156	688	228	5,000	2,384	362

where it was absolutely impossible to interview a designated resident were substitutions made. The substitute was the next in line on a similarly selected list, who was of the same sex, marital status, and having the same household composition as the original designate. For the most part, only about 15 percent of the original 100 designated at each site had to be replaced.

Table 46-II summarizes the background characteristics of the residents sampled in the six sites (as well as of the matched controls, who will be discussed in a later section). To summarize the sites in general, marital status at four of the sites shows primarily widows and other singles, with women predominating, while at the two villages with younger residents, most were married couples (6 respondents had grown children in the household). Residents at each of four sites have an average age of about seventy-five years, while residents at the other two sites average about sixty-eight years. The median income demonstrates a financial progression of the six sites, with residents of the fifth site having a rather high median income for persons of this age group. Education corresponds quite closely, and occupation, using the Hollingshead and Redlich (1958) scale, shows a similar trend. Most of the persons interviewed were retired at the time of the interview (with retirement status based on husband's status if respondent is a married woman), although at the Manor Village, approximately 20 percent were still working. Nearly 90 percent of all residents were born in the United States, and the median number of years lived in California ranged from twenty at the Apartment Tower and Purchase Village to forty-six at the Manor Village. The median length of residence at the site ranged from seven months at the Manor Village to $3\frac{1}{2}$ years at the Life-care Home. About three quarters of all site residents

were Protestant and 12 percent were Catholic. Provided with 600 site respondents, the next task was to assemble a control group.

Matching and Interviews with Control Respondents

Matching Variables

Ten variables were designated: sex, working status, marital status, age, income, education, occupation, present rental versus ownership of dwelling unit, household composition, number of children.

Pool of Potential Matches

Several months earlier, the study staff had investigated many possibilities of existing lists, such as the census, but no ready-made list of a population of this type was available. However, a large pool of names collected by a local newspaper was located. The pool was sorted and cases were assigned to broad typologies from which to select those corresponding to the types of persons at the sites.

Interviewers were assigned to conduct interviews (using the dispersed form) with such potential matches.

Matching on most of the items required identical matches within the category ranges specified, although even at the outset, adjacent category matches were permitted on a few items. However, especially as matching proceeded and certain groups in the newspaper pool become depleted, some additional adjacent category matching was tolerated, recognizing that systematic and cumulative errors might make for ultimate inequality between the groups. Early tabulations, however, revealed no cumulative biases.

A Screening Interview

Before long, a shortage of certain types became apparent: the newspaper pool did

TABLE 46-II

INITIAL COMPARABILITY ON MATCHING VARIABLES OF TOTAL WAVE I SAMPLES

	Retirement Hotel		Rental Village		Apartment Tower		Purchase Village		Manor Village		Life-Care Home	
	Site	Dsp.	Site	Dsp.	Site	Dsp.	Site	Dsp.	Site	Dsp.	Site	Dsp.
% female	54	54	69	69	78	78	41	41	51	51	83	83
Marital status (%)												
Married	1	1	32	32	21	21	92	92	82	82	21	21
Divorced, separated	28	21	12	10	12	11	0	1	3	2	6	0
Widowed	52	55	54	57	59	59	7	6	13	14	45	50
Never married	19	23	2	1	8	9	1	1	2	2	28	29
Mean age	75.7	74.6	75.8	74.9	73.5	73.4	67.8	68.1	67.8	68.3	77.8	76.9
Median income (dollars)	2013	1817	2390	2140	3129	2725	5700	5388	10595	8500	5615	4928
Median education	9th–11th	9th–11th	7th–8th	7th–8th	HS Grad.	HS Grad.	HS Grad.	HS Grad.	HS Grad.	HS Grad.	Coll. Grad.	Some[a] Coll.
Median occupational score[b]	4	5	5	5	3	3	3	3	2	2	2	2
% retired	94	94	98	98	91	91	87	87	80	80	90	89
% renting dwelling	100	96	100	95	100	97	0	0	0	3	9[c]	14
% living alone	100[c]	89	67	64	76	73	6	7	16	17	76[a]	58
Mean No. of Children	1.01	1.07	2.19	2.05	1.30	1.28	1.52	1.31	1.57	1.67	1.11	1.25

Note: N equals 100 in each group.

[a]$p < .01$ (χ^2).

[b]Hollingshead occupational scale ranges from 1: Higher Executives, Large-Concern Proprietors, Major Professionals to 7: Unskilled Employees.

[c]$p < .001$ (χ^2).

not contain enough upper-middle-class, married persons (of this age group); that is, matches for the last three of the six sites. Another group for which there was a scarcity was single men, rather poor, living alone, primarily matches for the first site and, to some extent, the second. To obtain a larger pool of subjects of these two types, door-to-door screening procedures were initiated. Four suburban census tracts were chosen for the first group, and six downtown tracts were chosen for the second. As the interviewer went door-to-door in the designated census tracts, the screening interview was administered to whoever answered the door. This person was to respond to questions on the ten matching variables for each person living in the household. The interviewer was to use all households with three or fewer people, (the maximum size of households in the test cases), with at least one resident fifty years of age or older, and with no occupant twenty-five years of age or younger. Data from the screening questionnaires were then matched to the site respondents. If a match was found, an interviewer was sent back to administer the full dispersed interview.

Toward the end of interviewing, in order to minimize wasted interviews and to locate other members of a household who might be a better match, before undergoing the complete interview, persons in the newspaper pool were prescreened with the screening interview. If a match to a site respondent was found, the interviewer was sent back to complete the full interview.

Completion of Matches

Matching was an open-ended task, since it was difficult to estimate when all 600 site cases would be matched. In order to obtain 600 matched controls, it was necessary to complete 945 full control interviews and 889 screening interviews.

TABLE 46-III
WAVE II MOBILITY AND ATTRITION: SITE AND DISPERSED

	N	%
Completed interviews	(934)	(78)
Still at site (disp. addr.)	(815)	(68)
No move	791	66
Within-site move	24	2
Moved in-state	(119)	(10)
To site	27	2
To dispersed	92	8
Completed mail questionnaires:	(18)	(2)
(Moved out-of-state)		
To site	3	1[a]
To dispersed	15	1
No Wave II interview:	(248)	(20)
Possibly eligible for Wave II		
Refusal	64[b,c]	5
Away until after field work, or moved in Calif. & unable to reach	6[d]	1[a]
Moved, no forwarding address	23	2
Inelegible for Wave II		
Too ill, phys. handicap, hospitalized	16[e]	1
Nursing or convalescent home, sanitarium	27	2
Deceased	112	9
Total	1200	100

[a] = % less than 1 have been rounded up to 1.
[b] = Includes out-of-state mover who did not return mail questionnaire.
[c] = 49 were still at Wave I address.
[d] = 3 were still at Wave I address.
[e] = 8 were still at Wave I address.

Table 46-II shows comparability data on the matching variables. The only significant test-control differences were at the Life-care Home on education, own vs. rent, and household composition; and at the Retirement Hotel on household composition. For all other sites, and for all sites on the other seven matching variables, there were no significant test-control differences.

Wave II Interviews

The Wave II interview took approximately one hour to administer. A portion

TABLE 46-IV

INITIAL COMPARABILITY ON MATCHING VARIABLES OF REMAINING NONMOVERS

	Retirement Hotel		Rental Village		Apartment Tower		Purchase Village		Manor Village		Life-Care Home	
	Site	Dsp.	Site	Dsp.	Site	Dsp.	Site	Dsp.	Site	Dsp.	Site	Dsp.
N	(38)	(62)	(64)	(63)	(63)	(59)	(80)	(74)	(78)	(82)	(79)	(73)
% female	50	60	67	65	84	81	42	41	53	49	85	86
Marital status (%)												
Married	2	0	27	38	14	22	91	91	80	83	20	18
Divorced, separated	16	18	12	13	10	14	0	1	3	2	6	0
Widowed	58	61	59	47	65	56	8	7	14	13	46	51
Never married	24	21	2	2	11	8	1	1	3	2	28	31
Mean age	79.0	74.3[a]	75.1	74.5	73.3	72.8	67.9	68.1	67.7	68.3	76.8	76.2
Median income (dollars)	2266	1916	2320	2133	2911	2727	5944	5600	10781	8636	5818	4600
Median education	HS Grad	9th-11th	7th-8th	7th-8th	HS Grad	HS Grad	HS Grad	HS Grad	Some Coll.	HS Grad	Coll. Grad.	Some[b] Coll.
Median occupational score	4	5	5	5	3	3	3	3	2	2	2	2
% retired	97	90	97	97	89	95	88	84	77	79	87	90
% renting dwelling	100	94	100	94	100	98	0	0	0	4	0	11[c]
% living alone	100	89[b]	72	59	81	73	6	7	17	15	77	59[d]
Mean No. of Children	0.92	1.00	2.55	1.90	1.32	1.24	1.67	1.42	1.59	1.70	1.11	1.22

[a] $p<.005$ (t-test of mean age). [b] $p<.05$ (χ^2). [c] $p<.01$ (χ^2). [d] $p<.02$ (χ^2)

of the Wave I questions were repeated, and new questions were added. One group of questions was specifically directed to the issue of change.

Mobility and Attrition

Although the lengthy procedures undertaken in the first wave to select the samples, particularly the matched controls, did not have to be repeated, problems of mobility and attrition were encountered. The following procedures were initiated so as to reinterview every possible respondent from the Wave I groups (excluding those who had moved to nursing homes or hospitals). After all persons still living at the sites or in the Los Angeles area had been interviewed, interviewers were sent elsewhere in California to conduct interviews with those who had moved within the state. A brief mail questionnaire was sent to those who had moved out of California. If the usual questioning of neighbors, landlords, etc. did not locate a missing respondent, the field staff tried one or all of the following: asking the post office for a forwarding address; telephoning the respondent's child; checking with the telephone information operator; checking at the county health department for a death certificate. These procedures were largely successful and very few respondents could not eventually be located.

Table 46-III shows the final distributions of mobility and attrition. Similar figures were found within each site-dispersed pair for each category of attrition and mobility, although differences from site to site were noteworthy. Sixty-eight percent of the original 1200 respondents were interviewed at the same address as at Wave I. Another 10 percent were interviewed, but at a new address; 2 percent, who had moved out-of-state, returned mail questionnaires, bringing to 80 the percentage heard

from at Wave II; 12 percent were ineligible at Wave II. This means that only 8 percent of the original sample were possibly eligible at Wave II but could not be interviewed; only 5 percent were refusals.

Final Groups and Comparability

Checks were run to see that, after attrition, the remaining site and dispersed groups were adequately matched, and, in particular, that all site and dispersed nonmovers could be used, not just remaining matched pairs. The ten matching variables (Wave I data) were checked for remaining matched pairs only (N = 564, data not shown) and for all nonmovers (N = 815). As shown in Table 46-IV, with only one exception, the test-control matches including all nonmovers were as good as the original test-control matches of 1200 cases. Therefore, it was deemed appropriate to analyze all nonmovers in order to have the groups as large as possible.

Further checks were run comparing the site and dispersed groups on Wave II status of those matching variables which might have changed in the interim (working status, marital status, income, household composition, and number of children). Table 46-V shows that the site and dispersed groups were as comparable after two years as at the first wave.

Finally, checks were run comparing the remaining groups of nonmovers with their respective groups of those not interviewed at Wave II or interviewed at Wave II, but at a new address. In any longitudinal study, it is imperative to check for any systematic biases distinguishing those respondents remaining in the study throughout from those who have dropped out (in the present study most dropping-out was due to migration, mortality, or ill health, rather than to noncooperation).

The present paper presents data for

TABLE 46-V

WAVE II COMPARABILITY ON MATCHING VARIABLES OF SITE AND DISPERSED NONMOVERS

	Retirement Hotel		Rental Village		Apartment Tower		Purchase Village		Manor Village		Life-Care Home	
	Site	Dsp.	Site	Dsp.	Site	Dsp.	Site	Dsp.	Site	Dsp.	Site	Dsp.
N	(38)	(62)	(64)	(63)	(63)	(59)	(80)	(74)	(78)	(82)	(79)	(73)
Marital status (%)												
Married	3	0	23	33	14	22	89	85	74	80	17	18
Divorced	16	18	10	13	10	14	0	3	3	2	6	0
Widowed, separated	55	61	67	52	65	57	10	12	20	16	49	51
Never married	26	21	0	2	11	7	1	0	3	2	28	31
Median income (dollars)	2333	2305	2431	2125	2861	2833	5411	6000	9454	8500	5066	4312
% retired	100	90	94	86	94	97	86	86	80	82	97	94
% living alone	100	89[a]	75	60	81	73	10	14	23	16	81	58[b]
Mean No. of Children	0.83	0.90	2.15	1.80	1.32	1.24	1.63	1.35	1.53	1.67	1.10	1.17

[a]$p<.05$ (χ^2).　[b]$p<.01$ (χ^2).

TABLE 46-VI

INITIAL COMPARABILITY ON MATCHING VARIABLES OF NONMOVERS COMPARED TO MOVERS
AND NOT INTERVIEWED AT WAVE II

SITE

	Retirement Hotel		Rental Village		Apartment Tower		Purchase Village		Manor Village		Life-Care Home	
	NM[a]	M,NI[b]	NM	M,NI	NM	M,NI	NM	M,NI	NM	M,NI	NM	M,NI
N	(38)	(62)	(64)	(36)	(63)	(37)	(80)	(20)	(78)	(22)	(79)	(21)
% female	50	56	67	72	84	68	42	35	53	45	85	76
Marital status (%)												
Married	2	0	27	42	14	32	91	95	80	86	20	24
Divorced, separated	16	36	12	11	10	16	0	0	3	5	6	5
Widowed	58	48	59	44	65	49	8	5	14	9	46	43
Never married	24	16	2	3	11	3	1	0	3	0	28	28
Mean age	79.0[e]	73.7	75.1	77.0	73.3	73.8	67.9	67.4	67.7	68.3	76.8[d]	81.5
Median income (dollars)	2266	1852	2320	2469	2911	3346	5944	4600	10,781	9750	5818	4250
Median education	HS Grad.	9th-11th	7th-8th	8th-9th	HS Grad.	HS Grad.	HS Grad.	HS Grad.	Some Coll.	HS Grad.	Coll. Grad.	Some Coll.
Median occupational score	4	4	5	5	3	3	3	3	2	2 – 3	2	2
% retired	97	92	97	100	89	95	88	85	77	91	87	100
% living alone	100	100	72	58	81	68	6	5	17	14	77	71
Mean No. of Children	0.92	1.06	2.55	1.56	1.32	1.27	1.67[e]	0.90	1.59	1.50	1.11	1.10

DISPERSED

	Retirement Hotel		Rental Village		Apartment Tower		Purchase Village		Manor Village		Life-Care Home	
	NM[a]	M,NI[b]	NM	M,NI	NM	M,NI	NM	M,NI	NM	M,NI	NM	M,NI
N	(62)	(38)	(63)	(37)	(59)	(41)	(74)	(26)	(82)	(18)	(73)	(27)
% female	60	45	65	76	81	73	41	42	49	61	86	74
Marital status (%)												
Married	0	3	38[f]	22	22	20	91	96	83	78	18	30
Divorced, separated	18	26	13	15	14	7	1	0	2	0	0	0
Widowed	61	45	47	73	56	63	7	4	13	22	51	48
Never married	21	26	2	0	8	10	1	0	2	0	31	22
Mean age	74.3	75.1	74.5	75.6	72.8	74.3	68.1	68.0	68.3	67.9	76.2	78.6
Median income (dollars)	1916	1647	2133	2100	2727	2667	5600	4812	8636	7500	4600	5667
Median education	9th-11th	9th-11th	7th-8th	7th-8th	HS Grad.	HS Grad.	HS Grad.	HS Grad.	HS Grad.	11th-12th	Some Coll.	Some Coll.
Median occupational score	5	5	5	5	3	3	3	4	2	2—3	2	2
% retired	90	100	97	100	95	85	84	96	79	83	90	85
% renting dwelling	94	100	94	97	98	95	0	0	4	0	11	22
% living alone	89	89	59	73	73	73	7	8	15	28	59	56
Mean No. of Children	1.00	1.18	1.90	2.30	1.24	1.34	1.42	1.00	1.70	1.56	1.22	1.33

[a] NM signifies nonmovers (between Wave I and Wave II).

[b] M signifies movers (between Wave I and Wave II); NI signifies not interviewed (at Wave II).

[c] $p < .01$ (t-test of mean age).   [d] $p < .001$ (t-test of mean age).   [e] $p < .05$ (t-test of mean age).   [f] $p < .05$ (t-test of mean number of children).   [g] $p < .05$ (χ^2)

demographic variables, i.e. those variables that were used in matching. No systematic biases were found on matching variables in the present study. Table 46-VI shows the distributions on matching variables for the nonmovers compared to the movers and those not interviewed at Wave II. The only statistically significant differences were as follows: Among residents at the Retirement Hotel the nonmovers were older than the dropouts, while among residents of the Life-care Home and nonmovers were younger than the dropouts. Nonmovers at the Purchase Village had more children than did dropouts. Among controls for the Rental Village, the dropouts had a higher percentage of widows than did the nonmovers. None of these differences appears to be systematic in any way and it is concluded that the nonmovers, for each site and control group, do not constitute a biased subsample of the original groups.

Summary

This paper has described the methodology employed in a longitudinal study of residents of special housing facilities for the well-elderly. One hundred persons were interviewed at each of six widely varying retirement housing sites, and their interviews were compared to interviews with 600 matched controls living in conventional dispersed housing. A large proportion of the original 1200 were reinterviewed two years later. Interviews covered such areas

as age-integration vs. segregation, provision of leisure activities and supportive services, motivation, morale, physical health, and demography. The present paper described selection of the sites and residents therein and interview construction. Particularly emphasized were matching procedures and methods used to minimize attrition.

REFERENCES

Carp, F. M. *A future for the aged: Victoria Plaza and its residents.* Univ. of Texas Press, Austin, 1966.

Donahue, W. Housing and community services. In E. W. Burgess (Ed.), *Aging in western societies.* Univ. of Chicago Press, Chicago, 1960.

Hollingshead, A. B., and Redlich, F. C. *Social class and mental illness.* Wiley, New York, 1958.

Mumford, L. For older people: Not segregation but integration. *Architectural Record*, 1956, *119*, 191-194.

Rosow, I. *Social integration of the aged.* Free Press, New York, 1967.

Sherman, S. R. The choice of retirement housing among the well-elderly. *Aging & Human Development*, 1971, 2, 118-138.

Walkley, R. P., Mangum, W. P., Jr., Sherman, S. R., Dodds, S., and Wilner, D. M. *Retirement housing in California.* Diablo Press, Berkeley, 1966.

Wilner, D. M., and Walkley, R. P. Psychosocial factors in housing for the aged. Unpublished NIMH Project Grant Description, School of Public Health, Univ. of California, Los Angeles, 1963.

Chapter 47

TOWARD PERSON/EN-VIRONMENT TRANS-ACTIONAL RESEARCH IN AGING

ARTHUR N. SCHWARTZ AND
HANS G. PROPPE

O NE IRONY OF OUR times is the marked disparity between the rhetoric about the happy, "golden" years of life and the decline in quality of life for many of our elderly. On the one hand, we hear about idealized retirement plans, promises of increased medical care and support, options in housing and feeding, proposals for more meaningful postretirement roles, and the like. On the other hand, we see large segments of the social environment of our aged disrupted, their life-space contaminated, their meaningful roles degraded, and their confidence and self-esteem declining.

It is clear that scientists document in embarassing detail the deficits and degradations of the elderly. At the same time, gerontologists appear unable to translate current research into the kind of broad-scale action needed to make life better for the older person.

Several crucial questions confront us. How much contemporary research by social scientists, especially gerontologists, aims at reversing the contaminated, polluted, blighted, impoverished, and often degraded circumstances in which many of our older

Reprinted by permission from the *Gerontologist*, 1970, *10*, 228-232.

citizens are caught? To what extent do gerontological studies relate to the questions inevitably asked by our society's social planners and decision-makers? If we agree that the aged are generally devalued, then is it possible that some aging research may actually, though inadvertently, contribute to the devaluation process? If so, to what extent? Finally, will the research training being given to the new generation of investigators eventually help correct the appalling conditions frequently suffered by the elderly? Or, are we teaching our young colleagues how to busily contribute to "the literature" while giving them little expertise in how to attack the problems of the aged?

Most traditional and much contemporary research on aging seems to be engrossed with either (a) the machinery of research, or (b) investigating processes in the aged person (mainly physiological but also psycho-social) occurring over time or associated with late maturity. Unquestionably, such studies are valid and frequently are not only illuminating and interesting but also useful. Nevertheless, their relevance to the critical needs of the aged remain, at best, problematic. Certainly we cannot resolve the problem of achieving a successful late maturity by insisting, even implicitly, that we pursue the genetic or biological search for "the secret of aging." There will be no moratorium on the steadily declining circumstances of the aged while we take up Ponce de Leon's quest. We frequently hear people ask what "causes" aging. What they are really asking is that we *do* something about all the deficits and decrements associated with old age. The study of environmental factors contributing to the incompetence of aged people constitutes a more pertinent inquiry.

Our essential point is that social action

research, particularly related to gerontology, remains at a premium. While advances have been made in this respect, many of these "advances" have contributed far too little toward helping the aged enhance the quality of their lives. Some familiar examples of this would include: the proliferation of short-lived pilot projects, "ideal" assistance programs that go unfunded, well-written position papers pointing to improvements in some distant future, variations on traditional expertise resulting in continuation of the *status quo,* or obtaining grants to subsidize conventional, "academic" research. Meanwhile, one of the more vulnerable groups of humans, those in late maturity, often continue to experience loss of meaningful roles, diminished real income, loss of effectiveness within and control over their environment. The *consequences* of such degradations continue to provide a rich field of study. But understanding the *precipitators* of the same is yet confounded by a morass of traditional attitudes, policies, procedures, and even myths about the aged as if they were inevitable and irrevocable. Indeed, they seem to be neither.

This is not meant to discredit or minimize the importance of contemporary gerontological research. Rather we see it as an opportunity to help crystallize and facilitate increased interest in aging research strategies aimed at improving the quality of life for older people. Part of the truth is that much aging research is either not amenable to translation into policy terms, or is simply irrelevant to social action in terms consistent with available data.

It seems that much more than a modicum of gerontological research should, like nonpornographic literature, have some socially redeeming value. Concomitantly, if the objects of our studies are reduced to

mere dehumanized *"Ss"* then we will fall into the same trap as the "good people" of whom Coser (1969) speaks: "good people" who have essentially chosen to ignore the degradations of their fellows in the name of whatever rationale. Actually, investigators from many disciplines have reported numerous deficits and decrements of the aged. In so doing they documented the several dimensions and facets of loss of dignity, independence, and effectiveness within the environment. In sum, they document *loss of control* in some degree over one's internal and external environment.

To describe what is occurring "within" the personality is clearly a necessary task. But doing this with only casual attention to the environmental transactions and contributions to "deficits" and "decrements" apparently produces some misleading conclusions about the aging process. Studies of the adverse effect of institutionalization of "healthy" aged (Aldrich and Mendkoff, 1963; Lieberman, Prock, and Tobin, 1968) indicate an environmental or "transactional" dimension may be useful to describe the behavior and/or personality of the older person.

The study and specification of environmental events has been relatively neglected. This is all the more unfortunate since such events may offer the surest clues for developing social policies which provide ameliorating and compensating options to people whose life-space becomes increasingly constricted. For example, an older person begins to become "withdrawn" socially as his hearing acuity diminishes: he feels increasingly uncertain and uneasy in social situations and begins to avoid them. In terms of the "client analysis" suggested by Cohen (1968), it would seem beside the point to "shoe-horn" such an oldster into a psychotherapy situation to "treat" his depression when correcting the hearing deficit could improve his ability to become socially competent again. The implications of this with regard to the disengagement theory seem obvious.

The foregoing is a limited illustration of the kind of person/environment transactional approach Barker (1968) calls *"naturally occurring* individual behavior variation" which we feel needs greater emphasis in contemporary and future gerontological research. In addition, we propose: (*a*) a matrix in which our multifaceted empirical findings can be meaningfully assessed and interpreted *vis-à-vis* social action; (*b*) a point of view which can integrate the techniques of professions serving the aged without jeopardizing the primacy of the client's needs; and (*c*) a framework to attack the worst problems of the aged and to give greater weight to life-space factors. The parameters of environmental variability need to be explored, specified, and related to human behavior variations so that the product of such transactions can be effectively dealt with. We choose to characterize this viewpoint as the person/ environment transactional approach to aging research insofar as it derives from the following considerations:

1. Most of the so-called old age deficits and degradations now described in the literature may be subsumed under the rubric: "loss of control and effectiveness within the environment."

2. The emphasis is on "transactional," i.e. the initiating event(s) leading to loss of control may be internal (biological/ psychological) or external (environmental), but ultimately involve both.

3. Such loss of control seems to have at least three dimensions:
   a. It is usually so gradual as to be imperceptible. Vision, hearing, and energy gradually diminish except in extreme instances such as limb amputation, catastrophic financial loss, or confinement in a locked room.
   b. It is multifaceted. That is, it encompasses a potential multitude of events ranging from body-system function to external circumstances, e.g. loss of privacy options just as clearly constitutes some loss of control as much as losing eyesight or a hand.
   c. It is cumulative. While deriving from many sources such losses, if uncompensated, are continuing. For instance, an individual can be expected to respond quite differently when experiencing simply loss of hearing than he would to hearing loss, plus complete income loss, plus loss of privacy, etc.

4. Cumulative loss of control does not in most instances appear to be irreversible.

5. Loss of control seems highly correlated with both subjective and objective estimates of decrease in "successful" or "satisfactory" aging.

We believe it vital, not only to understanding but even more to helping the aged maintain competence, to specify the transactions resulting in loss of control. For therein lie the clues for reversing the effects of such loss by compensation. We are led, then, to the question: is it possible to manipulate or redesign the older person's environment so as to literally give back options, thus providing compensatory effectiveness and control? Clearly, positive responses to this question are available, even if quite limited.

Studies and explorations by Barker (1968), Ittelson, Rivlin, and Proshansky, (1966), Pawley (1969), Sommer (1969), and White (1961), to cite but a few, strongly suggest the appropriateness of controlling the environment as a point of departure and matrix of analysis for gerontological research. The authors (1969) followed this strategy in studying institutionalized aged by focusing on one kind of transaction, namely, perception of privacy. One conclusion was that the environment, by virtue of its design and use, can so constrict personal space and so violate the life-space as to reduce the individual's privacy options to a most primitive level. This in turn potentiates a continuously socially-impoverished and socially-fragmented environment.

Any gerontologist recognizes the instance of an elderly person living alone and impoverished in a tiny apartment, withdrawn and "inactive." The use of conventional psychological and sociological measures might readily "demonstrate" another example of the disengagement theory. Yet one might interpret the same data in terms of loss of environmental control and account for such disengagement phenomena by saying this oldster lacks transportation, some personal encouragement, or is simply "broke," or a combination of such loss factors. Once we "understand" behavior in these terms, it is not difficult to design an environment to compensate for such loss.

The assumption made by many scientists, as suggested by Lawton and Simon (1968), that for experimental purposes at least, environment may be viewed as fixed or static has led and will lead us into errors of judgment; at the very least into misinterpreting available data. We all agree that each child added to a family grows up in an environment "different" from that of his siblings. We are bound to give no less weight to environmental variations for aged persons. Considering the differential effects upon elderly people occasioned by changing residences (e.g. moving from their own to a nursing home), we cannot hope to "explain" such effects simply on the basis of differential personality traits. The Lewinian view represented in the work of

the person/environment transactional researchers clearly states that environment in its broadest sense is fluid and dynamic. The essence of the transactional approach, then, lies in the insistence that the behavior of the aged be viewed not as occurring in front of the backdrop of a fixed environment. Rather we must take into account how individual behavior contributes to the environment and is in turn influenced by it.

Out of the case of person/environment transactional research in aging there arises at least one implication regarding the roles of the various disciplines. Conventionally, each discipline tends to define the "problems" of the aged in terms of its own expertise, the psychologist, physician, biologist, sociologist, etc. each defines these problems in terms of what he is trained to do. This has often led to a kind of gerontological reductionism. One unfortunate consequence of this is a fragmenting of aging research. Out of the vast pool of research data available, who can put together an integrated, comprehensive, yet holistic theory of aging which will effectively enable our society to diminish the deficits and decrements of the aged? Kent (1966) observed, "Any policy statement which defines objectives or goals calling for social action must necessarily include some assignment of responsibility for that action. . ." Who then is "responsible" for such social action? Surely the various professional groups must share this responsibility. When social action is the goal, it appears that no member of any discipline, whether researcher or practitioner, can afford to claim primacy for a particular area of gerontology. More important is the imaginativeness and practicality with which each discipline addresses itself to designing and manipulating environments to minimize loss and at the same time give back compensatory options and controls. In this regard, each discipline faces great challenges. Medicine, besides improving the quality of service, must facilitate both the delivery and utilization of such service; social service can, among other things, concern itself with how to help the aged become more "attractive" clients; psychology can involve itself also in the issues of selecting and training helpers; architects could well address themselves to assessing the ways in which people actually use the space which they design; and so on.

This approach promises to make gerontologists relevant in the market-place. In terms of the questions raised earlier, this approach should aim gerontology at reversing the blighted, polluted, and degraded circumstances of the aged. Finally, this approach, rather than contributing to devaluation, might help maintain the aged person's sense of worth, effectiveness, dignity, and self-esteem.

REFERENCES

Aldrich, C., and Mendkoff, E. Relocation of the aged and disabled, a mortality study. *Journal of the American Geriatrics Society*, 1963, *11*, 185-194.

Barker, R. G. *Ecological psychology*, Stanford, Calif.: Stanford University Press, 1968.

Cohen, E. S. Toward a social policy on aging. Neota Larson Memorial Lecture presented at the 21st Annual Meeting of Gerontological Society, Denver, 1968.

Coser, L. A. The visibility of evil. *Journal of Social Issues*, 1969, *25*, 101-109.

Ittelson, W., Rivlin, L., and Proshansky, H. The use of behavioral maps in environmental psychology. *Report, Environmental Psychology Program*. New York: City University of New York, 1966. (mimeo)

Kent, D. P. Social issues and social policy. In J. C. McKinney and F. T. De Vyver (Eds.), *Aging and social policy*. New York: Appleton-Century-Crofts, 1966.

Lawton, M. P., and Simon, B. The ecology of social relationships in housing for the elderly. *Gerontologist*, 1968, *8*, 108-115.

Lieberman, M. A., Prock, V. N., and Tobin, S. S. Psychological effects of institutionalization. *Journal of Gerontology*, 1968, *23*, 343-353.

Pawley, E. Environment and aging: Notations for awareness. Lecture presented at Institute for Advanced Study in Gerontology, University of Southern California, Los Angeles, 1969.

Sommer, R. *Personal space*. Englewood Cliffs, N.J.: Prentice-Hall, 1969.

Schwartz, A., and Proppe, H. Personal perception of privacy among institutionalized aged. *Proceedings, American Psychological Association*. Washington: American Psychological Association, 1969.

White, R. W. Motivation reconsidered, the concept of competence. In D. Fiske and S. Maddi (Eds.), *Functions of varied experience*. Homewood, Ill.: Dorsey Press, 1961.

NAME INDEX

439

SUBJECT INDEX

449